Encyclopedia of SPORTS & FITNESS NUTRITION

Also by Liz Applegate

101 Miracle Foods That Heal Your Heart

Bounce Your Body Beautiful

Eat Smart, Play Hard

Eat Your Way to a Healthy Heart

Power Foods

Encyclopedia of SPORTS & FITNESS NUTRITION

LIZ APPLEGATE, Ph.D.

Foreword by Eric Heiden, M.D.

PRIMA PUBLISHING

Published by Prima Publishing, Roseville, California. Member of the Crown Publishing Group, a division of Random House, Inc., New York.

The material in this book is supplied for informational purposes only and is not meant to take the place of a doctor's advice. Before embarking on a regimen of diet and exercise you should first consult your own physician.

Interior design and illustrations by Mike Tanamachi
Author photo by Blanche Mackey

Library of Congress Cataloging-in-Publication Data
Applegate, Elizabeth Ann.
Encyclopedia of sports & fitness nutrition : everything you need to know about . . . / Liz Applegate.
p. cm.
Includes index.
ISBN 0-7615-1378-7
1. Nutrition. 2. Athletes—Nutrition. 3. Physical fitness. I. Title.
RA784 .A659 2002
613.2'03—dc21 2002029027

02 03 04 05 06 BB 10 9 8 7 6 5 4 3 2 1
Printed in the United States of America

First Edition

To Marlia Braun and Terry Zimmer—
great cyclists and even better friends

CONTENTS

FOREWORD

As an orthopedic surgeon, I see frustrated fitness enthusiasts every day. They come in with chronic knee or hip or heel or ankle or elbow or shoulder pain. And they generally feel helpless, as if their bodies have let them down.

I know about aches and pains both as their doctor and as a patient. Because of cartilage damage in my own knees, I know the frustration of having to give up some of the sports I love, including speed skating.

I also know—both as a doctor and as a patient—just how much of a role good nutrition can play both in exercise performance and in exercise recovery and injury prevention and treatment.

All of us must follow certain rules when it comes to reaching our optimal fitness potential. We must exercise wisely, pushing ourselves hard and taking enough rest. We must stretch and strengthen strategic muscles to avoid imbalances. And we must eat right.

I learned the importance of eating right early on. I've been active most of my life, beginning my fitness career during childhood as an avid soccer and hockey player. You probably know me better for my speed skating. After winning five gold medals in the 1980 Olympic Games at Lake Placid, I moved on to cycling, eventually competing in the grueling Tour de France.

For all of those sports, I followed specific nutrition plans that provided enough fuel for 5-hour workouts, helped my muscles repair themselves afterward, and kept my immunity and energy high.

I was fortunate to meet Liz Applegate many years ago. She was a professional triathlete and I was a sports commentator for ABC when I interviewed her about her accomplishments during a big race.

Later, after I completed my residency and began treating patients at the U.C. Davis School of Medicine Sports Medicine Program, I began crossing paths with Liz more often. As one of the lead physicians of our newly developed Sports Performance Program, I see all types of athletes—elite professionals as well as those interested in getting the most out of their workouts and staying fit no matter what their place in "the pack" may be. They all tell me that Liz has a knack for explaining complicated nutritional concepts in down-to-earth language.

Possibly more important, as an athlete herself, Liz walks the talk. Like me, Liz has been active most of her life, competing in a variety of sports, including Ironman-distance triathlons. You name a sport or fitness pursuit and she's probably tried it. She walks, runs, swims, hikes, and bikes. Her advice doesn't just come from research and basic nutrition; it also comes from personal trial and error.

You want to know the most nutritious, best tasting, and least-likely-to-melt-in-your-jersey foods to eat on a long bike ride? Just ask Liz. Want to know the foods least likely to upset your stomach before swimming or yoga? She's your woman. Have trouble eating right after exercise because the hectic nature of life gets in your way? Can't get your kids to eat anything but Goldfish crackers? She's been there. She has the answers.

The night before I won my fifth gold medal at the 1980 Olympic Games, I watched the U.S.–Soviet Union hockey game. The American victory was so uplifting that I had trouble falling asleep that night. I stayed up so late that I overslept the next morning. When I woke, I only had enough time to grab a few pieces of bread and eat them on my way to the rink.

Other nutritionists might balk at that paltry breakfast. Not Liz Applegate. As an athlete herself, she understands the mental as well as the physical aspects of competing. She knows about sleepless nights and stomach nerves. She knows about the importance of eating light—for some people and not others.

I wish every athlete and fitness enthusiast could be as lucky as my patients and the students at U.C. Davis who are blessed with the opportunity to sit down with Liz for a personalized food plan. That's why I'm so happy Liz put pen to paper and came up with a manual that everyone can use to fine-tune their diet based on their individual fitness needs, health background, and age.

Liz Applegate's *Encyclopedia of Sports & Fitness Nutrition* is the essential eating guide for people of all ages and all fitness backgrounds. I particularly like her seven customized food and activity pyramids, which target different age groups. The advice is specialized, yet simple. Best of all, it works.

—*Eric Heiden, M.D.*
five-time Olympic gold medalist,
orthopedic surgeon, and professor,
University of California, Davis,
School of Medicine Sports Medicine Program

ACKNOWLEDGMENTS

Writing and producing this book took the efforts of wonderful and supportive individuals who were willing to go above and beyond expectations. My deepest thanks go to Alisa Bauman, whose superb and creative writing skills along with her knack for keeping me on track made this book possible. Many thanks also go to Marlia Braun, nutrition expert supreme, who performed the nutrition analysis for the menus and recipes. My assistant, Jessica Callaghan, patiently handled every crisis, glitch, and "get-it-out-yesterday" request—she's the greatest and I thank her for all her fabulous help. Thanks also go to Denise Sternad and Marjorie Lery, my editors at Prima, who did a wonderful job pulling the book together. A tremendous thank-you goes to Dr. Eric Heiden, who graciously wrote the book's foreword. Thank you Grant, Natalie, and Mark for your support. And finally, a thank-you to the many athletes I have had the privilege of working with—I salute your dedication and enthusiasm.

INTRODUCTION

At the beginning of this millennium, scientists made a discovery that has revolutionized the way we think about sports and fitness nutrition. They mapped the human genome.

This unveiling of the human genetic blueprint led to a flurry of research, along with lots of media fanfare. For example, you may remember headlines celebrating the discovery of the genes that cause Parkinson's disease or obesity or Huntington's disease. These exciting discoveries led to new hope for millions of people as pharmaceutical companies poured their research dollars into finding drugs that turned off these disease-causing genetic mutations.

Throughout all of this media fanfare, however, another group of researchers was quietly at work trying to find the answer to a different question: How should our individual genetic blueprints affect our food choices? These researchers are just beginning to answer this question, and their findings are proving quite revolutionary.

For example, in the not-so-distant past, you may have felt confused as you read news stories that cautioned against eating salt. These stories were followed by others that said salt really wasn't so bad after all. Genetic researchers now are clearing up this confusion. They've found, for example, that some people possess a gene that makes their bodies particularly sensitive to sodium. When they eat salt, their blood pressure rises. Other people, who don't have this gene, can eat salt without a blood pressure jolt.

Another example: You may remember news stories during the 1980s that promoted a high-carbohydrate, lowfat diet as the answer for preventing heart disease. Then news reports during the 1990s claimed that these same lowfat diets *triggered* some forms of heart disease. Thanks to genetic researchers, we now know that people with a certain gene react to high-carbohydrate, lowfat diets with lower cholesterol levels whereas other people, with a different gene, react with *higher* cholesterol levels.

In addition to your health, your individual genetics also affect how your body responds to fitness. For example, given the same temperature and activity level, some people's genes cause them to sweat more profusely than others, increasing their fluid requirements. Some people even sweat out a higher amount of salt than others, causing them to need a sports drink when someone else can get by without one.

Your age, fitness goals, and individual sport or activity will also affect the best food choices for you. Tennis players need to follow a different eating plan than runners, and runners need to follow a different eating plan than yogis. Active children must eat differently than active teens, who must eat differently than the middle-aged.

And finally, someone who is fit must eat differently than someone who is sedentary. Active people need more calories, healthy fats, protein, carbohydrate, and vitamins and minerals than do couch potatoes.

In short, no one food plan works for all people. Our genes, lifestyle, fitness, activity, and age all affect our optimal food choices.

Someday, our doctors may be able to custom-fit a food plan to our individual genetic profile. Though that day is still many years away, you can customize your diet to some extent based on your family history of disease as well as your lifestyle and fitness background.

That's what this book is all about.

Rather than provide you with a one-size-fits-all food plan and eating tips, I've customized my advice based on your genetic health needs. For example, if you have a family history of heart disease, you'll find an entry ("Heart Disease") that lists the best eating *and* fitness strategies to outsmart your genetics. If you have a family history of cancer, you'll find completely different eating and fitness strategies (in "Cancer").

You'll also find seven separate food plans designed for different life stages: children ages 4 to 8, children ages 9 to 12, teens, people in their 20s, people in their 30s, people in their 40s and 50s, and people 60 and older. Your age makes a huge difference in the amount of fluids, calories, protein, vitamins, minerals, carbohydrate, and fats that you need. With these plans, you'll be able to eat healthfully during the hectic 20s, hold off weight gain at middle age, and live with vigor and health well past age 60.

Your fitness habits also affect your nutrition plan. That's why this book contains entries for 41 different topics, helping you to customize your eating for golf, tennis, basketball, running, soccer, and more. For example, in "Cycling," you'll read about great ride foods that travel well in your back pocket and won't give you sugar mouth. Or, in "Tennis," you'll learn what to eat between matches to maintain your energy level.

Because lifestyle may sometimes interfere with fitness or eating habits, I've also included entries for on-the-go people, vegetarians, those with an organic lifestyle, and more. You'll also find information about avoiding fitness barriers such as fatigue, gastrointestinal distress, exercise-induced headache, and PMS.

Finally, no fitness nutrition book would be complete without exploring the wonderful world of supplements, vitamins, minerals, sports products, and functional foods. You'll learn how to tell if you're deficient in any vitamin or mineral, as well as which supplements hold promise as performance boosters or weight loss aids and which ones do not. I have no "agenda" other than giving you the information you need to make sound nutrition decisions. I do not promote any products, and I'm not involved with any supplement companies. I'm not against supplements, nor am I a supplement "pusher." Instead, I give you the information you need to decide whether a supplement, be it a multivitamin or chromium picolinate, is right for you.

Throughout, my goal is simple and straightforward: to inform and guide you in making decisions about eating and exercising. Never before have consumers like you been so aware of the power that food has to affect your health and performance. But equally true, never before have consumers been so overwhelmed with nutrition information, much of it misinformation, creating conflict and confusion in making decisions about food choices.

In this book, I provide you with practical, scientifically sound, current information that will empower you in making smart eating and fitness decisions both for yourself and for your family.

Part I

THE FUNDAMENTALS OF FITNESS NUTRITION

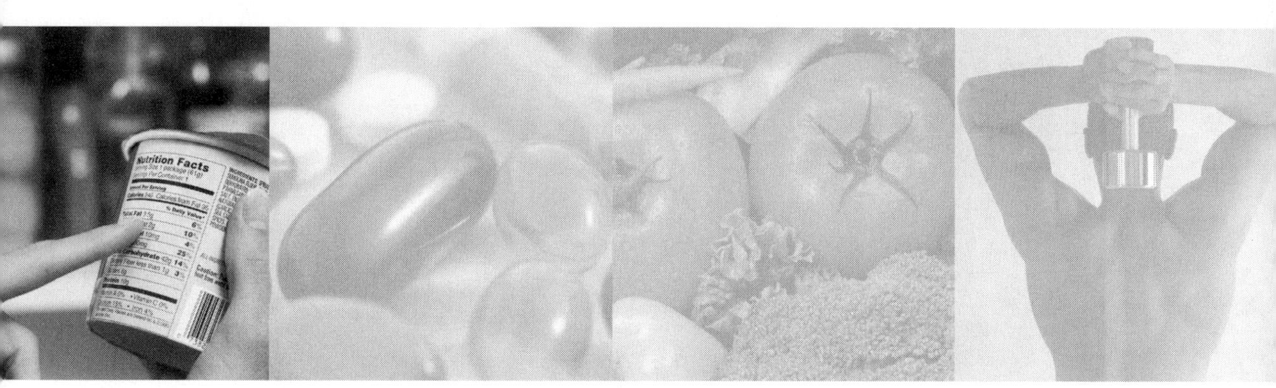

Chapter 1

FITNESS 101

Understanding your exercising body will motivate you to get and stay in shape.

During the late 1960s, when I was merely a little girl in elementary school, I did something that greatly worried my parents. I went to the high school track and ran laps.

At the time, people thought that running could be detrimental to girls, and even to women, which is what concerned my parents. I come from an academic family of nine brothers and sisters. In my parents' opinion, school was everything, and I was the only one of the nine Kirk children who dared to spend some of my free time playing sports and exercising rather than studying. One year in high school, Dad banned me from sports, saying that my studies were more important. He simply didn't want me to have any distractions.

To his dying day, Dad didn't understand my affinity for fitness. I remember one day in particular when I visited him in the hospital. I was wearing a sleeveless shirt. Dad took one look at my arms and shoulders—made muscular from swimming and pull-ups—and said, "When are you going to give up this exercise thing?"

I'm sure glad times have changed.

Today we know that physical fitness is one of the best ways to keep children in school and out of trouble. We know that exercise acts like a powerful therapy—for children and adults, for men and women—to stall the aging process, prevent disease, and increase well-being and energy.

However, you must work at fitness to achieve those benefits; I'll be honest with you.

For some people, fitness doesn't come as easily as it did to me. For many, the first few weeks on an exercise program—whether it be weight training, aerobics, or power yoga—can feel downright tough. And it's during those early weeks that many people stop exercising, claiming that they just aren't genetically suited to running or yoga or weight lifting or tennis.

Yet I am happy to tell you that you need only persevere a little longer to reach what I like to call the "fitness Promised Land." The hardest part about fitness is getting fit. Once you're fit, it's fairly easy to maintain your fitness. The awkwardness and discomfort of exercise melt away, and you're left with more amazing benefits than you can count.

I'll get to those amazing benefits in chapter 2, but first I want to show you how your body changes during those early weeks of a new exercise program. Understanding these adaptations will help you stay on track through that tough getting-in-shape phase. Whenever you ask yourself "Why am I doing this?" you'll have answers right here at your fingertips. These answers will help you to stay motivated and reach that fitness Promised Land.

With that in mind, let's take a journey deep inside your body, to your very cells.

IT STARTS ON DAY ONE

When you start an exercise program, your body transforms, starting during your very first workout. Though I knew this scientifically, I saw these results firsthand when I convinced my teenage daughter, Natalie, to try my abs workout. On the first day, she moaned, "Oh, I can't do this. This is too hard!"

After that first workout, cells in her body went to work, quickly trying to strengthen her abdomen. By the third workout, Natalie had doubled the number of repetitions she could perform of a particular abdominal exercise. Yes, she was sore, but she was amazed by her accomplishment.

And that's one of the most exciting aspects of starting a new exercise program: Gains happen rapidly, particularly in the beginning. For example, people who start a weight lifting program are usually amazed that they can increase the amount of weight they lift by their second workout. People who exercise aerobically by jogging or playing tennis find they last longer even during their first week of exercise. Those who start stretching find they can reach closer to their toes during their second or third stretching session.

That's because your body wants to work with you. Whenever you provide an effort to your body that your body must stretch to handle—for example, by lifting a heavy weight, walking farther than usual, or holding a stretch—your body performs numerous changes that make your next session that much easier. The most exciting aspect of all of this: Many of those same changes will help you shed pounds and boost your health and energy!

Here's a sampling of some of the positive changes that take place in your body within the early weeks of a fitness program, all of which help to make future exercise efforts much less of a struggle:

More "aerobic capacity." Your muscles power exercise with the help of a substance called ATP (adenosine triphosphate). You may remember learning about ATP back in high school or college biology class. ATP gives your muscles the energy they need to contract. Think of it as gasoline for the body.

Your muscles manufacture the vast majority of ATP from oxygen. However, if you exercise beyond your limit, your muscles can't always quickly extract enough oxygen from your blood to keep up with demands. When ATP production starts to fall behind, your muscles switch to a different form of ATP production, called anaerobic production, by burning either glucose or creatine phosphate. Though these fuel sources create a lot of needed energy quickly, they are not ideal, because your body can only sustain this rate of energy production for a few minutes.

The good news: As you become more fit, your muscles do a better job of extracting oxygen from your blood, boosting your aerobic capacity and allowing you to exercise at a higher intensity before your body must switch to anaerobic energy production.

Better waste removal. There are times when you must exercise anaerobically, for example, while sprinting or while weight lifting. When your muscles burn glucose to create ATP, however, they release by-products of lactic acid, heat, and hydrogen ions. Your blood usually can't clear these by-products as quickly as they are made. As lactic acid levels rise, your muscles lose their ability to contract, making you feel a burning sensation. However, the more fit you become, the faster you are able to clear lactic acid from your muscles, and the more lactic acid your muscles can withstand before they lose their ability to contract, allowing you again to go harder for a longer period of time.

Besides allowing you to sprint repeatedly on a running track, this also helps you in everyday life by allowing you to sprint up a flight of stairs for an important meeting.

More overall energy. As you become more fit, the mitochondria in your muscle cells multiply. Mitochondria break down fat and carbohydrate as a fuel source to produce ATP. The more mitochondria in a cell, the more energy, or ATP, that cell can produce. This not only gives you more energy during exercise, it also helps you feel energized all day long.

More confidence. Your mind plays a powerful role in how much you can accomplish. This is more easily seen in weight lifting, where beginners make huge gains—advancing in weight by 5 to 10 pounds at a time—simply because they feel more confident about the task at hand.

This confidence allows them to contract their muscles and tendons more fully, generating more force.

In other words, by your second session, your actual muscles may not have grown that much larger, but you will be able to lift a heavier weight because you employ more motor units within each muscle.

Bigger muscle fibers. When you provide a resistance to a muscle, the fibers break down and then build back up. When they build back up, they add a bit of girth in preparation to face that same resistance. This increased size results in a number of beneficial results. First, your body burns more calories. Your muscles burn a number of calories simply to maintain themselves. The larger your muscle fibers, the more calories a given muscle will burn. Also, these larger fibers give you that toned look that we all seek, giving shape to your abs, your buns, and your arms. And, of course, they give you more strength.

Other than larger muscle fibers, the protein content of your muscles also increases, and your connective tissues—tendons, cartilage, and ligaments—become thicker and stronger. This works together not only to give you more strength but also to prevent injuries.

More capillaries. These tiny vessels supply blood to your muscles, as well as your organs and other parts of your body. When you exercise, you grow more capillaries, boosting your blood-carrying capacity by 15 percent. More blood vessels means that more oxygen and nutrition can get to more parts of your body. That improves the functioning of just about every organ in your body, from your brain to your heart to your sex organs. You have more energy, you think more clearly, and your sexual interest heightens.

Better fat burning. Fat provides more calories than carbohydrate or protein. It's also much more abundant in your body and a more efficient fuel source. As you become more fit, there's an increase in the amount and activity of fat-burning enzymes, helping your body to mobilize fat faster. Your body also redistributes fat, storing more of it in your muscles as *intramuscular triglycerides* for easy access.

Finally, we all burn a combination of fat and carbohydrate for energy. In people who aren't fit, this combination is about 50-50. But in fit people, the ratio is closer to 70-30 with 70 percent of the calories burned as fat. This not only helps you shed flab, but it also preserves stored carbohydrate (called glycogen) in your muscles. You have a limited supply of glycogen, enough to last about 1½ to 2½ hours of endurance exercise. The more fat you burn during exercise, the longer your glycogen stores last and the more endurance you have.

MY FITNESS FORMULA

To get the most out of fitness, you need to perform three different types of exercise as explained here.

Cardiovascular Exercise

Also called aerobic exercise, cardiovascular exercise increases your breathing and heart rate, conditioning your heart and lungs. Types of cardiovascular exercise include power walking, jogging, tennis, cycling, and soccer, among many other types of exercise. Besides providing a number of health benefits that I'll describe in more detail in chapter 2, cardiovascular exercise burns off excess calories. For example, every mile you run or walk burns up to 100 calories, the equivalent of one banana, half an energy bar, one slice of whole grain bread with a tablespoon of jam, one cup of Healthy Choice vegetable soup, or a third of an apple spread with a tablespoon of peanut butter.

You may have heard that only lower-intensity exercises like walking burn fat and therefore help you lose body fat. That theory is overrated. While it's true that proportionately more fat than carbohydrate is used as fuel during low-intensity exercise, greater-intensity exercises such as hard running expend more calories overall per time spent, and collectively more fat is burned. But despite that, very high-intensity ex-

Your Cardio Goal

When it comes to exercise and fat loss, any exercise will do, as long as you do it! Low-intensity exercises are easier to do, especially as you start a fitness program. And as you become more fit, you can boost the intensity for greater calorie burning per minute. Here are some tips:

- Choose an activity—or several, for that matter—that you enjoy. The more different types of activities you perform, the better your fitness conditioning. More important, the better your motivation to stick with it.
- Aim for 20 to 30 minutes or more of cardiovascular exercise most days of the week.
- When crunched for time, break it up. You can break your exercise time into smaller chunks—for example, three sessions of 10 minutes. There's a common myth that you must exercise for at least 20 minutes before the message gets to your fat cells to release fat. It's not completely true. Yes, it takes a while for your body to start burning fat as a fuel, but to lose weight, you have to take in fewer calories than you burn. As long as you remain in a calorie deficit for the day, your body will eventually burn that fat, even if it's while you sleep.

ercises such as sprinting burn exclusively carbs as fuel, and in the long run you still lose body fat. This occurs after the exercise ends. The muscles recover and fat burning revs up as glycogen stores rebuild.

That doesn't mean you should spend all of your time exercising at a high intensity. In the final analysis, you want to exercise at an intensity that you can maintain, and one that doesn't make exercise feel dreadful. Let's face it—if you push yourself beyond your limits, are you going to feel motivated enough to stick with it?

Strength Training

This type of exercise—such as weight lifting—provides resistance to your muscles. Your muscles allow you to carry a heavy load of groceries from the car to the house, to hoist a three-year-old child over your head, and to push a baby carriage uphill.

Stronger muscles equal a faster metabolism and more calorie burning. Muscle is highly active body tissue and requires a lot of calories to maintain itself. Just 1 pound of muscle burns between 35 and 50 calories a day, even when it's not moving or working. The more muscle you have, the more food you can eat without gaining weight.

However, don't expect body-sculpting exercises designed for toning isolated muscle groups to cause fat burning in those specific areas. For the most part, spot reducing fails because energy is drawn from fat cells throughout the body to fuel the muscle that's working. On the bright side, more toned muscles will create a sleeker, leaner body, improving your overall appearance.

More muscle strength also gives you more coordination and helps you prevent injuries. You'll learn about even more benefits of strength training in chapter 2.

Flexibility Training

Just as a rubber band lengthens when you stretch it, so do your muscles. For example, when you bend over to try to touch your toes, your hamstrings—the muscles along the backs of your legs—stretch, growing longer from your knees to your hips. When you stretch consistently, the muscles remain longer.

This length allows you to bend farther, getting even closer to your toes. When you stretch a host of muscles consistently, particularly the ones around key joints such as your knees and shoulders, you increase your range of motion (your ability to move a joint in different directions).

Your Strength Goal

It doesn't matter what type of resistance you use. Your body weight, resistance bands, dumbbells, and exercise machines all work. Though I'm partial to exercise balls and bands because you can easily design a very effective at-home program, I want you to choose a resistance method that you enjoy. Again, the more you enjoy it, the more likely you'll stick with it.

Here are some other tips:

- Lift a weight that's heavy enough that you start to feel tired between 12 and 15 repetitions. If you can easily perform 15 reps or more, the weight is too light. Conversely, if you start to struggle on your fifth or sixth repetition, the weight is too heavy.
- Strength train your major muscle groups: your chest, your back, your abs, your upper arms (biceps and triceps), your shoulders, and your legs. Resist the urge to spot train only your trouble spots. You want overall body strength, not strength imbalances.
- Work strength training into your schedule two to three times a week.

This allows you to feel more balanced and agile as you walk or play sports. Research shows that flexibility programs such as yoga and tai chi help prevent falls in older adults. Increasing your flexibility will also lengthen your muscles, making them appear longer and leaner.

Target All Three Fitness Areas

Few forms of exercise target all three fitness areas. For example, weight lifting does a good job of improving your muscular strength, but not as good a job at increasing your flexibility or cardiovascular

Your Flexibility Goal

The most commonly tight muscles in the body include the front of the thighs, hip flexors, chest, and hamstrings (back of the thighs). Most people are also tight in their hips. Here are some stretches that target those areas. Hold each stretch for 20 to 30 seconds, and perform this series after your cardio exercise, when your muscles are warm.

Chest opener. Sit with your legs crossed in Indian style. Clasp your hands behind your back, with your knuckles facing the floor. Roll your shoulders up to the ceiling, then back to the wall behind you, then down toward the floor. Press your knuckles toward the floor. After holding for 20 to 30 seconds, relax and then reclasp your hands in the awkward position with the opposite thumb on top. Then repeat the stretch.

Hip opener. Still sitting in Indian style, bend forward from the waist. As you do this, keep your abs strong, pulling them in and up. Extend through the crown of your head, making your spine long. Relax and then switch the position of your legs (cross right over left or vice versa) before repeating.

Hamstring stretch. Unfold your legs from Indian style. Straighten your right leg and bring your left foot into your inner right thigh, so that your outer left thigh and calf touch the floor. Bend forward from the waist, lowering your torso to your thigh, keeping your abs strong and your back flat. Rise back to sitting, switch legs, and repeat.

Quad and hip flexor stretch. Roll onto your right side with your right leg extended. Bend your left leg at the knee, and hold the top of your left foot with your left hand. This may be all the stretch you need. If you need to increase the stretch, use your hand to guide your leg backward and up behind your torso. Switch sides and repeat.

endurance. Power walking, on the other hand, increases your cardiovascular endurance but does not do much for your muscular strength or flexibility. Some types of power yoga may target both muscular strength and flexibility but rarely also keep you cardiovascularly fit.

That's just one reason why no single exercise does it all, giving you a youthful, sleek body. Your ideal exercise combination will hit all three fitness areas, helping you to stay strong, balanced, flexible, and lean. When you target all three fitness areas, you'll achieve optimal fitness.

Chapter 2

THE BENEFITS OF FITNESS

Movement brings more rewards than you may realize.

I can tell if someone is fit simply by looking at his or her face. Exercise increases blood circulation all over your body, including to your skin. People who exercise have a healthy glow, whereas people who are overweight or who smoke tend to look ashen.

And that's only one of the many amazing benefits of becoming fit.

The going cliché among medical doctors and fitness experts is: "If I could harness the goodness of exercise and put it into a pill, I'd be a millionaire." Exercise is that good for you. You name just about any health problem, and you'll find that exercise helps prevent it or cure it. Exercise is the elixir of life.

You learned in chapter 1 about how your body adapts to training by creating new blood vessels, shifting its fat cell distribution, and creating easier ways to manufacture ATP. Those changes do more than simply help you get in shape and help make exercise feel more natural. They also create an exciting host of mental, physical, and emotional benefits.

As you get in shape, focus on these benefits. They'll help you stay motivated.

WEIGHT MANAGEMENT

You may already know that moving your muscles helps you burn more calories. However, if you solely concentrate on the number of calories you burn during a single workout, you can become depressed about exercise. It takes roughly a mile of running or walking to burn 100 calories. At that pace, you'd have to run or walk 35 miles before you burned a pound of fat. (A pound of fat equals 3,500 calories.)

Fortunately, exercise provides many more weight loss benefits than simply the calories you burn during your workout.

First, your metabolism stays high after your workout—particularly after a strength training workout—as your body goes to work repairing and resynthesizing muscle. This after-burn can last as many as 24 hours, boosting the number of calories you burn even during sleep. As I mentioned in chapter 1, weight lifting also boosts your metabolism by building muscle. Because muscle constantly breaks itself down and builds itself back up, it burns numerous calories just to maintain itself. Each pound of muscle in your body burns 35 to 50 calories. A typical person starting a strength program can add 1 to 5 pounds of muscle, creating a daily permanent metabolism boost of 35 to 100 calories or more.

As I mentioned in chapter 1, exercise also helps your body burn fat more easily. As you get fit, your body redistributes fat, storing more of it in your muscles for easy access. You also burn a higher proportion of fat during exercise, which is one reason why highly fit people tend to be lean.

Finally, regular exercise helps regulate your appetite, preventing you from overeating. When you become fit, your blood sugar levels, metabolites, and numerous other factors work together to tell you

The Weight You Want

Scientific fact: Muscle weighs more than fat. Muscle and other nonfat tissue in the body such as bone have a combined density of 1.1 grams per cubic centimeter, while body fat has a density of 0.9 grams per cubic centimeter.

That's one important reason why you can't entirely trust your weight on the scale to gauge your progress on a fitness program. For example, a fit, muscularly built man at 5 feet 10 inches may easily weigh more than 180 pounds, while an out-of-shape man of the same height sporting extra body fat may weigh less.

The most accurate way to gauge your body fat level? A technique that involves weighing yourself in water and comparing that to your weight out of water. Called *hydrostatic weighing,* this technique determines body fat values by computing your body's density, or weight per unit volume. Simply put, the less you weigh submerged under water, the more body fat you have (fat floats since it is less dense than water), and conversely, the more you weigh, the less body fat and more lean tissue you have (lean tissue sinks since it is more dense than water).

Though you can get weighed under water at some fitness centers and hospitals, I suggest using your clothes as a gauge. If you start dropping clothing sizes and your friends start telling you that you're looking fit, you know you're on the right track.

when and how much to eat. The result: You get hungry when your body needs calories, and you stop eating when your body doesn't, yet another reason why fit people tend to be lean. In less fit people, however, this appetite control mechanism doesn't function as well, making you hungry when your body doesn't need calories and neglecting to make you feel full on time. You end up eating more than your body needs and storing the excess as fat.

DISEASE PREVENTION

Exercise truly is a fountain of youth, reducing your risk for just about every age-related health concern you can name, from heart disease to diabetes to cancer.

Cardiovascular exercise strengthens your heart simply by making it beat harder and more often, giving it a needed workout. It also helps your blood and everything it contains move more easily through your arteries. It redistributes the lipoproteins that carry fat in your blood vessels, boosting the (healthy) high-density lipoproteins (HDLs) that carry cholesterol out of your bloodstream and reducing the (unhealthy) low-density lipoproteins (LDLs) that tend to get stuck along your artery walls, leading to heart disease and stroke.

Exercise also lowers blood pressure, powerfully. For example, a Duke University study of 112 people with high blood pressure found that exercise, particularly when combined with weight loss, could lower pressure significantly, even during periods of emotional stress.

Exercise also makes your muscle cells more sensitive to the hormone insulin. Insulin provides the key that allows glucose into your cells. However, the less fit you are, the less your cells respond to insulin, and the less blood sugar control you have. This can eventually lead to type 2 diabetes. If you already have type 2 diabetes, starting an exercise program may help you lower your medication dose or stop taking medication altogether. In fact, exercise is the number one prescription for people with type 2 diabetes.

Because fit people tend to have less body fat, they also tend to have a more desirable hormone level. Your body fat can produce some estrogen, so the less body fat you have, the less excess estrogen your body produces. This is important for prevention of certain types of cancers, such as breast cancer, that have been linked to high estrogen levels. Exercise also speeds the travel of waste through your system, getting carcinogens out faster. This may help to prevent intestinal cancers. Finally, as you become fit, your body produces more antioxidant enzymes. Oxidation is one of the primary reasons some cells turn cancerous. These antioxidant enzymes help prevent that type of cell damage.

All of those reasons are why a Yale University School of Nursing study found that women who jogged regularly were less likely to develop breast cancer as well as why a Norwegian review of the existing research found that regular exercise reduced overall cancer risk, particularly colon and breast cancer.

MENTAL HEALTH

Exercise creates a number of benefits for your brain. Those extra capillaries that I mentioned in chapter 1 may be responsible for getting more blood and oxygen to your brain. Exercise also boosts a number of beneficial brain chemicals responsible for putting you in a good mood, and the effects are powerful.

For example, a survey of 17,626 Canadians found that those who were more physically active were better able to deal with work stress than those who were not active. That same study found that physical activity also helped people remain positive during times of high stress.

These mood-boosting benefits translate into less risk of burnout at work, less depression, and better performance under stress. Research even shows that regular exercise can counteract the mood swings and lethargy that often accompany dieting.

And you don't have to run your brains out to make a difference. A University of Washington study of 112 women found that regular 20-minute walks combined with light exposure and a vitamin regimen increased mood, self-esteem, and general sense of well-being in mildly to moderately depressed women. Other research has found that some people with depression who start an exercise program can forgo their medication. The results also hold true in children.

Possibly most exciting: These mood-boosting benefits start during your first exercise session. A British study of 80 people found that just one aerobics class obliterated anger, confusion, fatigue, and tension, particularly in people who were depressed before the class.

INTELLIGENCE

Cardiovascular fitness helps your heart and lungs more easily get oxygen to your brain. That, in turn, helps you think more clearly.

For example, patients with poor lung function who participated in regular aerobic exercise for as little as three months considerably improved their cognitive functioning. Another study, published in *Medicine & Science in Sports & Exercise,* found that 132 adults who were aerobically fit performed better at tests of cognitive speed than those who weren't fit.

LONGER-LASTING YOUTH

As you age, you tend to lose muscle mass, which is one reason why many men in their 60s, 70s, and 80s develop "chicken legs."

This muscle wasting may not seem so important during your 30s, but over time, it can become dangerous. Low muscle mass is one of the primary reasons elderly people experience trouble with their balance and coordination. Losing your balance and falling when you're 60-plus—when your bones are not as strong as they were when you were younger—can result in debilitating broken hips and other fractures.

As I mentioned earlier, less muscle will also lower your metabolism, which is a huge reason why so many people in their 40s and 50s experience middle-age spread.

Fortunately, research has found that regular weight training can reverse this process. When researchers put women and men in their

70s on a resistance training program, they built back much of the muscle they had slowly lost over the years. That translates into better balance, a better metabolism, more vigor, and less frailty.

BONE HEALTH

Women aren't the only ones who need to worry about their bones. Men are now experiencing osteoporosis—a disease characterized by weak, brittle bones—at an alarming rate.

Weight-bearing exercise such as running, jumping rope, and weight lifting puts pressure on your bones. That pressure encourages your bones to hold on to more minerals. Because your bones are made of minerals such as calcium and magnesium, a higher mineral content equals stronger bones.

Any type of pressure can do the job. Even the repetitive movement of chewing gum can strengthen your jaw bone. Case in point: I'm a gum chewer and my dentist says I have the jawbone of a teenager!

In fact, exercise may even be more important than a daily calcium supplement when it comes to preserving bone mass. A Japanese study of 256 premenopausal and 585 postmenopausal women found that those with regular exercise habits had stiffer, denser bones and that exercise was even more important than diet at preserving bone density. An Australian study of 126 postmenopausal women found that strength training combined with calcium supplements increased bone density more than calcium alone.

JOINT HEALTH

Experts once thought that certain types of cardiovascular exercise were the cause of certain types of joint pain, particularly osteoarthritis. They reasoned that the pressure of certain types of exercise, such as running, wore away the cartilage that cushions joints, creating friction and pain.

Now we know better. Though a sudden injury—typically caused by sudden cutting movements in sports such as basketball and soccer—can become arthritic if left untreated, exercise definitely does more good than harm to your joints.

Both cardiovascular exercise and resistance training help make your joints stronger, and stretching helps improve your range of motion, enabling you to bend a joint farther in each direction. Research shows that regular exercise can lower the symptoms associated with both osteoarthritis and rheumatoid arthritis. In fact, doctors are now encouraging patients with all sorts of joint problems to get moving.

BETTER HABITS

Combine exercise's mood-boosting benefits with its appetite-control mechanism and you get a powerful bad-habit breaker. Studies show that people can more easily quit smoking if they start an exercise program. Additional research shows that fit people tend to make better food choices than less fit people.

For example, a University of Minnesota study of 2,111 people found that those who exercised regularly had an easier time adapting to a healthy diet that included more fiber and less fat than others who didn't exercise. Another study, of 10,412 adults done at the University of Texas-Houston School of Public Health, found that the more people exercised, the less fat and cholesterol they consumed, and the more fiber they consumed—automatically. People who exercised regularly were also more likely to follow national dietary recommendations than less fit people.

Finally, a British study of 78 smokers found that a short 10-minute bout of intense exercise on an exercise bike reduced the urge for a cigarette as well as withdrawal symptoms.

MORE ENERGY

Imagine how you'd feel if you had a container of pure oxygen to breathe whenever you felt the need. Every inhalation would result in massive amounts of energy as the heightened amount of oxygen coursed through your body, right?

That's one powerful reason why exercise boosts energy. It helps create better blood flow to the brain, delivering that energizing oxygen more easily. Exercise also boosts a number of beneficial brain chemicals that also create more energy.

People who exercise regularly also tend to sleep better. A Japanese study found that a short early afternoon nap coupled with evening exercise helped elderly people sleep better and longer, allowing them to boost their mental health. Another study, from the University of Nebraska, found that exercise and weight loss could reduce the severity of sleep apnea, helping subjects to sleep longer without reawakening and to feel more energetic during the day.

BETTER CHILDREN

Study after study has found that regular exercise does much more than simply keep kids in shape, healthy, and at an ideal weight.

Research shows that it also makes teenagers less likely to experiment with drugs and delays the age at which they become sexually active. Of course, this may partially be due to sports-minded kids not having the time or energy to get into trouble. However, it also may be a result of a better emotional outlook. For example, a study of 64 nine- and 10-year-olds found that 15 minutes of aerobic exercise increased positive moods and decreased negative moods compared to when the children watched a video, which had the opposite effect.

Even in children with developmental disabilities, exercise has a benefit. A University of California at Los Angeles study found that

How to Hit the Spot

You've probably seen numerous ads on television for all sorts of spot-reducing machines from thigh blasters to buns lifters. The reason most of these exercise gimmicks fail to live up to their claims is this: There's no such thing as spot reducing.

My teenage son, Grant, learned this firsthand during a recent quest for "six-pack abs." For a few months, he religiously performed crunch after crunch. Yet the six-pack never surfaced on his abdomen.

Finally, he started running 3 to 4 miles, three days a week. Soon those abdominal muscles popped, giving him the six-pack of his dreams.

Why did running work while crunches failed? Because, as I just mentioned, there's no such thing as spot reducing. When your muscles need calories to burn, they take calories from fat stores all over your body. As my son performed crunch after crunch, he sculpted six-pack muscles, but they were hidden under a layer of fat. Even if he had performed 6,000 crunches, he wouldn't have burned enough calories to burn off that layer of fat. When he began his running program and subsequently dropped a few pounds on the scale, that fat vanished, revealing the underlying six-pack that he had worked so hard to achieve.

developmentally disabled children who took part in sports and exercise were less likely to exhibit maladaptive behavior. The children also exhibited improved self-esteem and social competence.

SEXUAL PERFORMANCE

Last, but certainly *not* least, exercise can play a huge role in improving your sex life.

Because exercise keeps those arteries open, more blood flows to your sex organs, preventing age-related sexual complications such as impotence and lack of desire. This increased blood flow can also increase desire and sensation.

Those same chemicals that boost mood and energy in your brain can also boost your sexual desire. Also, each bout of exercise gives you a temporary boost in the hormone testosterone, which has been linked with sexual desire. That might be one reason why many people tend to feel frisky after an exercise session.

Finally, when you move your body, you feel better about your body. Improved body image can go a long way toward making you feel more comfortable and confident in the bedroom.

Chapter 3

REASONS TO EAT WELL

A healthful food plan combines with your fitness plan to create a better you.

I've met more than my share of athletes who think that they don't need to watch what they eat. Because they burn so many calories during their multihour bike rides or tennis sessions, their weight pretty much controls itself.

Yet, all fitness enthusiasts—from professional athletes to weekend warriors—should pay attention to the types of foods they eat. What you eat profoundly affects the way you feel and look. What you eat can fuel your workout, giving you more endurance, speed, or strength. It can also fuel your day, helping you perform better at the office or giving you more stamina for young children. It can even help your fitness plan fight off disease and aging.

Here are just a few ways a smart nutrition plan can boost your fitness as well as your quality of life.

Faster recovery after a workout. Have you ever felt that drained, dead muscle sensation the day after working out? That comes from not eating the right types of foods in the right amounts after a workout.

Your body craves two major nutrients after a workout: carbohydrate and protein. It uses the carbohydrate to restock fuel stores in your muscles. The protein helps repair any muscle damage and helps carbohydrate get to your muscles more efficiently.

When you don't eat the right foods—or worse, don't eat at all—your muscles often don't fully restock their fuel stores. The next day your gas tanks literally are running low—and you feel it. Your muscles burn simply when walking up steps.

More energy and motivation to move. Food truly is fuel. Feed your body the wrong fuel on a consistent basis—for example, by subsisting on too much fried chicken and French fries—and you'll start to feel sluggish. Also, a number of factors can conspire to make you find an excuse to not exercise. Physical hunger is the most common culprit. That's why I suggest fitness enthusiasts snack on small minimeals every few hours rather than eating two or three large meals a day.

Increased endurance. Your muscles run on a type of stored energy called *glycogen,* made from the carbohydrate that you consume in your diet. As you exercise, your body drains stored carbohydrate from your muscles. Unless you replace those stores by eating during your workout, your body will run out of this fuel within about 90 minutes. As your muscles pull sugar out of your bloodstream, your blood sugar plummets, setting off a chain of reactions in your brain that make you feel dead tired.

You can increase your endurance beyond 90 minutes, however, by eating the right foods the week before and the day of your endurance event or workout as well as by eating the right foods and drinking the right beverages during your event or workout. (You'll learn how to do just that in chapter 9.) Besides helping you stock more fuel into your muscles, the right diet will also increase your body's ability to handle lactic acid accumulation. It also might interact with various neurotransmitters in your brain, helping you simply to feel less fatigued.

More speed. High-intensity exercise burns the stored glycogen in your muscles at a very high rate, even if that high-intensity exercise only lasts the few seconds it takes you to run to first base. Though one short sprint may only drain your glycogen fuel tanks by 5 percent or so, multiple sprints, such as in a game of soccer or football or baseball, can eventually drain those tanks to empty. Just as it can help you exercise longer, the right diet can help you sprint over and over again, maintaining your speed for a longer period of time.

Better health. Fitness is only part of the better health equation. Sure, exercise will lead to all of those beneficial changes that I mentioned in chapters 1 and 2. Yet, to boost your overall health, you need to combine your fitness plan with an eating plan. Don't you want to live as long and as healthy as possible? The only way to do so is to eat right.

A ton of research in recent years has shown that whole foods—fruits, vegetables, and whole grains—contain important disease-fighting chemicals, called *phytochemicals.* These have long names such as resveratrol and 3-n-butyl phthalide, and they work together to protect you from heart disease, cancer, eye problems, joint problems, and more. What you eat can even affect how well you feel. New research is now finding that a high-fat diet and smoking can cause back pain by clogging the blood vessels that supply the back muscles.

Weight maintenance. As I said earlier, some people exercise so much that they can easily maintain their weight without watching the calories they eat. For the vast majority of us, however, this isn't the case.

Few of us exercise multiple hours a day. For the masses of us, 20 to 30 minutes a day of endurance exercise isn't enough to let us eat whatever we want, whenever we want. Of course, as I said in chapter 2, exercise certainly helps control weight by boosting metabolism, burning calories, and regulating appetite. But you must combine it with a healthful diet to see true results. That holds true whether you want to lose weight—or gain it.

To achieve these benefits, you need to eat the right types of foods—at the right times. In this chapter, we'll explore the six basic types of foods and nutrients that fit into a performance diet. In chapters 9 and

10, you'll learn how to customize your fitness diet to best suit your fitness needs.

FLUIDS

In all of the customized daily food and activity pyramids in chapter 10, you'll notice that fluids form the base of the pyramids. That's because no matter your age, fluids form the foundation of your fitness program—and most people build their fitness program on a shaky foundation.

Your body needs fluid to carry nutrients around your body, give cells their shape, maintain body temperature, lubricate your joints, manage food digestion, and rid waste products through the urine. Between 50 and 65 percent of your body is water, amounting to 96 pints for the average man and 70 pints for the average woman. (Because lean tissue is water rich and fat tissue is "dry," or water poor, the more body fat you have, the less water you have, which is why women have less water.)

Some of this water is concentrated in important parts of your body. For example, your blood is nearly 100 percent fluid. When you lose more water than you drink, your blood gets sticky and thick, moving more slowly and making your heart work harder to push it through your blood vessels. This allows less oxygen and nutrients to make their way to cells all over your body, which, in turn, results in fatigue. Also, a higher heart rate makes moderate tasks, such as walking, feel more vigorous.

Have you ever felt winded even though you didn't feel as if you'd done anything to cause your heart to beat faster? You probably were dehydrated.

Another important organ, your brain, is 75 percent water. When your brain runs low on fluid, it lets you know with a dull headache. Perhaps you've felt this type of headache from time to time during a busy workday, when you forgot to drink. Or perhaps you've felt it

Sweating 101

I'm often asked why some people sweat more or less than others, and my answer often surprises people. The average person sweats about 1 liter of fluid per hour during exercise. However, some sweat more, others sweat less based on the following factors:

Fitness. When you exercise, your muscles generate heat as they burn ATP for fuel. The more fit you become, the better your body rids that heat through your skin. As sweat evaporates, so does heat, cooling your body. So the more fit you are, the more easily and copiously you sweat to rid yourself of excess heat. This greater sweat rate helps you to continue to exercise on a hot day, whereas someone less fit would have to call it quits.

Body fat. Body fat insulates your body, trapping heat in and preventing it from evaporating. Since not as much heat can escape to your skin, you don't sweat as much.

Age. As you age, your sweat rate becomes impaired. Also, children have immature sweating mechanisms, causing them to sweat less and be more susceptible to heat illness.

Genetics. Some people dissipate heat more easily than others due to a genetically greater number of sweat glands, making them sweat more.

more intensely after an outdoor workout on a hot day, when you've lost a lot of body fluid by sweating.

As you can see, fluids can make the difference between success and failure at work and during your workout. When you get low on fluid, you'll feel dizzy, tired, headachy, impatient, thirsty, and weak. More serious dehydration can result in blurred vision, deafness, difficulty swallowing, rapid pulse, and even unsteady gait.

To stay hydrated, you need to replace the fluids you lose through sweating, respiration (your body uses fluid to humidify the air you breathe), and urination. On average, you exhale 2 cups of water per day, and water also evaporates from your skin to keep you cool. Added together, the typical day at work causes you to lose up to 10 cups of fluid. Sweating during your workout can double or triple that figure. Also, certain beverages, such as those that contain caffeine or alcohol, increase fluid loss in the urine.

If you follow the customized pyramid for your age in chapter 10, you'll consume the right amount of fluid for you. You'll also find more tips to help you remain hydrated in chapter 9.

CARBOHYDRATE

Next to fluids, carbohydrate is your most important ally for achieving peak stamina, energy, and endurance. Called *carbs* by athletes, these sugars supply fuel for your body to burn during exercise and even during your day at work.

When you don't consume enough carbohydrate, your gas tanks are constantly tapped and never completely full. That means you won't last as long at an endurance effort or at an intense workout that involves multiple sprints, and your muscles will tire faster and more easily. Particularly, you won't be able to perform back-to-back days, as your muscles don't get a chance to refuel. Have you ever crawled from bed the day after a hard exercise bout? That empty leg feeling was from lack of carbohydrate.

Carbohydrate can also help you during your workout. Studies show that consuming some form of carbohydrate ½ hour into your workout can help you exercise longer and more intensely, especially if your session will last 90 minutes or more. That's because carbohydrate keeps your blood sugar levels steady, which, in turn, helps your brain and muscles access more fuel. As an added benefit,

Carbohydrate 101

Carbohydrate comes in three different forms:

Simple carbs. A simple carbohydrate contains one or two ring-shaped molecules called *sugar units.* Examples include sugar, honey, and fruit. Many people erroneously think because your body doesn't have to break down simple carbohydrate that these types of carbs are "fast-release" carbs that supply quick energy. This isn't necessarily the case. Some simple carbs, such as white sugar, do enter your system quickly, whereas others, such as honey and fruit, do not. In fact, some complex carbs (see next carbohydrate form) get into your system faster than some simple carbs. Also, not all simple carbs are created equal. Some, like white sugar, contain nearly no nutritional value, whereas others, such as fruit, contain a wealth of beneficial nutrients.

Complex carbs. These contain a large chain of simple units and are often found in starchy foods, such as beans, potatoes, pasta, and rice. Though your body must first break complex carbs down into simple units, they do not necessarily move through your system any more slowly than simple carbohydrate. As with simple carbohydrate, some complex carbs, such as white bread and snack crackers, supply little nutrition, whereas other complex carbs, such as oatmeal, supply much more.

Glycogen. A form of complex carbohydrate, glycogen is only found in your body. You won't find it in any food. Your body converts carbohydrate you eat into glycogen and stores it in your muscles and liver for later use. When you run low on blood sugar during an endurance effort such as running a marathon, your body dips into liver glycogen reserves and supplies the blood and ultimately the brain with fuel. Your muscles then use up their own supply of stored glycogen. You have enough stored glycogen in your muscles to last about 1½ hours of vigorous exercise. When your muscles or your brain run low on glycogen fuel, you feel tired.

regular carbohydrate consumption also keeps your immunity high. (Some studies show immunity plummets with long, intense exercise such as marathoning and century bike riding unless you eat carbohydrate during exercise.)

If you follow the customized pyramid for your age in chapter 10, you'll consume all the carbohydrate you need. You'll also find some more carbohydrate fueling tips in chapter 9.

PROTEIN

Beyond making muscle, protein helps you fight disease, build, repair, and maintain all types of tissue in your body, and keep brain cells thinking and blood flowing.

Protein makes up about 20 percent of your body weight. Many different proteins with specific duties enable your body to function smoothly. Your body makes these proteins by breaking down bulk protein in the food you eat into its different components, called *amino acids*. Your body arranges those amino acids into different combinations to create each kind of protein needed to perform nearly everything you do.

Yet sporadic eating and less-than-routine work schedules make many of us low on this important macronutrient. Each day you lose protein in your hair, skin, and nails along with protein that is routinely broken down in the body. Because your body can't store protein as it can carbohydrate and fat, it must use it as it comes in.

When you eat protein, it goes to where it's needed most. In time of an energy crisis (when you are skimping on calories), your brain and muscles can use protein to burn as fuel when carbohydrate stores run low. This lowers your ability to fight infection and rebuild muscle. That's why very low-calorie diets cause you to lose muscle protein rather than body fat.

To keep up with demands, your body needs a daily supply of amino acids from food.

Protein 101

Protein can be broken down into 20 different amino acids. Because your body can manufacture 11 of them all by itself, only 9 of the 20 acids are considered dietary essentials.

A food that contains all 9 essential amino acids, in proportion to your body's need, is called a *complete* (or *high-quality*) *protein source.* All animal products are complete proteins. Soybeans are also a complete protein source. Many *incomplete proteins*—grains, beans, seeds, and nuts—can be combined to form complete proteins. For example, grains are low in the amino acid lysine, but beans have plenty of it. Beans are low in methionine, while grains are not. Eating grains and beans together during the same day forms a complete protein.

One word of caution: Too much protein can be as destructive as too little. Eating more steak will not necessarily help you build more muscle. Extra protein beyond what your body demands does not make extra muscle, grow stronger fingernails, or make you more resistant to illness. The liver and kidneys must process the nitrogen by-product of excess amino acids, which increases your fluid needs. It also may cause loss of calcium in the urine.

My customized pyramids in part III will help you get the right amount and type of protein for you.

FAT

A few years back, all fat was considered bad, and eating a lowfat diet was thought to be best for heart health. Times sure have changed.

Besides tasting great and helping you feel full, fat is just as important as vitamins and minerals. Besides keeping you healthy, the right fats in the right amounts may also keep you exercising.

Along with carbohydrate, fat serves as a vital fuel source during endurance efforts. Researchers have long noted that endurance training turns your muscles into better fat burners, and a handful of studies done at the State University of New York at Buffalo suggest a 30 percent fat diet makes more sense for fit people than diets of less than 20 percent.

In one of those studies, a group of men and women runners who averaged 40-plus weekly miles ate a 17 percent fat diet for four weeks and then switched to a 32 percent fat diet for another four weeks. At the end of each four-week segment, the participants ran to exhaustion during a treadmill test.

Result: The men ran 24 percent longer and the women 19 percent longer following the moderate-fat diet compared to the lowfat one.

In addition to providing fuel for your exercising body, certain types of fat can also keep you healthy. Special essential fats called *omega-6* and *omega-3* fatty acids found in nuts, vegetable oils, flaxseed, and fish are crucial for building a strong immune system, healthy skin, and nerve fibers.

Research suggests that our early ancestors ate much more of these omega-3 fats than we do. We instead eat mostly saturated and hydrogenated fats from animal foods and processed snacks. These modern-day foods provide hardly any essential fatty acids, particularly omega-3s. As a result, an array of chronic ailments may have developed including autoimmune diseases, heart disease, some cancers, multiple sclerosis, and skin conditions such as psoriasis—most of which were nonexistent thousands of years ago.

In fact, studies have found that eating up to 40 percent of your total calories from fat—as long as it's mostly monounsaturated fat such as olive oil—can cut cholesterol levels and heart disease risk. On the other hand, avoiding saturated fats and trans fats (found in processed foods) also helps keep your arteries clear.

In addition to boosting your health and exercise performance, fat can even help boost your mood. In a study from the nutrition and

Fat 101

To boost the right amounts of fats in your diet, you need to understand exactly where the right and wrong fats come from. Here's a simple fat primer:

Omega-3 fat. Your body cannot make this "good" essential fat, so it must be gleaned from your diet. Omega-3s help protect you from a host of age-related ailments, such as heart disease, certain cancers, immune disorders, arthritis, and possibly Alzheimer's and multiple sclerosis. We need just a few grams daily, but most of us skimp on these precious fats. Good food sources include fatty, cold-water fish like salmon, mackerel, and tuna along with flaxseed meal and oil (used as salad dressing but not in cooking). Nuts and canola and soybean oil also contain small amounts.

Omega-6 fat. As with omega-3s, omega-6s are also an essential fat type. However, unlike omega-3s, we typically have no trouble getting enough omega-6 fats, as we consume plenty of corn, sunflower, and other vegetable oils. While these fats are crucial for healthy skin and brain function, too much of a good thing can spell trouble. Getting no more than about a third of your total daily fat (about 20 grams or less) from vegetable oils is best for heart health; too much may lower heart-healthy HDL cholesterol levels.

Monounsaturated fat. This fat type, found in olive, canola, and peanut oil as well as in avocados, is definitely a "good" fat. Studies show that getting a majority of your fat from these sources helps lower cholesterol levels and drops heart disease risk. Aim for more than a third of your total fat intake as monounsaturated fat by using these oils in cooking and spreading avocado on breads and as a dip rather than using margarine, butter, or sour cream.

Saturated fat. Dubbed the "bad" fat for good reason, saturated fat bumps up cholesterol levels and raises risk for heart disease. Most of us chow down too much saturated fat in the form of butter, margarine, fatty meats, full-fat dairy

(continues)

Fat 101 *(continued)*

products, and fast foods, which are typically prepared with vegetable shortening or lard. Keep your intake to fewer than 20 grams daily.

Trans fat. This fat is formed when vegetable oils are hydrogenated. According to numerous studies, trans fats are as deadly to heart health as saturated fats. Avoid processed foods made with hydrogenated or partially hydrogenated vegetable oils, such as crackers, chips, margarine, and fast foods. A trans fat limit for the diet is not set but should be counted in with your saturated fat budget of 20 grams or less daily.

psychiatry departments of the University of Sheffield in the United Kingdom, ratings of anger and hostility increased in people who switched from a 40 percent to a 25 percent fat diet. Researchers suspect a diet too low in fat may alter brain chemicals that control mood and behavior.

Based on various studies and on American Heart Association recommendations, you should shoot for a diet that includes 30 percent of total calories from fat. The amount of fat, however, is much less important than the type. My customized pyramids in chapter 10 will help you eat the right amount and type of fat. You'll find additional tips for eating the right fats in the right amounts in chapter 9.

VITAMINS, MINERALS, AND PHYTOCHEMICALS

Food contains important nutrients that keep your body running smoothly. Vitamins, minerals, and phytochemicals are types of these nutrients. They are needed to feed your metabolism and rejuvenate your body's cells. Getting too little of any of them can sap your performance and compromise your health.

However, you can also go overboard. Many of these nutrients, particularly those considered fat soluble, can be toxic if taken above the recommended dose. Also, vitamins, minerals, and phytochemicals interact with one another. So taking too much of one can compromise your absorption of another.

Here's a rundown on these three types of nutrients.

Vitamins

From vitamin A to vitamin K, vitamins facilitate hundreds of biochemical reactions in your body. They also act as regulators that oversee processes like bone growth and the maintenance of healthy skin. Without them, you would not be able to process the carbohydrates you need for stamina, your body's protein metabolism would fall apart, and you would slowly degenerate, becoming weak and unable to think clearly.

Many of us fall short on vitamins due to poor food choices. They are found most abundantly in fruits, vegetables, and whole grains, not in soda, potato chips, and cookies. You'll learn more about the 13 vitamins in chapter 5.

Minerals

Minerals keep your metabolism clicking along by assisting in chemical reactions. Minerals also keep you in balance by controlling your body's pH (acid level) and water balance. Unlike vitamins, minerals give your body shape by providing structure to bones and teeth. And unlike any other nutrient, minerals are inorganic, simple elements that originate from the earth's soil and water. Minerals are so simple in their nature that your body does not metabolize them—that is, it doesn't arrange their chemical structure as it does other nutrients. You'll learn more about 15 essential minerals in chapter 6.

Phytochemicals

Foods also contain a host of other important nutrients known collectively as phytochemicals. Found predominantly in whole foods such as vegetables, fruit, and grains, they are also sometimes called *nutraceuticals.* Besides fighting off age-related disease such as cataracts, heart disease, and cancer, phytochemicals may also power your exercising body. They may help repair the nicks and dents made to your muscles during a tough exercise bout, forestalling postexercise soreness. They may also give your immunity a boost during long efforts, and they may even improve lung function.

Though these nutrients have undergone much research in recent years, experts still are not at the point where they can pinpoint a healthy dose or intake for any of them. However, that hasn't stopped supplement makers from packaging them into pills for you to take. You'll learn more about phytochemicals in chapter 8.

ELECTROLYTES

These foreign-sounding nutrients will come up again when you read about sports products and supplements in chapters 4 and 7. Put simply, electrolytes are merely a handful of minerals—sodium, potassium, magnesium, and calcium, to name a few—that carry an electrical current when dissolved in water.

For example, if I took a beaker full of pure water and tried to pass an electrical current through it, I wouldn't get anywhere. Water doesn't carry a current. However, if I take that same beaker of water and add a pinch of salt—presto!—now it carries a current. That's one reason why water boils faster when you add a pinch of salt.

This becomes important in your body because much of your body survives on electrical impulses. Electricity is what forms your nerve impulses and makes your heart beat. Positive and negative charges help your body balance fluid in and out of cells and allow all different processes in life to occur.

You need a delicate balance of calcium, potassium, sodium, and magnesium to do everything from regulating your blood pressure and water balance to allowing your muscles to contract correctly. During exercise, you lose two important electrolytes—sodium and chloride—through your sweat. Under most circumstances, you don't lose enough to make you deficient in either nutrient. But during an endurance effort such as a marathon, a century bike ride, or an adventure race on a hot, humid day, you can lose enough sodium to run dangerously low.

When this happens, you set off an electrolyte imbalance, leading to a serious problem called *hyponatremia.* The condition can trigger seizures, coma, and even death. Initial warning signs include confusion and disorientation, muscle weakness, and vomiting.

Women and slower, beginner endurance exercisers are most at risk. According to a study from the New Zealand Ironman Triathlon, 18 percent of the finishers were hyponatremic, with three times as many women suffering as men. I saw this firsthand when working the medical tent at an Ironman a number of years ago. The winner crossed the finish line, stumbled, collapsed, and then started convulsing. It took a sodium IV drip for 1 hour before he returned to consciousness.

Fortunately, only ultraendurance athletes need to worry about such complications. Most of the rest of us have more than enough salt in our bloodstream from eating salt-rich processed foods. Following my eating tips in chapter 9 as well as the customized daily food and activity pyramid for your age will help you keep your electrolytes in optimal balance.

Part II

THAT EXTRA EDGE

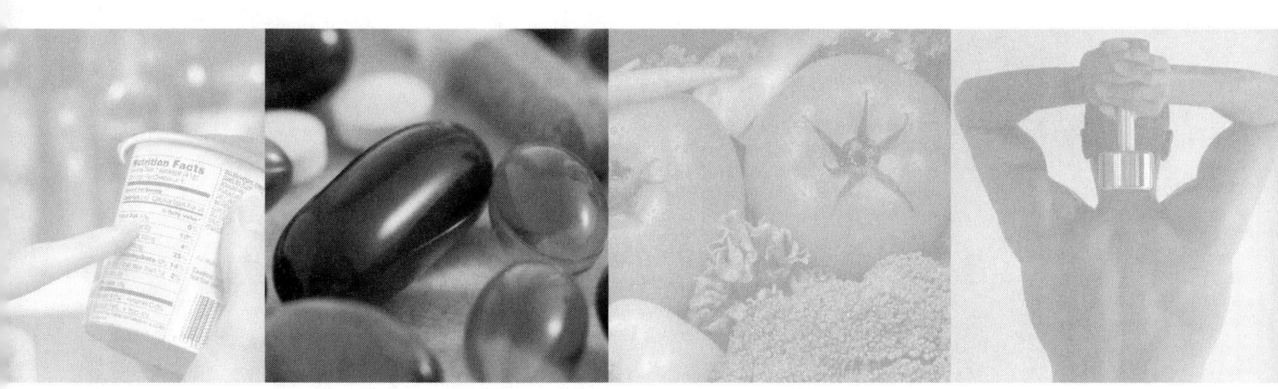

Chapter 4

SUPPLEMENTS

Find out what works, what doesn't, and what might even harm your health.

With flashy packaging, company-produced "research," and compelling claims, marketers often seduce us into believing that dietary supplements provide the secret weapon against everything from low energy to stubborn fat deposits to frequent colds to lagging endurance or sprint performance. For years, the vast majority of consumers have looked to supplements rather than conventional over-the-counter or prescription medication as a cure-all for just about every ill.

Fortunately, that's beginning to change. As more and more discoveries are made about drug interactions, health consequences, and the effectiveness—or lack thereof—of certain supplements, consumers are now beginning to ask questions before buying.

The government does not regulate dietary supplements by the same strict laws that it uses to regulate foods. That means, for the most part, that what supplement makers claim on a bottle or on their Web site doesn't necessarily have to be true. In fact, supplements currently don't even have to contain the actual ingredients that they list on the label. They can also include extra ingredients and contaminants *not* listed on the label, such as lead or steroids.

The government allows supplement manufacturers to make what are called *structure-function claims* on labels, such as "boosts energy levels" or "promotes healthy blood cholesterol." Unlike prescription or over-the-counter drugs, supplement manufacturers don't even need to provide scientific proof to back up such claims unless the FDA demands it. The FDA rarely does so unless a significant number of complaints or safety issues arise.

These loose regulations add up to some simple advice: Know what and why before you buy. Just because a supplement is for sale doesn't mean it lives up to labeling claims, contains what it states on the label, or is safe. Also be aware that many dietary supplements, particularly herbal products, may interact with medications you may be taking. Taking excessive amounts of some supplements may lead to liver damage, birth defects, and even death.

Here are a few ground rules to shop by:

- No one nutrient or substance determines good health. Don't look to any one supplement as a cure-all for a health problem. For example, strong bones are "built" through adequate calcium along with protein, vitamins D and K, and other minerals including magnesium and boron. This mix of ingredients must be stimulated by plenty of weight-bearing exercise to produce results.

- Many of the studies done on particular supplements were done on the foods that contain them, not on the supplements in isolation. It's likely that nutrients interact with other substances found in food that together promote good health rather than a nutrient acting in isolation. In other words, when you remove a nutrient from a food and put it in a pill, it may lose some or all of its healing powers.

- Read the labels and uncover as much information about a supplement as you can. (See sidebar, "Do Your Own Detective

Work.") If you compete on the semiprofessional or professional level, you must closely examine your supplements, as many contain extras such as glandular extracts, which can cause you to fail a drug test.

- Consult with your physician, especially if you are using any over-the-counter or prescription medications. Your local pharmacist may also help you pinpoint potentially risky combinations of supplements.

THE SUPPLEMENT LOWDOWN

Technically, dietary supplements include vitamins, minerals, amino acids, herbals, and more. However, I discuss vitamins in chapter 5 and minerals in chapter 6, so here I'll be dealing with herbs, amino acids, and other substances that are neither vitamin nor mineral.

This is in no way an exhaustive list of supplements. I could write an entire book about what you might find on the shelves at a health food or vitamin store. In this chapter, I've chosen the 20 most popular supplements that claim to bolster fitness by helping you to run faster, lose weight, build muscle, or heighten energy or immunity. I chose these supplements based on how well they sell at health food stores, making sure to include the top-selling fitness and weight loss supplements, as well as the ones I receive the most questions about from friends, students, and athletes.

ANDROSTENEDIONE

"Andro" made headlines a few years ago when baseball slugger Mark McGwire mentioned that he took it, along with the supplement creatine, to build muscle mass. At that time, andro quickly sold out as scientists tried to find out whether the supplement worked and whether it was safe.

Do Your Own Detective Work

Because supplement marketers often make sweeping and unsubstantiated claims on their packaging and because they list ingredients that aren't always in the bottle—and don't list others that are—you must do your own sleuthing to find out if a supplement works, is safe, and contains what it claims.

This actually isn't a hard or time-consuming process. You can find just about everything you need to know on the World Wide Web. Here are some good sites to check:

To find out if a supplement contains what appears on the ingredients list: Go to www.consumerlab.com. This independent lab tests vitamins, minerals, herbs, and other supplements for potency and purity, making sure each bottle of particular brands contains what the label lists without hidden contaminants. For example, in a recent testing on chromium supplements, the lab found that some contained less than 5 percent the amount stated on the label. Another contained a form of chromium thought to be toxic in the body.

To find out if a claim made on a supplement's packaging has been scientifically studied: Do what I do when I am researching a supplement—go to the National Library of Medicine's online database of medical studies at http://www4.ncbi.nlm.nih.gov/entrez/query.fcgi. When you type the name of the supplement in the site's search engine, you'll receive a list of studies. Click on any that look interesting to read an abstract of the study and what it found.

To find out about adverse side effects or drug interactions of a particular supplement: The National Institutes of Health's National Center for Complementary and Alternative Medicine offers a wealth of information about supplements at its Web site: http://nccam.nci.nih.gov/health. The site includes the latest FDA danger alerts, the latest research on drug interactions, and more.

Fortunately, much of the andro hype has faded—and for good reason. The supplement not only doesn't work, but it's dangerous to your health.

The Claims Manufacturers claim androstenedione, a hormone secreted by your adrenal glands, boosts levels of the hormone testosterone, helping to build muscle mass.

The Research When scientists tested this theory in the lab, they found that andro did not boost testosterone or improve muscle mass or body composition.

The Dangers In studies, supplemental andro has lowered the healthy (HDL) cholesterol, increasing risk for heart disease. One study published in the highly respected *Journal of the American Medical Association* even found that andro boosted estrogen, which is dangerous for men. Among other things, the supplement may increase the risk of male breast enlargement, cancer, and heart disease.

My Recommendation If you seek bigger muscles and less fat, invest in a gym membership rather than wasting your money on this dangerous supplement.

BRANCHED-CHAIN AMINO ACIDS

Branched-chain amino acids (BCAAs) have been a hot topic for years, and they show promise for endurance athletes. Several well-designed studies suggest that supplemental BCAAs may improve your exercise performance and help prevent the muscle damage that can occur with heavy training.

The Claims BCAAs, along with 17 other amino acids, make up the building blocks that form all of the protein in your body. The three

BCAAs (L-leucine, L-isoleucine, and L-valine) are found primarily in muscle. During 2 or more hours of exercise, your body breaks down these amino acids and burns them for energy, causing your muscle protein supply to dwindle. Taking a BCAA supplement helps bolster your muscle protein pools, preventing muscle damage during heavy exercise. This in turn speeds your recovery.

The Research In a study done at the University of Tasmania in Australia, cyclists took either a placebo or 12 grams of BCAAs daily for six days. (This amount is about double what you normally consume from dietary sources such as meats and beans.)

On the seventh day, subjects cycled hard for 2 hours. After this exercise bout, researchers took blood samples every hour for several hours, then once a day for four days. The researchers then measured muscle-tissue damage based on various enzyme levels in the blood.

Compared to the placebo group, cyclists who took BCAA supplements showed decreased muscle damage, leading researchers to believe that supplementation may have helped replace the BCAAs lost during exercise.

The Dangers While those in the study had no adverse side effects from BCAA supplementation, six days isn't enough time to determine long-term side effects.

My Recommendation Branched-chain amino acids show promise, especially for distance runners, cyclists, and other endurance athletes. Nevertheless, wait for more research to determine the safety of this supplement before popping one every day. Instead, make sure you are eating enough protein—75 to 100 grams a day—because the best way to maintain adequate muscle tissue is by eating food with enough calories and protein.

CAFFEINE

Few of us think of caffeine as a dietary supplement. However, this stimulant finds its way into numerous products, including many supplements designed to bolster energy or aid weight loss. In such products, caffeine is sometimes disguised as guarana, the name of a plant that contains caffeine, or green tea extract.

Many of us—myself included—use caffeine to wake up in the morning or to give us a little jolt before a workout. Many of my college students take caffeinated "uppers," such as GNC's Super Guarana Energy Rush, NoDoz, or Vivarin, when trying to stay up all night to study for an exam.

The Claims Bolstered energy, clear thinking, and improved physical performance.

The Research Simply put, caffeine works. It wakes us up, clears our heads, and may even bolster our physical performance. Countless studies show that taking about 200 to 300 milligrams of caffeine (the equivalent of 2 to 3 cups of coffee) improves feelings of alertness and reaction time and even makes an exercise session feel less strenuous.

The Dangers Side effects are minimal at levels less than 300 milligrams daily. However, when combined with other stimulants such as ephedra (see "Fat Burners" on page 59) or in higher doses, caffeine may cause a racing heartbeat, weakening your heart.

My Recommendation If using caffeine in pill form, check the label for amounts, as the dose may exceed the 200 to 300 milligram limit.

CHROMIUM

Chromium picolinate remains a hot-selling supplement for people interested in losing body fat and beefing up muscle size. While it may sound exotic, chromium picolinate consists of the mineral chromium combined with what's referred to as a *chelating agent,* picolinate, which helps in the absorption and transport of chromium into body cells.

In the body, chromium plays a vital role in the operation of the hormone insulin, which is responsible for processing carbohydrates from foods. After you eat a meal, chromium makes insulin's job possible, helping carbohydrates (sugars) make their way into your body cells for use. Protein and fat metabolism also rely on proper functioning of insulin.

The Claims Both manufacturers and body builders hype chromium supplements as a quick way to shed fat and get a "cut" look. Several weight loss products tout chromium as their secret fat-burning ingredient. Manufacturers also promote this supplement as a way to control blood sugar if you have diabetes.

The Research Research clearly shows that a low intake of chromium from the diet may hamper the body's ability to use sugar or glucose. This means that after a meal, levels of glucose become elevated beyond normal for an extended period of time. Referred to as *glucose intolerance,* this is a warning sign of diabetes. In some people, high blood glucose levels (called *hyperglycemia*) improve with chromium supplements.

Research also shows that the body's ability to handle sugar is improved with supplements of chromium in the amount of 200 micrograms. But this benefit may simply reflect a poor intake because of a highly refined diet.

Though chromium may benefit those with diabetes or those prone to diabetes, no research shows that it bolsters fat burning. Several well-controlled studies done on athletes have shown that chromium supplements do not boost performance, help lower body fat, or boost muscle size. In one study, wrestlers took either 200 micrograms daily of chromium or a placebo for 14 weeks while participating in a weight training and running program designed to enhance muscle strength and endurance.

Both groups of wrestlers became fitter and stronger with the program, but there was no difference between groups. Both the placebo and the chromium group lost equal amounts of body fat and gained the same amounts of muscle during the exercise program.

While most research has failed to support chromium for fat burning or muscle building, the supplement may boost sprint performance. In a study done at the University of Dayton in Ohio, cyclists worked out for an hour while they drank either a carbohydrate beverage similar to a sports drink or the same beverage with added chromium. They consumed about 60 grams of carbohydrate (240 calories) and about 200 micrograms of chromium (equivalent to the daily recommended intake).

At the end of the hour ride, cyclists pedaled as hard as they could for just under a minute. Researchers measured the amount of work performed during the sprint and found that the chromium-fortified drink boosted sprint performance by 7 percent compared to the plain carbohydrate drink. Blood sugar levels were also slightly lower with the chromium beverage, suggesting greater glucose uptake by the muscles.

The Dangers Taking a chromium supplement is safe at levels of 200 micrograms. In large amounts—hundreds of times the estimated need—chromium supplements may become toxic. One study found that high amounts caused chromosomal damage, a possible connection to cancer. If you consume too much chromium, which could only happen via supplementation, you can hamper your absorption of iron and zinc.

My Recommendation Many people fall short of the recommended 50- to 200-microgram chromium intake. Also, you may sweat out small amounts of chromium during heavy training. So, you might

Where to Find Chromium

The following foods are all high in chromium:

- Apples
- Beer
- Brewer's yeast
- Brown rice
- Chicken
- Mushrooms
- Oysters
- Peas, cooked
- Red wine
- Shredded Wheat (and other whole grain cereals)

improve your carbohydrate use and possibly your performance by increasing your daily chromium intake. Also, as type 2 diabetes has now become a national epidemic with serious health implications, taking steps to get enough of this mineral makes sense.

However, you don't need to buy a supplement to do so. You'll get 50 to 60 micrograms of chromium from a cup of refried beans, two microbrewed beers, a cooked chicken breast, or a cup of peas. To keep chromium levels optimal, beware of eating too many refined foods, such as white bread and sweets, which are not only low in chromium but also may boost your need for it (to help process carbohydrates).

CONJUGATED LINOLEIC ACID (CLA)

This fatty acid found in whole milk and beef is starting to show up in pill form on supplement shelves, with much commotion. It seems not a day goes by that one of my students doesn't ask me about this supplement's slimming powers.

The Claims Makers produce the supplement form of CLA from safflower and sunflower oils. Products such as EverSlender and Tonalin claim that supplemental CLA aids in weight loss by encouraging the body to store extra calories in muscle rather than in fat cells. Other products claim it boosts immunity. Manufacturers say this fatty acid should be required in the diet, and some scientists agree. So far, however, the government has not set a daily recommended intake.

The Research Because CLA acts as a cell messenger that helps turn on and turn off different prostaglandins responsible for signaling the production of immune cells, the immunity-boosting theory makes sense. One study has found that 1 to 3 grams of CLA a day enhances immune function. Though no one is quite sure of the mechanism, other preliminary research has found that the supplement may indeed increase muscle mass and decrease body fat.

The Dangers So far, no health risks have been uncovered. In fact, a few animal studies show CLA may bolster health by lowering cholesterol levels and inhibiting cancer cell formation.

My Recommendation Usually I recommend that you get the substances you need from food. However, because beef and whole milk contain artery-clogging saturated fat, I can't do so in this case. Because human trials are only now getting under way, I suggest waiting until more research is done before trying this expensive supplement. Instead, focus on increasing your consumption of healthy fats, such as the omega-3 fatty acids found in fish and nuts, as these beneficial fats have been shown to produce the same effects.

CREATINE

Creatine is a proteinlike substance that your body makes daily. You also consume plenty of it if you eat beef, fish, and other meats.

Creatine's most notable activity takes place in your muscle tissue. It acts much like cylinders in your car's engine helping to fire up your muscle. Remember when I mentioned ATP in chapter 1? During sprint performance or weight lifting, your body switches to anaerobic energy production, using either creatine or glucose to make more ATP. The more creatine in your muscles, the better your ability to create ATP and the longer you can last without fatigue.

The Claims Load up with creatine from a supplement, about 20 to 25 grams for five to seven days, and you boost the number of cylinders (creatine levels) in your muscles by some 20 to 30 percent. According to manufacturers' labels, this in turn boosts muscle strength and size and sprint performance.

The Research Research shows that creatine supplements do translate into more strength and a greater ability to do single or repeated bouts of high-effort exercise such as sprinting. However, there is one catch: You have to train. You can't take creatine and then go sit on your couch for a few days expecting your muscles to grow. You must hit the weight room.

As an added benefit, creatine supplements taken over several weeks may boost levels of good (HDL) cholesterol.

So far, research only shows that loading up on creatine helps during weight lifting and during brief, high-intensity exercise typically lasting less than a minute. Dosing with creatine has not been shown to have any performance-enhancing powers for longer efforts, especially continuous exercise such as long-distance running and cycling. In fact, creatine loading in swimmers does not appear to boost sprint performance and may even have a negative impact since weight gain can change body position in the water.

The Dangers Few studies have looked at the supplement's long-term safety, especially in adolescents who are growing. One recent study showed that creatine dosing did not alter liver and kidney function, a good sign since these two organs are involved with clearing creatine from the body. Additionally, another study, looking at long-term creatine supplementation in strength athletes, such as football players, did not show that supplementation had adverse effects such as cramping.

My Recommendation If you're interested in pumping up the size of your muscles, or if you want to run sprints, give creatine a try. But if you've been trying to keep your weight down for the next marathon, stick with your high-carbohydrate diet. The dose for creatine is 25 grams daily for five to seven days, followed by a maintenance dose of 2 to 5 grams daily.

FAT BLOCKERS (CHITOSAN)

Made from chitosan, a type of sea fiber from shrimp and crab shells, "fat-blocking" supplements such as Chroma Slim, GNC's Optibolic, and Twinlab's Diet Fuel claim to stop your intestines from absorbing fat, which lowers your caloric consumption.

The Claims Sometimes touted as "marine fiber," chitosan's large, bulky chemical structure acts much like a sticky piece of Velcro that traps small amounts of fatty substances in your intestine. The chitosan, along with the fat and cholesterol, doesn't get absorbed by your intestines but instead ends up in your stool. End result: Calories get sucked out of your body before they can be absorbed.

The Research Over several weeks, researchers fed laboratory mice a high-fat diet that was about 10 to 15 percent chitosan by weight. The animals gained significantly less fat than control mice eating the same fat-laden diet. This may sound promising, but the mice ate large amounts of chitosan (much more than the recommended amount on many product labels).

Studies done on people are few and far between, and results are less promising than those on mice. In one group, men were given 3 to 6 grams of chitosan a day, the approximate dosage recommended on product labels, for a few weeks. According to that study, chitosan binds to, at most, 3 to 4 grams of fat per meal. That amounts to a mere 30 calories, the amount in less than a teaspoon of butter. That's hardly a situation where you can eat anything you want and still lose weight.

The supplements, however, may be more promising for your heart health. While the men in the study didn't lose weight, their blood cholesterol levels fell significantly. Levels of the good (HDL) cholesterol rose. This suggests chitosan may have some potential as a cholesterol-lowering supplement.

The Dangers These supplements may lower your absorption of fat-soluble vitamins such as vitamin E and cause intestinal yeast overgrowth. Also, like the fat substitute olestra, high amounts of chitosan may cause steatorrhea, an uncomfortable and embarrassing involuntary leakage of fat-laden waste.

My Recommendation The pills cost about $10 for a one-week supply. Spend your money on something more worthwhile, such as a grocery cart full of fresh produce.

FAT BURNERS (INCLUDING EPHEDRINE, MA HUANG, CAFFEINE, AND GUARANA)

Log on to the Web, flip through a fitness magazine, or cruise the supplement aisles in a health food store, and you're bound to see a staggering array of supplements that claim to speed your metabolism and shed unwanted fat.

Many of these products contain a Chinese herb called Ma Huang (also called ephedra) or a synthetic version called ephedrine. Caffeine is also a common ingredient. So is guarana, a substance from a plant that also contains caffeine, in amounts up to four times that of a typical cup of coffee. Some also contain green tea extract, which is just a healthful-sounding way to say "caffeine."

Some supplements pack all of these stimulants into one pill, creating quite an adrenaline jolt.

The Claims These products, such as Metabolife and XtremeLean, claim increased calorie burning by boosting the basal metabolic rate. These stimulants increase heart rate and blood pressure as well as cause your body to waste heat energy, boosting calorie burn.

The Research These ingredients do show promise as weight loss aids, but at a high health risk.

A few studies show that manufacturers' claims are valid when these supplements are combined with a low-calorie diet. When combined with caffeine, ephedra supplements do enhance fat loss, suppress appetite, and stimulate fat burning beyond what would normally happen when you restrict calories. In one recent study, people lost 36 pounds during the six months that they took a daily caffeine and ephedrine supplement, compared to 29 pounds for the placebo group.

Can a Dieter's Tea Help You Lose Weight?

So-called dieter's teas usually contain senna, cascara, aloe, buckthorn, or other natural laxatives from plants. Marketers claim that the increase in bowel movements as a result of drinking the teas will prevent the absorption of some calories and fat—an effortless way to lose weight.

Yet, trying to lose weight through the use of laxatives is anything but effortless. Using these products on a regular basis or in excessive amounts can result in diarrhea, vomiting, nausea, stomach cramps, chronic constipation, fainting, and even death. It also doesn't work. Research shows that laxatives work on the colon, not the small intestine, where calories get absorbed.

When faced with such side effects and dismal benefits, you will find that exercise keeps looking better and better as a weight loss tool.

The Dangers The dose that you need to produce this effect is 60 milligrams of ephedra and 600 milligrams of caffeine, the amount in 6 cups of coffee. Many people who take the supplements report a speeding heart rate, dizziness, sweating, and other symptoms of nervousness. The U.S. Food and Drug Administration has been notified of more than 800 adverse side effects, including heart attack, stroke, tremors, and insomnia. More than 80 deaths are suspected from use of the supplement.

My Recommendation I, along with the FDA, recommend avoiding these products. The FDA is trying to limit the amounts of ephedra and caffeine in these products to 8 milligrams of ephedrine per serving and a maximum daily dosage of 24 milligrams. A warning label on these supplements may eventually tell you to limit your usage to only seven days.

FIBER

I didn't want to lambaste every weight loss supplement without giving you at least one that worked, which is where fiber comes in. Yes, that roughage in whole grains, vegetables, and fruits fills you up and helps squelch your appetite.

Fiber is easy to get from foods, but on those days you may not be eating your veggies and whole grains, a fiber supplement made with vegetable or grain fiber can help fill in the gaps.

The Claims Often sold as tablets, powder drink mixes, and candy-like bars, fiber supplements are available at grocery stores, at pharmacies, and on the Internet. They advertise many purposes. Here are the three main types:

Laxatives. These fiber supplements claim to relieve constipation and promote regular bowel movements. Most powder mixes contain psyllium, a husk from a seed that acts as a laxative. Capsule versions often contain polycarbophil, a synthetic fiber that absorbs water.

Cholesterol lowering. Typically sold as tablets or in "food" form such as a cookie or bar, these products contain oat bran, fruit pectin, or psyllium, which are all great sources of water-soluble fiber. This fiber type helps trap cholesterol and by-products of cholesterol in the intestinal tract so that this fatty substance doesn't get into the circulation.

Appetite suppressing. Sold as wafers and capsules, these products consist primarily of water-soluble fibers from fruits, beans, or psyllium that form a gel in the stomach and help make you feel full.

The Research In general, laxative products do what they say: bulk up fecal mass and relieve constipation. But you have to check the label for dosage. Some contain only a few grams of fiber and may not be effective as a laxative.

Studies also show that oat fiber is a very effective means of lowering risky levels of cholesterol and cutting heart disease risk. The amount of fiber shown to have positive effects on blood cholesterol is 6 to 15 grams daily. Be sure to check product labels as many provide only a fraction of this in a recommended serving.

Finally, studies also support that water-soluble fiber may be helpful in weight loss efforts, but only along with efforts to cut calories and increase physical activity. Studies show that people who eat the recommended 25 grams of fiber or more daily weigh less than those who eat a low-fiber diet.

The Dangers When using these products, you may also experience flatulence, abdominal rumbling sounds, and even cramping or diarrhea. You must take these products with plenty of water. Fiber bulks up in the intestinal tract, and water is needed to keep things "moving." Insufficient fluid intake could cause blockage in the intestinal tract and require medical attention.

My Recommendation In general, these products vary in fiber content, contributing anywhere from less than 10 percent to more than 100 percent of the Daily Value (DV, the recommended amount of a nutrient for a typical consumer eating a 2,000 calorie diet) for fiber of 25 grams.

Instead of only reaching for a fiber supplement, however, try real food first. Start your day with a high-fiber cereal in the morning (one that has at least 5 to 10 grams of fiber), and then top this with dried fruit (raisins, apricots, figs, cranberries) for even more fiber (the dried fruit counts as a serving of fruit). At lunch, bring along a ready-to-eat package of baby carrots or other cut-up vegetables. Or if there is a juice bar nearby, opt for a fruit smoothie for lunch. Then follow up with a big salad at dinner.

FISH AND ALGAL OIL

You may have already heard that a type of oil found in fish—called *omega-3 fatty acids*—can lower blood cholesterol. But as a fitness enthusiast, you may be more interested in fish oil for its anti-inflammatory action. A typical omega-3 fatty acid supplement of 1 to 1.5 grams a day may reduce joint pain and rheumatoid arthritis symptoms and may even help those with psoriasis and inflammatory bowel disorders. Think of it as a natural painkiller for your sore, overworked muscles.

The Claims Supplement makers say fish oil lowers heart disease risk, as well as a host of other age-related diseases such as rheumatoid arthritis. Some omega-3 supplements are made from algae (algal oil), which also contains this fat.

The Research Fish oil may work by affecting the prostaglandin levels in your body. Different types of prostaglandins signal different bodily responses. Some tell your tissues to swell up; others tell those same tissues to calm down. Researchers suspect that years of eating too much of one type of fat (omega-6 fatty acids) and too little of another (the type found in fish) may bring on inflammation.

Omega-6 fats are not bad fats. Found in vegetable oils, they can be quite healthful. Problem is, most of us are out of balance. Scientists suspect the more healthful ratio of these fats is four omega-6s to every one omega-3. Sounds easy until you learn that the typical American diet contains about 10 omega-6s to every one omega-3.

The Dangers Taking lots of fish oil supplements can have not-so-nice side effects such as bad breath, body odor, and diarrhea. They also thin the blood, so avoid them if you are taking anticoagulant medication. Look for enteric-coated, delayed-release capsules, which will help offset those side effects, and put the focus on real fish rather than only on supplements. Also, some scientists worry that these supplements may be contaminated with mercury, dioxins, or PCBs, though testing has failed to find those contaminants in actual supplements.

My Recommendation For fish oil to work, you need to increase it while decreasing other fats such as the saturated fats found in butter, the trans fats found in processed foods, and the omega-6 fatty acids found in vegetable oil. So, as you supplement with up to 2 grams a day of omega-3s, cut back on other less healthful fats. And bump up your intake of fish and flaxseed meal or oil to two servings a week.

GINSENG

You'll find ginseng just about everywhere these days, in sports drinks, iced tea, herbal supplements, and energy gels. Used for thousands of years by the Chinese, ginseng is an herb traditionally taken for chronic fatigue, nervous disorders, low sex drive, and forgetfulness.

The Claims In terms of exercise, ginseng has been said to boost energy levels and performance and to speed workout recovery. Asian (also called *Panax,* Chinese, or Korean) ginseng accounts for the most common herbal type. However, some products contain American ginseng, said to be a milder form of the herb. Others contain Siberian ginseng, which costs less to grow and make.

The Research Wayne State University exercise physiologist H. J. Engels, Ph.D., tested ginseng on a group of female athletes. Each athlete took either a placebo or 200 milligrams of ginseng extract daily for eight weeks. The women then pedaled to exhaustion on a stationary bike while being monitored for performance factors during and immediately after exercise. Result: Ginseng provided no performance benefit, nor did recovery rate improve.

In another study, Engels looked at whether ginseng improved mood state and/or lowered perceived exertion. Again, researchers used an eight-week supplementation period and the same bike test. Yet again, the herb provided no mood benefit, nor did the subjects feel they were pedaling more easily.

On the other hand, ginseng might help you somewhat if you play a sport that requires a lot of hand-eye coordination. In one small study, researchers tested the reaction time of soccer players who had supplemented with 350 milligrams of ginseng or a placebo for six weeks. They asked the soccer players to strenuously ride a stationary bike. During the workout, the soccer players who had taken the ginseng had faster reaction times than those who had not.

The Dangers These supplements may be contaminated with pesticides or heavy metals. Some tested samples have contained a pesticide called *pentachloronitrobenzene,* a possible carcinogen that may be toxic to the liver and kidneys, at up to 20 times the allowable amount. Testers have also found lead in some of these supplements.

My Recommendation Ginseng has a long history as a medicinal herb, but it hasn't been scientifically shown to provide any performance benefit. Save your money for something more worthwhile.

GLUCOSAMINE AND CHONDROITIN SULFATE

In the past few years, orthopedists and other physicians have increasingly advised patients to take both glucosamine and chondroitin sulfate to ease the inflammation and pain of osteoarthritis, a degenerative joint condition that accelerates with age as well as with excessive use. One of the hallmarks of osteoarthritis is an erosion of the cartilage that cushions your joints. Cartilage often only slowly repairs itself and, with injury, may fail to grow back fully.

Chondrocytes—the cells in your joints that make cartilage—need glucosamine to function optimally. Think of this amino acid as a "food" for cartilage cells. It also acts as the structural component of tendons, ligaments, and cartilage. Chondroitin is an important structural component of cartilage found in all of your joints.

The Claims Marketers claim that the supplements when taken together protect joints and tendons and relieve osteoarthritis pain.

The Research According to several studies, supplemental glucosamine and chondroitin—around 1,500 milligrams of each daily—helps soothe pain possibly by stimulating cartilage growth. Animal studies also suggest that supplemental glucosamine may speed repair to injured joints.

Compared to nonsteroidal anti-inflammatory drugs (such as aspirin and ibuprofen), the supplements eased pain comparably but also improved joint function as measured by range of motion. In addition, glucosamine helps produce substances in ligaments, tendons, and joint fluids called *glycoproteins.* So it may speed healing in those areas as well, though research has yet to test that theory.

The Dangers So far, studies show that glucosamine and chondroitin are well tolerated, with fewer side effects than anti-inflammatories, which often result in stomach upset and even bleeding. Follow your doctor's advice and keep him or her informed of your symptoms and any side effects. In one small study, a group of people with diabetes who took glucosamine experienced lower insulin sensitivity and blood sugar control.

My Recommendation While glucosamine and chondroitin won't prevent an injury, they may help in recovery from cartilage injuries brought on by overuse. Take 1,500 milligrams of each daily (divide into three 500-milligram doses over the course of the day). Know that pain reduction and improvement of symptoms will take several weeks as your chondrocytes repair eroded cartilage.

GLUTAMINE

This nonessential amino acid found abundantly in your muscles and blood plasma serves as fuel for your immune cells, possibly helping to prevent the drop in immunity that tends to occur with heavy endurance training.

The Claims Because physical stress and heavy exercise deplete this amino acid from your plasma, some researchers suspect that taking supplemental glutamine may ward off colds and muscle soreness induced by endurance exercise.

The Research While few studies have been done on this supplement, research does suggest that supplemental glutamine improves your immune function and response to infections. One study published in the *Journal of Applied Physiology* found that the addition of glutamine to a carbohydrate beverage (such as a sports drink) could increase total body carbohydrate storage after a workout. In other words, you recover faster. Other research has found 2 to 10 milligrams of the supplement taken after exhaustive exercise such as a marathon could cut in half the risk of catching a cold.

The Dangers Supplements may flood your body with higher amounts of this amino acid than you could ever consume in your diet. Theoretically, this could block certain other amino acids from passing through the blood-brain barrier into your brain, influencing your brain chemistry.

Can a Juice Fast Help You Lose Weight?

When I was in the middle of writing this book, the Hollywood Celebrity Diet two-day juice fast ranked as one of the top-selling "supplements" for weight loss. Marketers claimed that the special juice was the "best kept secret of Hollywood stars," that you could "lose up to 10 pounds in two days," and that the drink contained special botanical extracts that would cleanse, detoxify, and rejuvenate your body.

The juice fast is just one of a number out there, some of which you concoct yourself at home out of orange or grapefruit juice. Do they do what they claim?

Well, sure, after two days on a juice fast, you will lose weight. But this is nothing magical. A juice fast results in weight loss from pure, old-fashioned calorie deprivation.

For example, the Hollywood Celebrity Diet juice fast has you drink 4 ounces of the juice mixed with cold water three times a day. Other than drinking eight glasses of regular water, you're not allowed to eat or drink anything else while on the fast. Each day your calorie intake totals 300 calories. Essentially, you're starving your fat off.

As for the "detoxifying" and "cleansing" effects, such a juice fast would only do the opposite. When your body runs low on calories, it begins to burn muscle for fuel, which slows your metabolism and dumps a load of by-products into your bloodstream. Your digestive process also shuts down, allowing waste products to stagnate in your intestines.

As for these "special botanicals," they are nothing more than juice—orange, pineapple, white grape, apple, plum, and lemon—sprinkled with some vitamins and minerals, as well as some green tea extract for a caffeine jolt.

My Recommendation Glutamine comes in pills, in powder, and in combination with other types of protein. Take 5 to 20 grams after endurance exercise such as a 4-hour bike ride or 2-hour run. This supplement, however, is no substitute for rest and a proper recovery diet. Also, lots of research shows that simply ingesting some form of carbohydrate—such as a sports drink—during endurance efforts provides the same immunity boost as glutamine.

HYDROXYCITRIC ACID (HCA)

You'll find this extract from the fruit *Garcinia cambogia* in many weight loss products.

The Claims Manufacturers of Xenadrine, Xtreme Lean, Hydroxycut, and others say HCA inhibits an enzyme involved in energy metabolism, halting new fat from being made.

The Research Study results conflict. A few experiments using large amounts of HCA, some with animals, seem to indicate that this compound may aid with weight loss efforts in people who are overweight. But a recent study shows that HCA provides no benefit beyond what simple calorie cutting can do.

The Dangers Many of these products also contain ephedra, which may weaken your heart. Those that do not are considered safe.

My Recommendation This supplement is expensive and hasn't been shown conclusively to work. You're better off spending your money on a pair of walking or running shoes.

L-ARGININE

This nonessential amino acid found in protein foods and made by the body is a precursor to anabolic growth hormone.

The Claims Manufacturers claim that bolstering your pools of L-arginine will in turn bolster amounts of growth hormone, causing more muscle to grow.

The Research Though the theory makes sense, it just doesn't pan out. I'm happy for that, as extra growth hormone can hurt your health by damaging the heart and bones.

Though L-arginine may not pump up the size of your muscles, it may improve heart functioning. L-arginine does bolster levels of nitrous oxide, which in turn dilates blood vessels.

The Dangers L-arginine is safe in amounts available in most supplements (100 to 1,000 milligrams). In excessive amounts, L-arginine can hamper the use of other amino acids.

My Recommendation You don't need a supplement. You can easily consume enough L-arginine by eating meat and fish.

L-CARNITINE

This amino acid, made in your body, helps stimulate fat burning. L-carnitine sits on the cell's inner membrane, helping to escort fatty acids into the cell's mitochondria, a hotbox compartment that burns fat. Without enough carnitine, fat burning slows.

The Claims Since you need carnitine to burn fat, manufacturers claim that consuming more of it will stimulate fat burning even more. They also state that the supplement boosts endurance performance because fat is a major fuel source during a long run, bike ride, or swim.

The Research Unfortunately, studies show that this supplement does not increase fat burning or weight loss. Fat burning aside, this supplement may offer a benefit to people with compromised immunity and other health disorders. For example, research shows that people with AIDS, chronic fatigue syndrome, or heart disease reduce their symptoms when they take this supplement.

The Dangers As with any amino acid, taking too much may block other amino acids from getting into your brain, influencing your brain chemistry.

My Recommendation Wait for more research before taking this supplement.

PROTEIN POWDERS

Every part of your body contains protein, from your muscles, blood, and immune cells to tendons, ligaments, skin, and hair. Sedentary people need 50 to 70 grams of protein a day to keep them going. Fit people need more—a good 25 to 50 percent more—to take care of muscle repair and increased energy requirements.

The Claims Manufacturers claim that an extra dose of protein goes straight to muscle building, and that more is always better. With the high-protein diet craze, others look to this macronutrient as a way to squelch hunger and lose weight.

The Research As with all substances, more isn't always better. If you are already consuming 70 or more grams of protein a day, an extra dose in the form of a protein powder shake has not been shown to boost muscle building. As for those high-protein diets, most of them work because they are also extremely low in calories, not because they are low in carbohydrate or high in protein. That said, protein does slow digestion, so including some protein with each meal has been shown to delay hunger by slowing stomach emptying.

Despite what many manufacturers claim, the type of protein found in powders is not better absorbed than the type found in real food. Most protein supplements come from soy or milk proteins, which are well used by the body. But of course, you are paying more for the protein in a can than you would for virtually the same protein from a tofu stir-fry or carton of yogurt.

The Dangers You can easily consume more protein than your body needs. Your kidneys must process the extra protein, which if not needed by the body, gets burned as fuel or converted to fat and stored for later use. People with kidney disease should avoid extra protein.

My Recommendation Here's the dilemma with protein: The very people who need more of it (endurance exercisers) are often the ones who don't get enough. The reason, basically, is because runners, cyclists, hikers, and swimmers tend to eat less meat than sedentary people and body builders, and meat is one of the best sources of protein.

Skimping on protein can cause fatigue and slow recovery from injuries and infections, so be sure you're getting enough from high-quality sources such as lean meat, soybeans (in the form of tofu, soy milk, or soy protein), fish, and lowfat dairy products.

Each day, try to include 5 to 6 ounces of lean meat or two to three servings of soy products, plus two to three servings of lowfat or nonfat dairy products and several servings of grains along with legumes (two to three servings of grains and legumes if you're a vegetarian who doesn't consume dairy). Unless you're a vegan vegetarian who is allergic to soy, you probably don't need to supplement with protein shakes or energy bars.

PYRUVATE

This end product of carbohydrate metabolism occurs naturally in your body. Supplement makers say pyruvate acts like a potent antioxidant and speeds up energy metabolism and calorie burning.

The Claims Claims on bottles of pyruvate are stunning: "increases endurance by 20 percent" and "promotes 47 percent greater fat loss."

The Research According to well-done studies from a few years back, pyruvate taken in fairly hefty doses of 20 to 25 grams daily appears to boost endurance performance and assist in weight loss. According to one recent study, pyruvate taken daily boosted endurance in a group of men riding stationary bikes. While this sounds promising, it's important to point out that these men did not exercise regularly. So these results may not apply to someone who exercises on a regular basis.

Pyruvate may, however, show more promise as a fat burner. Preliminary studies on obese subjects on a very low-calorie diet showed that the supplement did enhance fat loss. But some aspects of the study design are suspect, especially the way the researchers measured fat loss.

In one study, exercise physiologist Rick Kreider, Ph.D., from the University of Memphis, compared a 10-gram daily dose of pyruvate to a placebo in a group of sedentary, obese women who were beginning a six-week walking and weight lifting program. The women lifted weights and walked three times a week for 30 minutes at a time. The women taking the placebo lost no weight over the six weeks, while the pyruvate-supplemented women lost about a pound of fat. The dosage used in his study was 15 to 30 times more than recommended on the product label.

The Dangers Study subjects who took pyruvate suffered a drop in levels of the good (HDL) cholesterol, increasing their risk for heart disease.

My Recommendation Thus far, research showing any promise for pyruvate as a fat burner involves daily doses that greatly exceed recommended dosages printed on most product labels. Manufacturers recommend approximately a 1- to 2-gram daily dose, but there's no evidence it works at such a low dose.

SODIUM BICARBONATE

Taking a few spoonfuls of sodium bicarbonate (commonly known as baking soda) several hours before intense bouts of exercise may improve staying power. That's because sodium bicarbonate acts as a buffer in the body, decreasing the lactic acid levels that lead to muscle fatigue.

The Claims During high-intensity exercise—such as sprinting—your body uses pure carbohydrate, and no fat, as a fuel source. When your body burns carbohydrate for fuel, it creates a by-product, called *lactic acid,* which is normally cleared away and subsequently used as an energy source itself. However, if your body produces lactic acid faster than it clears it, you feel the burn and your muscles fatigue. As it accumulates, lactic acid begins to hamper muscle contractions, and you soon get that heavy feeling in your legs.

The Research Several recent studies have shown that a dose of sodium bicarbonate can delay that burning feeling, thus improving performance during short exercise bouts.

The Dangers Large doses (20 grams or more) may cause severe intestinal cramping, bloating, and diarrhea.

My Recommendation Sodium bicarbonate's fatigue-busting powers come into play only for short-duration, high-intensity exercise, such as sprinting.

WHEY PROTEIN

A lot of hype surrounds whey protein. In fact, many of the athletes I counsel snatch it up and use it to make shakes.

Whey protein is nothing mysterious, however. It comes from milk, representing about 20 percent of the total milk protein, with the rest coming from casein. It's also very common, as it's a by-product of cheese production. Manufacturers have a large, inexpensive supply of whey at their disposal.

The Claims These supplements claim that whey builds muscle mass better than other proteins.

The Research Research on people fails to support these claims.

The Dangers Some of these supplements contain glandular extracts that can make you fail an athletic drug test.

My Recommendation Until studies find any promise for this supplement, save your money, and, instead, consume your protein from foods such as soy, seafood, eggs, lowfat dairy products, or lean meats.

Chapter 5

VITAMINS

How to tell when you're getting enough and when you're getting too little.

First came the dizzying array of scientific studies that claimed certain vitamins prevent aging, life-threatening diseases, and even birth defects as well as beautify your looks and keep you mentally alert and energized. Then came the follow-up scientific reports that flip-flopped earlier claims, warning us that these same vitamin supplements may be dangerous. Vitamin A, for example, was said to ward off age-related maladies; now research suggests that supplements of this antioxidant may actually increase cancer risk in some people.

Giving your body the vitamins it needs shouldn't be so confusing, which is why I've provided the answers right here.

Let's start with what vitamins actually do. Your body needs 13 of them to facilitate hundreds of biomechanical reactions in your body, acting as regulators that oversee processes like bone growth and the maintenance of healthy skin. You need vitamins to feed your metabolism, rejuvenate your cells, process the foods you eat, and keep your muscles healthy.

Vitamins are generally split into two camps, the water-soluble type and the fat-soluble type.

Water-soluble vitamins are found in the watery parts of cells and include vitamin C and the eight B vitamins. They assist enzyme-driven chemical reactions. Because your body can't store water-soluble vitamins, they get broken down and excreted from your body within 24 to 48 hours of eating. Overdoing it on any of these usually only results in what scientists like to call "expensive urine."

The fat-soluble vitamins—A, D, E, and K—are found in the fatty parts of body cells. They act as metabolic regulators. For example, vitamin D is in charge of directing calcium into your bones. Unlike water-soluble vitamins, fat-soluble vitamins can be stored in the body for later use. For example, your liver has a one- to two-year supply of vitamin A. If you don't consume enough of a particular fat-soluble vitamin, your body will take what it needs out of storage. However, because these vitamins accumulate in your body, they can easily become toxic if you take them in supplement form.

Because your body can't make most vitamins (or minerals, but we'll get to them in chapter 6), you must consume them in the food you eat. Consuming too few of any of them will drain your energy and hurt your health, yet overdosing on any of them can bring on a host of bad changes from skin changes to hair loss to death.

How do you know when you're getting too much and when you're not getting enough? For each vitamin entry, I've given you signs of not getting enough, as well as signs you're getting too much. Keep in mind that it's very rare for someone to experience a vitamin deficiency. Deficiency problems happen when you routinely fall more than 20 to 30 percent below the Recommended Dietary Allowance (RDA, the recommended intake for vitamins and other essential nutrients to meet the needs of most healthy people based on age, gender, and condition, such as pregnancy). Even if a stressful period at work forces you to live for a few days on fast and processed foods, you still won't become deficient. It's usually only alcoholics, chronically malnourished people

Stay in the Safety Zone

Taking a multivitamin with 100 to 150 percent of the RDA is safe. But popping vitamins in amounts several times the RDA can pose real health risks. The fat-soluble vitamins (A, D, E, and K) get trapped or stored in fatty tissue and organs when taken in excess. Medical reports show that vitamins A and D are particularly toxic, causing liver damage and bone deformities when taken in amounts just five times the RDA.

In contrast, the water-soluble vitamins (B vitamins and C) flush out of your body in the urine if you consume them in excess, either through diet or a pill. Because of this, scientists generally view water-soluble vitamins as safe in amounts greater than the RDA. However, you still shouldn't take any side effects lightly. Vitamin B_6, for example, has been shown to cause nerve damage when taken in excess (100 times the RDA).

Besides supplements, you should also pay attention to how much fortified foods boost your intake. If you look at any box of cereal, you'll notice that numerous vitamins and minerals have been added. This fortification turns many breakfast cereals into caloric multivitamins. Beyond cereal, numerous other products from energy bars to orange juice are now coming fortified with various vitamins and minerals. As with supplements, you don't want to overdo it.

Besides getting a possible vitamin-mineral "OD," reaching for an antioxidant-fortified food bar instead of a naturally antioxidant-packed orange or carrot may shortchange your health. According to cancer and heart disease researchers, it may be the unique interaction of these antioxidants and other nutrients found in perfect balance only in produce and a few other real foods that helps reduce cancer and heart disease risk. Once you take these nutrients out of their natural form and process them into a pill, shake, or bar, they may lose some of their healing properties.

To make sure fortified foods don't overtake your diet, follow these tips:

- Reach for real food first. Eat a minimum of five fruit and vegetable servings (eight or more servings daily if you want to ward off high blood pressure or heart disease), and at least eight to 10 servings of whole grains daily.
- Vary selections of cereals, fortified beverages, and other vitamin-boosted foods and feel free to go for nonfortified foods as well.
- If you eat fortified breakfast cereal or other vitamin-boosted food daily, then skip your vitamin-mineral supplement.

such as those with anorexia, those on medications that might alter absorption, or those with altered nutrient requirements, such as pregnant or lactating women, who experience deficiencies. You're more likely to run into problems of vitamin excess if you routinely take supplements that supply well over recommended levels.

Let's take a look at the four fat-soluble vitamins first, and then the water-soluble vitamins.

VITAMIN A

Vitamin A actually encompasses numerous molecules called *retinoids*, which is why the well-known wrinkle cream made primarily out of vitamin A is called Retin-A.

You need vitamin A for normal vision in dim light. It also maintains the normal structure and function of mucous membranes as well as aids the growth of bones, teeth, and skin.

But what makes this vitamin stand out from others is that it acts as an antioxidant when eaten in a plant form called *provitamin A carotenoids*. Antioxidants such as carotenoids help prevent the formation of free radicals, substances that damage cell membranes and promote the formation and growth of cancer and heart disease.

Beta-carotene (the primary plant precursor to vitamin A) gives many fruits and vegetables their yellow to red color and is converted to vitamin A inside your body, specifically in the wall of your digestive tract. Diets rich in beta-carotene and vitamin A have been shown to lower cancer risk. Besides beta-carotene, there are numerous other carotenes that give fruits and vegetables color, including the red of tomatoes. Though these other carotenes perform important functions in your body, they are not converted to vitamin A as well as beta-carotene is.

Researchers have recently noted that not as much beta-carotene gets converted to vitamin A as once thought, which means all of us probably could consume more beta-carotene-rich foods.

Best Food Sources Yellow-orange fruits and vegetables, dark-green leafy vegetables, fortified milk, eggs, liver.

How Much You Need 800 micrograms of retinol for women and 1,000 micrograms for men daily.

When to Supplement Because vitamin A is a fat-soluble vitamin, it can easily build up in your body and become toxic, which is why supplements are not recommended.

However, it is nearly impossible to overdose on vitamin A from food. Your body only converts as much beta-carotene to vitamin A as it needs. So, no matter how many carrots you eat, you simply can't overdose on this vitamin.

Signs You're Not Getting Enough Night blindness, anemia (fatigue), depressed immunity (frequent colds), hard and white hair follicles.

Signs You're Getting Too Much Nausea, appetite loss, dry cracked skin, hair loss, joint pain, severe headache, blurred vision.

VITAMIN D

Even though your body can make vitamin D through an interaction with sunlight, it is becoming more important to make sure you get enough of this vitamin from your food. Due to the risk of skin cancer, we now keep much of our skin covered with clothing and sunblock when outdoors, preventing the body from interacting with sunlight to make vitamin D. For younger adults, this doesn't seem to cause deficiency, probably because it only takes 10 to 30 minutes of sun a day on your hands and face for your body to make enough D. However, studies show many of those age 60-plus are deficient in this vitamin, possibly because they spend little time outdoors.

The Right Time to Take a Vitamin

Some people erroneously think that they can take a vitamin supplement just before an activity—such as running—to help make that activity go better. This simply isn't the case.

Your muscles do need these nutrients, such as thiamin and niacin, for using carbohydrates and fats as fuel to drive muscle contraction and movement. But these nutrients are already available for quick use inside your muscle cells. Additionally, it takes some time—anywhere from 20 minutes to hours—for the vitamins and minerals in a pill to get distributed throughout your body.

The best time to take a multivitamin supplement? With a meal, so there's food in your intestinal tract. Several vitamins are better absorbed when they accompany food. For example, fat-soluble vitamins such as A, D, and E need fat for absorption. It's best to take your vitamins at the same time every day. That will make it part of your routine so you're less likely to forget.

A few things to consider, though, when taking your vitamins: If you take a calcium supplement, take it at a meal when not taking a multivitamin. High doses of calcium can hamper the absorption of iron as well as cause constipation. Also, check the label of any prescription medication you take for information or ask your pharmacist about your medications since many may interfere with vitamin and mineral absorption. And last, avoid coffee, tea, or wine when you take your multivitamin. These beverages contain tannins, substances that block absorption of minerals like iron or zinc.

Your body needs vitamin D for calcium absorption, making it an important vitamin for proper growth of bones and teeth. Deficiency may also play a role in diabetes, according to recent research done in Finland, where people get much less sunlight, and therefore less vitamin D than in the United States.

Best Food Sources Fortified milk, eggs, fish, liver.

How Much You Need 5 micrograms for both men and women daily, increasing to 10 micrograms for those over age 50 and 15 micrograms for those over 70.

When to Supplement If you are older than age 60 and spend little time outdoors, talk to your doctor about supplementation. Do not take vitamin D supplements without a physician's supervision, as they can become toxic in high doses.

Signs You're Not Getting Enough Retarded bone growth and stunting in children, poor formation of teeth, soft bone fractures in adults, muscle spasms.

Signs You're Getting Too Much Growth retardation, calcium deposits in soft tissue, kidney damage.

VITAMIN E

Of all the antioxidant vitamins, E is perhaps the most important—as well as the least consumed.

When you eat vitamin E, it makes its way to your cells, positioning itself on their surfaces, acting much like a cell bodyguard that's armed and ready to fight off attacks by rogue molecules called *free radicals*. Vitamin E comes armed with extra electrons that it lends to these free radicals, neutralizing them, preventing them from damaging not only that cell but any cell in your body.

Many researchers believe this powerful antioxidant protects us from age-related ailments such as heart disease and cancer. As with vitamin C, studies also show that vitamin E supplementation—often at the level of about 400 international units (IU) a day—may help protect you from the oxidative damage caused by endurance exercise. This free-radical-induced damage is what, in part, causes muscle stiffness and soreness.

Increased exposure to air pollution and other environmental contaminants may call for additional vitamin E to combat the damaging effect of these substances. Also, some studies show that vitamin E status may be diminished with exercise, particularly at high altitude. Age-related changes such as cataract formation have also been linked to low vitamin E intake.

Unfortunately, because E is found primarily in oils, nuts, and other high-calorie foods, many of us don't consume enough of this important vitamin.

Best Food Sources Almonds, vegetable oils, green leafy vegetables, wheat germ, whole grain products, fortified breakfast cereals.

How Much You Need 15 milligrams (30 IU) for men and women, but many people argue that you need much more, as much as 400 IU (more than 13 times the recommendation).

When to Supplement You have to eat a lot of food—particularly high-calorie food—to meet the recommended intake. Elderly people, young women, and anyone restricting calorie intake probably aren't getting enough. If you want to take vitamin E supplements, look for those that contain no more than 1,000 IU. Take your supplement with a meal, since your body needs a small amount of fat to break it down.

Look for supplements with the natural form of vitamin E rather than the synthetic, as research shows that natural E is more biologically active in the body. Natural E supplements list d-alpha-tocopherol rather than only dl-alpha-tocopherol as an ingredient.

Signs You're Not Getting Enough Anemia, weakness, muscle pain.

Signs You're Getting Too Much Fatigue, nausea, blood thinning (impaired ability to make a blood clot).

Maximum Vitamin Power

To ensure you get the widest array of vitamins that you need, follow these tips:

Eat a wide variety of whole foods. All food contains vitamins, from very small amounts to very large amounts. However, whole foods such as fruits, vegetables, and whole grains contain more vitamins than processed foods contain. Try to eat many different types of whole foods, rather than just your usual staple, to vary the nutrients you consume.

Use vitamin-safe cooking methods. High temperatures and long cooking times can zap vitamins from food. Light can also destroy some nutrients. To retain more vitamins (and minerals and phytochemicals) in your food, cut vegetables and fruit into larger pieces rather than smaller, steam or microwave rather than boil, store produce whole rather than in pieces, and keep juice in airtight containers and freeze whenever possible.

VITAMIN K

At birth, babies are usually given a shot of this blood-clotting vitamin because their bodies can't yet make their own and because they don't usually get enough from breast milk. The vitamin shot helps give boy babies enough K for proper clotting during circumcision.

However, besides clotting, vitamin K is often overlooked as an important bone builder.

Your body needs vitamin K for chemical reactions that bring about bone formation. Usually older people who experience bone problems as they age may be deficient in this vitamin as well as vitamin D and calcium.

Your body does make some K all by itself by intestinal bacteria; however, we've recently learned that the bacteria doesn't make as much K as we once thought. I used to tell my students that you get half of the K you need from bacteria, but it's really less than 30 percent.

Best Food Sources Cabbage-family vegetables, green leafy vegetables, vegetable oils (but not hydrogenated oils, as vitamin K is destroyed during processing).

How Much You Need 65 micrograms for women and 80 micrograms for men daily.

When to Supplement You probably don't need to supplement with this vitamin. However, avoid using mineral oil as a laxative, as it can trap K in your intestine, preventing absorption.

Signs You're Not Getting Enough Inability to clot blood.

Signs You're Getting Too Much Very rare, though too much can cause jaundice.

THIAMIN (B_1)

This important B vitamin is involved in breaking down carbohydrate as a fuel source.

Thiamin deficiency used to be much more common a century ago, particularly when people began switching from whole grain foods to refined grains. When grains are refined, the protective outer covering gets removed, simultaneously removing much of the fiber and nutrients of the grain, including thiamin.

When grains first were refined, no one realized that this was problematic. As more and more people began switching from whole to refined grains, a strange condition called *beriberi* began showing up in eastern Asia. When translated from Senegalese, *beriberi* means "I cannot. I cannot." Thiamin deficiency was hampering sugar from being used properly by the nervous system in affected people, causing paralysis. To test if someone were developing the condition, doctors at the time asked people to sit into a squatting position and stand up. Those with beriberi would squat and then say "beriberi" because they could not stand up.

In the 1930s and 1940s, the United States eliminated the problem when it began adding thiamin and other vitamins back into grains that were processed. Today, alcoholics fall prey to thiamin deficiency due to poor intake and increased losses in the urine as a result of excessive alcohol consumption.

Best Food Sources Pork, liver, whole grain and enriched grain products, beans, nuts.

How Much You Need 1.1 milligrams for women and 1.2 milligrams for men daily.

When to Supplement Not necessary.

Signs You're Not Getting Enough Weakness, fatigue, painful muscles, hallucinations.

Signs You're Getting Too Much Not currently known.

RIBOFLAVIN (B_2)

The only experience most people have with this vitamin is its listing on cereal boxes and supplement labels. Yet it does perform an important job.

You need riboflavin for protein, fat, and carbohydrate metabolism as well as for healthy skin. In particular, riboflavin helps transform protein into neurotransmitters, chemicals in your brain that allow thinking and memory to occur.

Riboflavin also works with an antioxidant enzyme that helps to prevent heart disease and cancer. Other B vitamins also use riboflavin to chemically change into the correct form inside the body.

Best Food Sources Dairy products, whole grain and enriched grain products.

How Much You Need 1.1 milligrams for women and 1.3 milligrams for men daily.

When to Supplement Because cereals are fortified, it's rare to not get enough.

Signs You're Not Getting Enough Skin rash, bright red tongue, cracks at the corners of the mouth, eyes sensitive to light, fatigue.

Signs You're Getting Too Much Bright yellow urine.

NIACIN (B_3)

If you've ever taken a niacin supplement before, then you're probably familiar with one of its main attributes—vasodilation. This widening of the blood vessels can give your skin a reddish glow. But it also does something even more important. When taken under the direction of a doctor, niacin may help slow the progression of heart disease by widening those same blood vessels and by interfering with cholesterol production in the liver. But a doctor's direction is a must. Too much of the wrong type of niacin can cause liver damage.

You also need this vitamin for protein, fat, and carbohydrate energy metabolism as well as for nervous system function.

Do You Need Organic Vitamins?

Vitamin scientists agree that it makes little difference to the body if a vitamin is made in a test tube or "naturally" by plants or bacteria. Synthetic and natural vitamins are absorbed equally as well and perform the same duties once inside your body—with one exception. Natural vitamin E, or d-alpha-tocopherol, is slightly more potent than the synthetic version, dl-alpha-tocopherol.

Best Food Sources Meats, milk, eggs, poultry, whole grain and enriched grain products, nuts.

How Much You Need 14 milligrams for women and 16 milligrams for men daily.

When to Supplement Take only under the supervision of your doctor.

Signs You're Not Getting Enough Diarrhea, severe cracking and darkening of skin, weakness, delirium.

Signs You're Getting Too Much Flushing and itchy skin, irritability, headaches, intestinal cramps, nausea, diarrhea.

BIOTIN

Biotin is involved in numerous reactions that help process carbohydrate, protein, and fat.

Though an important vitamin, you don't hear about it much because deficiency is extremely rare. Recently, an abnormal processing of biotin has been observed in some pregnant women and may be linked to birth defects. The bacteria in your intestinal tract can actually manufacture a small amount of biotin, which may explain why even people who subsist on marginal diets rarely display a deficiency.

Best Food Sources Found in many foods, including eggs, milk, and cereal.

How Much You Need 30 micrograms for both men and women daily.

When to Supplement No need.

Signs You're Not Getting Enough Muscle pain, weakness, fatigue, hair loss.

Signs You're Getting Too Much There's no upper limit set for this vitamin—excess is excreted in the urine.

PANTOTHENATE

In Greek, *pantothen* means "from every side." It's fitting because we consume this vitamin in just about every food we eat. It truly comes at us from every side, in everything.

Because so many foods contain pantothenate, deficiency is almost never seen except in alcoholics, who usually don't eat well and don't fully absorb the food they eat.

Toxicity is also unheard-of, making this innocent little vitamin not guilty of causing a single problem in the body.

Pantothenate is needed for the normal metabolism of carbohydrate, fat, and protein. It may also play a key role in detoxifying harmful synthetic compounds such as pesticides and drugs.

Best Food Sources Found in all sorts of food, including whole and enriched grains, vegetables, and meats.

How Much You Need 5 milligrams for both men and women daily.

When to Supplement Not necessary.

Signs You're Not Getting Enough Appetite loss, depression, fatigue, insomnia, cramping.

Signs You're Getting Too Much Occasional diarrhea, but there's no upper limit set for this vitamin.

VITAMIN B_6

You need B_6 for protein metabolism as well as for normal growth. Along with riboflavin, this B vitamin helps make neurotransmitters in the brain that help you think and remember important events. Vitamin B_6 also helps clear a dangerous circulating metabolite that may lead to heart disease.

However, one of its most important functions involves transferring nitrogen, a by-product of protein metabolism, out of your body. That's one reason why protein consumption and B_6 needs are so closely linked. The more protein you eat, the more B_6 you need.

Because B_6 doesn't get added back into grains when they are refined, it's not as naturally prevalent in our diets as some of the other B vitamins. In fact, most of us probably consume a marginal intake at best.

Best Food Sources Meats, fish, poultry, beans, grains, green leafy vegetables, oranges, liver.

How Much You Need 1.5 milligrams for women and 1.7 milligrams for men daily.

When to Supplement You may be low in B_6 if you eat more than 100 grams of protein a day or if you are age 60-plus.

Because this vitamin is involved in making the brain chemical serotonin, B_6 supplements were once touted as a way to control depression and PMS. However, subsequent research has failed to find a beneficial link. In fact, supplements may be dangerous. Research shows that too much B_6 may cause nerve damage and paralysis.

Signs You're Not Getting Enough Anemia, skin rash, muscle spasms, convulsions, kidney stones.

Signs You're Getting Too Much Headaches, numbness, bone pain.

FOLATE (FOLIC ACID)

You may have heard of this important B vitamin as it relates to pregnant women, who are encouraged to take it to prevent birth defects.

However, this vitamin is also an important heart disease fighter. It seems to lower levels of a dangerous blood chemical called *homocysteine,* which can damage artery linings. It may also prevent certain cancers, including cervical, lung, and colon.

Folate is also needed for red blood cell development and helps fight off a severe form of anemia, which can make you drag through your workouts.

Best Food Sources Green leafy vegetables, lentils, fortified cereals, citrus fruits.

How Much You Need 400 micrograms for both men and women daily.

When to Supplement While folate is relatively scarce in foods, the U.S. Food and Drug Administration's (FDA's) folate-fortification program requires all enriched grain products (breads, cereals, pastas) to be folate-fortified. So including any of those products daily will help you meet your daily quota. Only take supplements when directed by your physician, as excess folate may mask a more serious deficiency of vitamin B_{12}.

Signs You're Not Getting Enough Antibiotics, over-the-counter painkillers, and oral contraceptives may decrease your absorption of folate. Deficiency symptoms include anemia, diarrhea, fatigue, depression, and smooth, bright red tongue.

Signs You're Getting Too Much Masking of vitamin B_{12} deficiency that may lead to paralysis.

VITAMIN B_{12}

Along with folate and B_6, vitamin B_{12} is vital in keeping blood levels of homocysteine in check, preventing heart disease. It's also involved in red blood cell production and new tissue growth.

However, its largest and possibly most important role is as a nerve protector. This vitamin is needed to produce myelin, the sheath that insulates nerve fibers, helping your nerves continue to send messages throughout your body.

Best Food Sources Animal products, including fish, poultry, meat, and dairy. Vitamin B_{12} is not found in fruits, vegetables, beans, or grains.

How Much You Need 2.4 micrograms for both men and women daily.

When to Supplement Because B_{12} is found in meat, vegan vegetarians risk deficiency. Also, those age 50 and older lose their ability to absorb B_{12} from food, and certain antibiotics may decrease your absorption of B_{12}. If you suspect you aren't getting enough, take a multivitamin and mineral supplement that contains 100 percent of the DV for this vitamin.

Signs You're Not Getting Enough Anemia, fatigue, nerve degeneration that progresses to paralysis, memory problems, confusion, impaired pain perception, loss of balance, numbness.

Signs You're Getting Too Much Not known.

VITAMIN C

Linus Pauling first brought fame to this important antioxidant in the 1970s, crediting the vitamin for preventing numerous diseases, bolstering immunity, and improving skin health. In turn, vitamin C supplements began flying off the shelves. In particular, people began taking as much C as they could when they felt a cold coming on, believing that more and more and more of the vitamin must be better.

Here's what's true—and what's not:

You do need vitamin C for building collagen, the material that holds cells together. Collagen is needed for just about every body tissue, from healthy gums to teeth to blood vessels. This standout vitamin also acts as an antioxidant, helping to protect your body from oxidative damage caused by exercise and other stresses such as air pollution and secondhand cigarette smoke. Vitamin C is also critical for maintaining a strong immune system, which sometimes can be taxed by endurance exercise.

In one study, done at the University of Cape Town Medical School in South Africa, runners took 600 milligrams of vitamin C a day (nine times the RDA) for three weeks prior to an ultramarathon. After the race, their incidence of upper respiratory tract infections was significantly lower than those who had been taking a placebo.

Do You Need a Stress Formula?

Stress can wreak havoc on your body, triggering tension headaches, back pain, rashes, yeast infections, and digestive problems such as diarrhea or constipation. Unfortunately, "stress formula" vitamins, which usually consist of an array of the B vitamins in megadose amounts, provide little ammunition against your body's reaction to the stressful situations in your life. Research shows that the body doesn't need more vitamins beyond what your diet or a multivitamin would provide.

Instead, find ways to handle as well as decrease the amount of stress you face. First, recognize that stress is not in your head but is affecting your entire body. Then find ways to lessen stress. Ask family members to handle more of the household duties. Delegate tasks at work. Try to reduce tension both at home and at work by talking about conflicts rather than avoiding them. Also, find ways to cope with your stress, such as through leisurely physical activity (such as walking the dog or playing in the park with your children). Learn relaxation techniques through stress-reduction courses or from your family health care provider. And of course, eating a balanced diet will help keep you in balance.

High intake of vitamin C is also linked to a decreased risk of certain types of cancer as well as decreased incidence of cataract formation (the leading cause of blindness in those older than 65).

However, there's really no need to look to supplements to get your C. You can get plenty of vitamin C from food. For example, an orange and a kiwifruit each supply about 100 percent of the RDA. Many other fruits and vegetables (strawberries, green peppers, and tomatoes, to name three) contain more than 50 percent of the RDA per serving.

Best Food Sources Citrus, peppers, cabbage, strawberries, tomatoes.

How Much You Need 75 milligrams for women and 90 milligrams for men daily.

When to Supplement If you take supplements, keep your intake below 2,000 milligrams. Anything above that level may increase your risk for kidney stones.

Signs You're Not Getting Enough Bleeding gums, pinpoint hemorrhages under the skin surface, weakness, joint pain, impaired wound healing, depression, scurvy.

Signs You're Getting Too Much Nausea, diarrhea, kidney stones and other urinary tract problems.

Chapter 6

MINERALS

From the soil to your dinner plate, learn which of 15 minerals you most need to power your fitness.

This is still hard for me to admit, but when my daughter, Natalie, was nine months old, my doctor informed me that she was anemic. Of course, I was embarrassed. As a nutritionist, I hold myself to a higher standard. I never expected to rear a child with a mineral deficiency!

Then it happened again, but this time with my son, Grant. I had been giving both of my children fluoride supplements to help ensure their teeth grew in strong and cavity-free. However, little did I know, Grant was swallowing his toothpaste rather than spitting it out. This resulted in more fluoride than his five-year-old body needed. The result: His first permanent tooth came in chalky. Fortunately, I recognized the symptoms of fluoride overdosing. I eased up on the supplements and began monitoring his toothbrushing, watching to make sure he spit out the paste. Eventually the excess fluoride made its way out of his system.

I tell you these stories for one reason—to let you know that nobody's perfect. Mineral deficiencies and overdoses even happen to nutritionists!

Fortunately—for me and for you—it's relatively easy to ensure that you get most minerals in the right amounts. Though mineral presence in foods is minuscule, you need very small amounts of minerals in your body.

However, your body absorbs minerals poorly, with about 5 to 60 percent of the minerals in the food you eat actually getting inside your body. Fiber in whole grains, tannins in coffee, and oxalate found in spinach can all inhibit iron's entry, for example. That's why some foods stand out as better sources of particular minerals, not only because of the actual amount of the mineral in the food but also because of how well the body absorbs the mineral from that particular food. For example, about 30 percent of the iron in red meat can be absorbed, as opposed to less than 10 percent of the iron in grains.

Despite this low absorption rate, few of us run low for most minerals because our bodies can store minerals for later use as well as increase the absorption of particular minerals when needed.

Minerals are grouped into two categories, major and trace, based on how much of a particular mineral is present in your body and needed in the diet. The major minerals—calcium, chloride, magnesium, phosphorus, potassium, and sodium—are present in the body in amounts greater than 0.01 percent of body weight and are required in amounts greater than 50 milligrams per day. Trace minerals are present in the body in amounts less than 0.01 percent of body weight and are required in amounts less than 50 milligrams per day.

For example, you have about 1,000 grams (about 2 pounds) of calcium in your body and need about 1 gram daily. On the other hand, if I scraped together all of the trace minerals from your body, they would fit into a tablespoon. Also, your daily requirement for these trace minerals adds up to a tiny fraction of your calcium requirement. That's one reason why supplement packagers often create separate calcium supplements. They can't fit all the calcium you need into a neat, tiny multivitamin small enough for you to swallow.

Who Should Supplement

Because minerals come from rocks and soil, many consumers wonder how much actually ends up in foods. In fact, some mineral supplement makers capitalize on this fear and claim that farmland soils have become depleted of minerals due to overuse, though nutrient analysis of vegetables, fruits, and other foods shows no mineral depletion over the years.

However, some minerals, such as iron, are harder to absorb than others, making it difficult to get an optimal amount. A number of factors can make you more likely to experience deficiency in a mineral—or even a vitamin. They include:

Dieting. If you restrict your food intake to fewer than 1,200 calories, you're probably missing out on important nutrients.

Lactose intolerance. If you don't do dairy, you'll have a tough time getting enough calcium and riboflavin.

Food allergies. If you can't eat particular foods such as wheat and fruit, you'll have a tougher time getting the nutrients you need.

Vegetarian diet. If you don't eat meat, you'll have a tough time getting enough iron and zinc, especially if you're female. You also may come up short on riboflavin and vitamins B_{12} and D.

Pregnancy. If you're pregnant, supplement with iron and folic acid or eat fortified cereals.

In addition to these factors, many of us don't follow the best diet all the time. Processed foods such as white rice, white bread, candy, and baked goods simply don't contain as much nutrition as whole foods such as fruit, vegetables, and whole grains.

But this still doesn't mean you need to take large amounts of separate vitamin or mineral supplements. Because different minerals interact with each other—with too much of one type lowering absorption of another type—your best strategy is to take a multivitamin and mineral supplement that contains 100 to 150 percent of the DV of all the vitamins and minerals listed in this chapter and chapter 5.

The one exception is a calcium supplement. Calcium is a bulky mineral that's needed in large amounts. It simply doesn't fit neatly inside of a multivitamin and mineral supplement. Take your calcium supplement at a meal when you are not taking a multivitamin. High doses of calcium can hamper the absorption of iron as well as cause constipation.

You need minerals to bolster your metabolism as well as control your body's pH (acid level) and water balance. Minerals also provide structure to bones and teeth.

Here's a rundown on the 15 minerals your exercising body needs, starting with major minerals (calcium through sodium) and then moving on to trace minerals.

CALCIUM

You may already know that calcium helps build strong bones. What you may not know is that calcium is just as important for men as it is for women. Men are developing osteoporosis—the weakening of bones—at an alarming rate. Truly no one is immune from this disease.

Calcium and other minerals such as magnesium help strengthen bones by filling in holes between the collagen that forms the bone structure. The more porous your bones, the more easily they break. The higher your bone mineral content, the less porous your bones.

As a fitness enthusiast, you're already giving your bones a helping hand. Any repetitive exercise that tugs and pulls on your bones can strengthen them. But an overuse injury such as shin splints can turn into a stress fracture, especially with poor calcium intake and menstrual irregularities that reflect low levels of the female hormone estrogen, which in turn lead to bone mineral loss.

Besides protecting your bones, calcium also regulates blood pressure, prevents colon cancer, and even may aid weight loss. It is also involved in muscle contraction, blood clotting, and healthy nerve function.

Best Food Sources Milk and dairy products, green leafy vegetables, sardines with bones, tofu, calcium-fortified orange juice, cereal and other fortified foods.

How Much You Need Aim for 1,000 to 1,500 milligrams daily, the amount in three to five glasses of milk a day.

When to Supplement If you don't drink milk; are taking antibiotics, diuretics, or laxatives (which all cause your body to excrete excess calcium); have been diagnosed with amenorrhea; or have a hereditary risk of osteoporosis, a daily 500-milligram supplement is a good option. Take the supplement with dinner, the lowest-calcium meal for most people. That will ensure optimal absorption.

Signs You're Not Getting Enough Poor bone growth, brittle bones.

Signs You're Getting Too Much Constipation, poor absorption of other minerals—iron and magnesium—and kidney stones in susceptible individuals.

CHLORIDE

You hardly ever hear about this mineral without the word "sodium" in front of it. When you add the two minerals together—as in sodium chloride—you get table salt. Sodium and chloride balance one another with positive and negative charges, working together to maintain fluid balance throughout your body.

Though this mineral certainly serves an important job, you need not worry too much about it. Because most of us eat quite a bit of table salt—either straight from the salt shaker or hidden in processed foods—we consume much more chloride than we need.

Best Food Sources Table salt and anything that contains it, including most processed foods.

How Much You Need You only need 700 milligrams daily, yet most of us consume 4,500 milligrams.

When to Supplement Never.

Signs You're Not Getting Enough Very rare. Dizziness, muscle cramps, convulsions.

Signs You're Getting Too Much Because the body does a good job of excreting excess chloride, this, too, is rare. The worst damage that too much chloride can cause is fluid retention.

MAGNESIUM

For years, researchers have known that magnesium plays a critical role in endurance performance. Magnesium mainly exists inside the cells of muscles and bones, where it assists with muscle contractions and energy metabolism.

Because the mineral is involved in nerve and muscle contraction all over the body, magnesium supplements have been credited with everything from preventing heart disease, easing PMS, and lowering high blood pressure to reducing the incidence of muscle cramps, lowering the severity of asthma, and even preventing kidney stones.

Epsom salts—discovered in Epsom, England—are made of magnesium sulfate and are known to draw water from inflamed muscles.

Studies with people and lab animals show that magnesium deficiency reduces endurance and that low blood levels of magnesium are associated with decreased aerobic capacity. Extreme endurance events such as the marathon can deplete magnesium from your body.

Researchers believe that low magnesium levels reduce production of a substance called 2,3-DPG (for our purposes, simply DPG), which is essential for oxygen delivery to exercising muscles. So, theoretically, increasing magnesium intake should boost DPG level, thereby improving oxygen delivery and in turn boosting aerobic capacity and performance.

Best Food Sources Green vegetables, beans, nuts, cocoa and chocolate, whole grains, molasses.

How Much You Need 420 milligrams for men and 320 milligrams for women daily.

When to Supplement Because oversupplementation can cause diarrhea and can interfere with calcium absorption and metabolism, try to get your magnesium from food. Also, magnesium interacts with calcium, and too much calcium can cause your body to excrete magnesium. Few people consume more calcium than they need, but it's something to check. Also, some asthma and heart medications can rob your body of magnesium. If you take such medications, talk with your doctor about possible deficiency issues. Cut back on alcohol and caffeine, which also can lower magnesium levels in your body.

Signs You're Not Getting Enough Nausea, muscle weakness, irritability.

Signs You're Getting Too Much Lethargy, nausea, diarrhea.

PHOSPHORUS

Phosphorus combines with calcium to form healthy teeth and bones. Phosphorus is also used in energy metabolism and is part of every cell's genetic material.

Thanks to soft drinks, most of us consume more than enough phosphorus. In fact, the only people who might have to worry about a deficiency are those who chew antacids all day long, as if they were candy. Antacids can bind phosphorus, preventing it from getting where it needs to go in your body.

On the other hand, plenty of us get too much of this mineral, particularly teenagers and children who drink a lot of soda, which contains phosphorus. Too much usually isn't a problem unless you're not consuming enough calcium. The ratio of calcium to phosphorus is important. Too much phosphorus and too little calcium can actually weaken bones as well as cause fatigue.

Best Food Sources Meat, fish, poultry, milk, beans.

How Much You Need 700 milligrams daily for both men and women.

When to Supplement There's no reason to supplement with this mineral.

Signs You're Not Getting Enough Poor bone growth and development. However, we get so much from a typical diet that these results are extremely rare.

Signs You're Getting Too Much Weakened bones, low energy, and in extreme cases kidney damage.

POTASSIUM

Go to any endurance race and look at the food tables after the finish line. You'll almost always find bananas being served to the finishers, and potassium is why.

You need potassium for proper muscle contraction and nerve impulse transmission throughout the body. Without enough of it or with an imbalance in your body, you could experience muscle cramping or weakness, which definitely doesn't help your exercise efforts.

Potassium is also an important mineral that helps regulate blood pressure. Potassium attracts water into your cells, whereas sodium attracts water to the blood outside your cells. In some people, a sodium and potassium imbalance can cause too much fluid to stay in your blood, overexpanding your blood volume. This increases the pressure in your arteries in the same way a sudden rainstorm causes a river to

Do You Need Colloidal Minerals?

Makers of colloidal mineral supplements extract decomposed plant matter from shale and then turn it into a mineral supplement. The result is suspension-like mixtures of some 60 to 80 or more different minerals—everything from essential minerals such as iron and calcium to deadly minerals including lead and mercury.

Colloidal mineral manufacturers claim that getting your minerals from this "organic" source allows the minerals to be better absorbed into the body than those from regular foods and other supplements.

The claims are not only a bunch of hogwash, they can be downright dangerous. Colloidal supplements provide a wide array of minerals, many of which have not been determined to be essential for humans and others that are known to be toxic, such as aluminum and arsenic. Also, the amount of each mineral present in these supplements has no bearing on human requirements. For example, calcium levels may be present at a fraction of the requirement, yet levels of selenium may exceed needs, a concern since this mineral is toxic in amounts contained in these colloidal supplements. In fact, the FDA has warned several colloidal mineral manufacturers against making such false claims on their packaging.

Worse, some scientists have expressed concern that radioactive compounds may exist in these preparations since these suspensions are made from shale and sold without purification. And chemical analysis of some preparations has revealed that what's in the bottle frequently doesn't match amounts stated on the label or in product literature. Colloidal preparations pose other risks such as overexposure to minerals not typically consumed, for example, silver, which may cause neurological damage and a permanent blue-gray discoloration of the skin.

flow with more pressure. Potassium may also help keep pressure low by helping blood vessels stay wider and more supple.

Many people don't eat as much potassium as they should, and most of us consume more sodium than needed. Fortunately, this doesn't mean you need to give up all of your favorite salty foods. Rather, research shows that the best approach is maximizing potassium-rich foods. In other words, focus more on eating the right foods and less on restricting the wrong ones.

Best Food Sources Whole foods, vegetables, fruits, meats, milk.

How Much You Need 2,000 milligrams daily for both men and women.

When to Supplement Your body better tolerates potassium from food than it does from supplements. Aim for six to 10 servings of fruits and vegetables a day, all of which are naturally high in potassium.

Signs You're Not Getting Enough Muscle weakness, numbness, tingling in limbs, nausea, irritability.

Signs You're Getting Too Much Muscle weakness, tingling in the hands, feet, or tongue, slow or irregular pulse.

SODIUM

You've probably only heard bad things about this mineral, so let's first talk about its benefits.

Sodium is vital for fluid balance and normal nerve function. It also works with potassium to regulate blood pressure and maintain the permeability of your cell walls. During exercise, a small amount of sodium—for example, in your sports drink—serves three important functions. It makes you thirsty, which encourages you to drink more; helps you retain water, preventing dehydration and annoying potty stops; and replaces some of the sodium you lose through sweat.

Now, for the bad news. Thanks to sodium-rich processed foods as well as the salt shaker, most of us consume more than we need of this mineral. Though sodium doesn't raise blood pressure in all people, some people are sodium responders. Sodium and the mineral potassium work in concert in your blood to regulate fluid balance in and out of your cells. Potassium brings fluid into your cells, whereas sodium draws fluid out of your cells and into the surrounding blood.

In most people—no matter how much sodium they consume and how little potassium—this process works smoothly, balancing water in the right portions in your blood and in your cells. However, in about 20 percent of people, a sodium and potassium imbalance can cause too much fluid to stay in your blood, overexpanding your blood volume.

Just as too much sodium can cause problems, so can too little. When you sweat profusely and don't replace the sodium lost in your sweat, you can run low on blood sodium, which throws off fluid balance and results in a host of symptoms including low blood pressure, dizziness, muscle cramps, and, in a worst case scenario, coma. However, you must sweat a lot for a long period of time for this to occur. The only people who are susceptible are usually Ironman athletes, ultramarathon runners, and sometimes football players or those in the military who spend a lot of time outside in the heat while wearing lots of clothing.

Best Food Sources Salt, processed foods, soy sauce and other seasonings.

How Much You Need For good health, don't exceed 2,400 milligrams daily for both men and women.

When to Supplement There's no reason to supplement with salt tablets. However, if you are attempting a long-endurance effort in the heat, you should consume some sodium during the effort. The easiest way to do this is by consuming a sports drink that contains 100 to 110 milligrams of sodium per 8-ounce serving or other foods with added sodium such as pretzels or soda crackers.

Signs You're Not Getting Enough Dizziness, low blood pressure, vomiting, muscle cramps, convulsions.

Signs You're Getting Too Much Water retention, high blood pressure.

CHROMIUM

You need this trace mineral for the proper operation of the hormone insulin. Insulin is a messenger that knocks on the door of your cells to let them know blood sugar is trying to get in. For insulin to do its job, it needs chromium.

This explains why blood sugar levels improve in diabetics who are given extra chromium in their diets. If you don't consume enough of this important mineral, you end up with high blood sugar and high insulin levels.

Because chromium helps blood sugar get to where it needs to go, the mineral has been rumored to help burn body fat and build muscle size and strength. Besides shuttling sugar into cells, insulin also helps manufacture new proteins, which is why some people think chromium supplements may speed the muscle-building process.

And though that theory does sound reasonable, it just doesn't pan out. Much of the chromium craze is based on a slew of flawed studies showing that chromium supplements (in the form of chromium picolinate) improve muscle gains during strength training. Yet in a recent, well-designed study on football players, those who weight trained four days a week while taking 200 micrograms daily of chromium saw no increase in muscle mass compared to a placebo group.

While most research has failed to support chromium for fat burning or muscle building, the supplement may show promise in another area. New research may prove this supplement useful for boosting sprint performance. It makes sense that an extra shot of chromium during exercise could help shuttle more carbohydrate into muscle cells for a sudden sprint to the finish line.

Researchers from the University of Dayton in Ohio tested this theory on a group of trained cyclists. On two separate occasions, cyclists worked out for an hour while they drank either a carbohydrate beverage similar to a sports drink or the same beverage with added chromium. They consumed about 60 grams of carbohydrate (240 calories) and about 200 micrograms of chromium (equivalent to the daily recommended intake).

At the end of the hour ride, cyclists pedaled as hard as they could for just under a minute. Researchers measured the amount of work performed during the sprint and found that the chromium-fortified drink boosted sprint performance by 7 percent compared to the plain carbohydrate drink. Blood sugar levels were also slightly lower with the chromium beverage, suggesting greater glucose uptake by the muscles. More research is needed for a definitive answer to chromium's role in sprint performance.

Best Food Sources Refried beans, wheat germ, microbrewed beer, chicken, peas, grains, vegetables, organ meats, brewer's yeast, grape juice. Note: To keep chromium levels optimal, beware of eating too many refined foods, such as white bread and sweets, which are not only low in chromium but also may boost your need for it (to help process carbohydrate).

How Much You Need 50 to 200 micrograms daily for both men and women.

When to Supplement You can easily meet your daily quota by drinking two microbrewed beers or eating a cup of refried beans. Taking supplements can easily oversupply your system with chromium, which can decrease your absorption of iron and zinc as well as cause cancer-causing free radicals to form in your body. Get more chromium through food, not through supplements.

Signs You're Not Getting Enough Many endurance athletes do fall short of the recommended intake. Also, you may sweat out more chromium during heavy training. In some people, a marginal chromium intake combined with genetic predisposition, lack of exercise, and a high amount of refined foods can trigger a pre-diabetic state of high blood sugar levels.

Signs You're Getting Too Much If you stick to real food, you can't overdo it. The only people who suffer from chromium toxicity are usually painters, who tend to inhale it. Signs of toxicity include ulcers and kidney damage.

COPPER

Copper helps hold together collagen and elastin, found throughout the body, helping to build new tissue. This mineral also helps keep your muscles, nerves, and immune system functioning.

A deficiency can show up anywhere in the body from a weak heart to bad blood vessels to weak bones to weakened immunity. Copper also interacts with iron, so lower levels can lead to anemia.

Studies indicate that many of us don't get as much of this important mineral as we should. That's not good, as studies have also shown that a chronically low copper intake can weaken your body's disease-fighting cells. Because your body easily excretes excess copper in your bile and to your stool, it's very rare to overdose. However, in extreme cases, a high copper intake—usually only possible with supplements—can lead to liver damage.

Best Food Sources Grains, shellfish, organ meats, legumes, nuts, beans.

How Much You Need 900 micrograms daily for both men and women.

When to Supplement Copper can be toxic in high amounts. It's okay to take a multivitamin that contains no more than 3 milligrams of copper. However, it's best to try to get your copper from food.

Signs You're Not Getting Enough Anemia, growth problems in children.

Signs You're Getting Too Much Very rare.

FLUORIDE

As I mentioned earlier, my son used to swallow toothpaste, which gave him an overabundance of fluoride.

Too much of this trace mineral generally becomes a cosmetic concern. It causes a chalky appearance to the teeth called *fluorosis*. That's how we learned Grant was getting too much, when his first adult tooth grew in hard and chalky.

In extreme cases—for example, when a child eats an entire tube of toothpaste—fluoride can be toxic, which is why the toothpaste tube contains a warning to seek medical attention if ingested.

However, short of children eating toothpaste, most of us underdo this important mineral. Well water, municipal water, and, of course, fluoridated water all tend to contain fluoride. However, bottled water tends not to. If you drink bottled water all day long, chances are, you're not getting enough fluoride.

Some people have argued that fluoride is not essential to the diet, but that's simply not true. Your body cannot make this mineral, so your only access to it is through the water you drink and the paste you use to brush your teeth.

Mineral Water Versus Tap: Which Is Better?

Since water trickles through rocks and soil, it picks up the naturally occurring minerals, such as calcium, magnesium, and fluoride, allowing those minerals to make their way into your well or tap water.

However, more and more of us are switching to bottled water, mostly for the purer taste. Many bottled waters are distilled or purified, making them void of minerals. The trouble with drinking mineral-free water is that your body may be missing out on what it needs.

For example, for most of us, drinking water is our major source of fluoride, a mineral crucial in keeping your teeth resistant to tooth decay. And for folks drinking hard water (mineral rich), a day's supply of tap water may contribute 10 to 25 percent of calcium and/or magnesium needs. If you opt for distilled water, make sure your diet supplies these minerals and that you use fluoridated toothpaste and get regular dental checkups.

Also, read labels on bottled waters. Some purified water brands add back a few minerals after distillation, making them a better choice for your health.

When you ingest fluoride by drinking fluoridated drinking water, it makes its way into your saliva, where it constantly bathes your teeth. This is important because not only does fluoride make your teeth stronger, it also inhibits bacterial growth in your mouth that can cause tooth decay and gum disease.

And for those of you who think teeth are not all that important, think about it this way: When you age into your 70s and 80s, a good set of teeth will help you continue to eat a wide variety of foods, helping you to get the nutrients you need to stay healthy. When you don't take care of your teeth and they subsequently fall out, you'll have trouble chewing. You could eventually die from a nutrient deficiency because of your lack of teeth. You see, eventually, fluoride deficiency can be fatal! Fluoridation of water costs $1 per person per year—well worth it when you compare it to all the dental costs that you save.

Best Food Sources Water containing fluoride, fish, tea.

How Much You Need 3 milligrams daily for both men and women.

When to Supplement If you drink bottled water, consider a fluoride supplement of no more than 3 milligrams a day.

Signs You're Not Getting Enough Increased susceptibility to tooth decay, possibly associated with the development of osteoporosis.

Signs You're Getting Too Much Chalky appearance to the teeth (dark stains in extreme cases).

IODINE

We wiped out iodine deficiency in the United States with the introduction of iodized salt. However, more than 200 million people worldwide, mostly in undeveloped countries, experience marked deficiencies in this important mineral because their locally grown food does not naturally contain enough iodine.

Iodine, more accurately *iodide* the ion, is essential for proper function of your thyroid gland, which makes a deficiency in this mineral an extremely serious problem. Your thyroid gland uses iodide to make hormones that direct energy use to every single cell in the body, in turn regulating calorie burning, body temperature, breathing rate, and muscle production and tone. How many calories you burn each day is largely dependent on proper thyroid function. Too little iodide and your metabolism slows, and you gain weight. In order to grab more iodide from your blood, your thyroid gland enlarges, causing a noticeable swelling in the front of your throat, called a *goiter.*

Some supplement companies have capitalized on this physiology by manufacturing a weight loss patch that secretes iodide through your skin. However, adding more iodide to your body will only boost your metabolism if you are deficient to begin with, which is very rare in the United States.

Best Food Sources Milk, grains, iodized salt, processed foods.

How Much You Need 150 micrograms daily for both men and women.

When to Supplement There's no need to supplement, thanks to iodized salt.

Signs You're Not Getting Enough Enlarged thyroid gland, sluggishness, weight gain.

Signs You're Getting Too Much Getting too much is rare. The only way to do it is to live on a diet of seaweed, which contains iodide. Too much iodide will suppress thyroid hormone, causing the same symptoms of getting too little: fatigue, weight gain, and goiter.

IRON

Iron forms hemoglobin, the stuff that helps your red blood cells transport oxygen. You need adequate amounts of iron in your blood to get oxygen to your muscles. When you don't consume enough iron, not enough oxygen gets to where it needs to go, eventually resulting in iron-deficiency anemia. You feel fatigued, can't perform up to expectations (at work or during your workout), and, oftentimes, complain of chills even when the temperature isn't all that chilly.

Iron is also an important mineral for your immune system, which is why too little iron can result in frequent colds.

Some experts estimate that as many as 20 percent of us are deficient in this mineral. If your iron stores dip slightly below normal, your energy can plummet, even if you're not technically anemic.

Best Food Sources Red meat, poultry, fish, green leafy vegetables, whole grains, legumes, iron-fortified breakfast cereals.

How Much You Need 8 milligrams daily for men; 18 milligrams for women 50 and under; 8 milligrams for women over 50.

When to Supplement Since you may be losing some iron in your sweat and urine, and because exercise itself can hamper your ability to absorb the mineral, you need to pay careful attention to your intake. Antibiotics and aspirin can also cause loss of iron.

Before you start taking supplements, however, try consuming more iron in your diet. Meat is your best source because it contains heme iron, which is the most readily absorbable form of iron. Eating a 3-ounce serving of red meat three to four times a week will help supply you with plenty of iron, as will eating other good sources including iron-fortified cereals, lentils, and broccoli. Eat a vitamin C–rich food (such as strawberries or bell peppers) with your nonmeat iron source, as vitamin C significantly improves iron absorption.

If you do supplement, stay away from products that contain more than 20 milligrams of iron; too much iron can hamper your zinc absorption, making you just as tired.

Signs You're Not Getting Enough Anemia, fatigue, decreased physical performance.

Signs You're Getting Too Much Constipation, diarrhea.

MANGANESE

You need manganese for bone and connective tissue formation as well as for carbohydrate and fat metabolism. Manganese helps form molecules called *mucopolysaccharides,* which are used to form collagen, the material that builds tissues and bone. Collagen is the scaffolding that holds calcium and other minerals in your bones. Without it, the minerals would have nowhere to attach themselves.

Manganese is also important for proper brain function.

Best Food Sources Spinach, pumpkin, nuts, legumes, tea.

How Much You Need 2.3 milligrams for men and 1.8 milligrams for women daily.

When to Supplement There's no reason to supplement with this mineral. We need so little of it, an amount easily obtainable through our diet. However, manganese can be toxic in high doses. If you take a multivitamin and mineral supplement, make sure the amount of manganese is no more than 100 percent of the recommended intake.

Signs You're Not Getting Enough Deficiency is rare. Manganese deficiency has been produced in animals, resulting in disordered brain function.

Signs You're Getting Too Much Most people who overdose on this mineral do it by drinking contaminated well water. Too much will result in psychosis as well as Parkinson's-type symptoms including trembling and shuffling.

MOLYBDENUM

You need molybdenum primarily for nitrogen metabolism. It's a component of three separate enzymes that get chemical reactions started in your body. One of those enzymes is sulfite oxidase, which helps detoxify sulfites found in protein and processed foods. The two other enzymes, xanthine oxidase and aldehyde oxidase, are both involved in the production of genetic material and protein.

Best Food Sources Unprocessed grains and vegetables.

How Much You Need 45 micrograms for both men and women daily.

When to Supplement Not necessary.

Signs You're Not Getting Enough Though extremely rare, too little can cause mental confusion and increased heart rate.

Signs You're Getting Too Much Also rare, too much can cause weight loss and anemia.

SELENIUM

Along with vitamin E, selenium works with an enzyme that helps protect your cells from damage caused by oxidation (from air pollution, cigarette smoke, and everyday metabolism).

Antioxidants act like fire extinguishers, stopping rogue molecules called *free radicals* from damaging cells. These fire extinguishers put out little fires all over your body, protecting you against numerous age-related diseases, including cataracts, heart disease, and cancer. They also may even help protect your muscles from soreness after a tough workout.

In addition to its antioxidant role, selenium binds with toxic substances to make them less harmful, and it bolsters immunity.

Best Food Sources Grains, meat, fish, poultry, Brazil nuts (two nuts supply the recommended intake).

The Truth About Hair Analysis

On various sites on the Web, some labs are advertising "hair analysis." They claim that nutrients in your body make their way into your hair, which can then be analyzed to check for deficiency, health status, or toxicity.

Sounds compelling, but hair analysis simply doesn't hold water.

For a recent study published in the esteemed *Journal of the American Medical Association,* scientists sent identical hair samples to different analysis labs across the country. Each lab came up with different results, some claiming a person was deficient in a nutrient that another lab found to be in good supply.

Why the conflicting results? Your hair simply isn't an accurate gauge of nutrient status. Research shows that a person can be very deficient in zinc, yet a hair sample will suggest adequate zinc status. Also, regular everyday elements that you expose your hair to—such as shampoo and air pollution—can alter the nutrient content of your hair, making it seem as if you are suffering from toxicity when you're not.

Most important, however, is that your body does an extremely good job of keeping levels of vitamins and minerals constant. When you are deficient, it pulls vitamins and minerals out of storage, from your fat, your bones, and other parts of your body. You could be eating a calcium-poor diet, for example, but a blood test for calcium would reveal normal levels because your body will rob calcium from your bones to make up for the shortfall.

So how do you find out if you are deficient? First, find the most qualified expert to help. You might ask your family physician to refer you to an internal medicine specialist, as these doctors generally have more training in nutrition. Your doctor should take the following into account:

Your symptoms. Certain types of deficiency will show up in specific ways. For example, a deficiency in iron, zinc, or any of the B vitamins will make you feel fatigued.

The Truth About Hair Analysis *(continued)*

Your diet. Keep a food diary (and be honest!) for three days of each week for three weeks. This will help your doctor to determine if you regularly skimp on certain nutrients.

Your bodily fluids. Though testing blood or urine for specific vitamins and minerals will offer misleading results, your doctor can look at a host of other factors that indicate your nutrient status. For example, levels of certain blood proteins will be affected by deficiency in certain nutrients. Also, your actual blood cells will take on a different color or shape based on your nutrient status. The actual count of your red and white blood cells as well as the status of certain enzymes can also reveal a good picture of your health.

Finally, your doctor may also perform a few functional tests to see how well various systems of your body are functioning. A skin patch test will reveal your immune status, for example. Your doctor may also test your hand-grip strength.

Only by putting all of these factors together—not by taking a quick sample of your hair!—will your doctor get a good idea of your nutritional status.

How Much You Need 55 micrograms for both men and women daily.

When to Supplement Not recommended because as little as two times the recommended dose can be toxic.

Signs You're Not Getting Enough A rare type of heart disease called Keshan disease.

Signs You're Getting Too Much Hair loss, garlic breath, metallic taste in mouth, dizziness, streaked fingernails, vomiting, nervous system disorders.

ZINC

Though you have only about 2 grams of it in your body, zinc works in tandem with more than 100 different enzymes, many of which participate in energy metabolism. Zinc is also essential for a healthy immune system. Plus it makes wound healing and injury recovery possible and is vital for male sexual functioning.

Despite its importance, studies have shown that most people don't consume enough of this mineral. Since you sweat out small amounts of it each time you exercise, you can quickly run the risk of a zinc deficiency. In one study, athletes had twice the zinc loss through urine following a 6-mile run compared to when they didn't exercise.

Up to 40 percent of athletes may have below-normal levels of zinc in their blood. Part of the problem is that many fit people tend to shy away from the best sources of zinc—oysters, clams, liver, and several other meats—because of the relatively high fat content. That's understandable, but you can also get zinc from lowfat foods such as wheat germ, fortified breakfast cereals, and nuts.

Best Food Sources Seafood, meats, nuts, legumes, wheat germ.

How Much You Need 11 milligrams for men and 8 milligrams for women daily.

When to Supplement Your body absorbs zinc best from beef, poultry, pork, lamb, and seafood, so getting enough zinc can be tricky if you don't eat meat. Vegetarians should look to fortified cereals for zinc, as they come with anywhere from 25 to 100 percent of the RDA per serving.

Supplementation may be the best way to ensure you get enough zinc. Look for a vitamin or mineral supplement containing no more than 11 milligrams for men and 8 milligrams for women. High-fiber foods and the tannins found in coffee, some teas, and wine can hamper zinc absorption, so take your supplement at a time when you won't be consuming those foods or beverages.

And remember, more isn't better. Too much zinc blocks the absorption of copper, which in turn hampers iron absorption. Also, oversupplementation with zinc has been shown to lower "good" (HDL) cholesterol and raise "bad" (LDL) cholesterol.

Signs You're Not Getting Enough Delay in sexual development, poor wound healing, depressed immunity, frequent colds.

Signs You're Getting Too Much Nausea, diarrhea, increased blood fat levels.

Chapter 7

SPORTS PRODUCTS

The right performance fuel can help you go the distance. The wrong one can spell performance disaster.

Not long ago, fitness enthusiasts had just three sports products from which to choose: sports drinks, sports gels, and sports bars. Made primarily of carbohydrate, these products were designed to digest easily, fuel endurance exercise, fit in a pocket, and remain intact during gym bag, fanny pack, and pocket transport and storage.

Today, however, you have many more choices, with convenient products that not only fuel your muscles during exercise but also help you recover faster afterward, keep you energized at work, fuel weight loss, build muscle, and even serve as a handy meal on the days you're too busy to cook.

To find the best product for you, you must first define your needs. Are you looking for a great recovery product or one to nibble during a workout? Do you want a snack that helps to boost your protein intake or one that replaces an entire meal?

Here's a rundown on 11 types of performance products. To help you sort through each product type, I've provided a summary with each entry that lists how much you need, what type of exercise and fitness enthusiasts most benefit from the product, and common real foods that also work just as well. You can further evaluate these products with the comparison tables included in each section.

CARBOHYDRATE BARS

PowerBar, the first true "energy" bar on the scene, in the mid-1980s, was designed with an endurance athlete's high-carbohydrate needs in mind. Since then, many others, such as Clif and Gatorade Energy Bars, have followed.

When these bars first hit the market, some fitness enthusiasts and researchers turned their noses, claiming that only the liquid carbohydrate from a sports drink could digest easily during exercise. However, several studies have looked at the solid versus liquid carbohydrate question. They show that for a particular carbohydrate (glucose, for instance), it doesn't matter if it's in solid or liquid form, as long as you consume it with enough water.

A true carbohydrate bar supplies about 200 to 260 calories, with more than 70 percent of those calories coming from carbohydrates. Sugars (such as corn syrup or brown rice syrup) and grains (such as oats or rice) serve as the major ingredients, with some bars (such as Clif and Odwalla) also using dried fruit. All serve as easily digestible fuel for working muscles.

Most bars in this category also are fortified with an array of vitamins and minerals, as much as in a bowl of fortified cereal. This extra boost of nutrients may help if you eat sporadically or avoid eating nutritious fruits, vegetables, and whole grains. Also, extra antioxidants, including vitamins C and E and beta-carotene, may help prevent oxidative damage caused by exercise.

But if you also eat fortified breakfast cereal and other foods or take a multivitamin, you don't need extra fortification.

Beyond vitamins and minerals, some bar makers add extras such as herbs, amino acids, and specialty ingredients that you otherwise wouldn't expect in an energy bar. For the most part, the amounts of these specialty ingredients are too small to provide a benefit.

Best For Endurance fitness enthusiasts (cyclists, runners, rowers) who need a convenient source of easily digestible calories before, during, and after exercise.

What to Look For Aim for 120 to 240 calories per hour of exercise. During exercise, opt for bars with no more than 8 to 10 grams of protein and 4 or fewer grams of fat per every 230 calories, as any more may slow digestion and make you feel nauseous. Too much fiber may also slow digestion and may trigger the urge to defecate, so choose bars with 5 or fewer grams of fiber.

Good Food Sources Fig bars, bananas, honey sticks, and bagels all contain easily digestible and portable carbohydrate.

How to Use It These bars make great preworkout snacks, particularly when on the road. Eat one about 1 to 2 hours prior to exercise, and make sure to drink 16 ounces of water with your bar. During a

Comparing Carbohydrate Bars

	Calories	Protein (g)	Carbohydrates (g)	Fat (g)
Clif Bar	240	10	41	4
Gatorade Energy Bar	260	8	46	5
Odwalla Bar	250	7	38	7
PowerBar Performance	230	10	45	3
Tiger's Milk	140	7	18	5

workout, eat about one energy bar per hour (aim for 30 to 60 grams of carbohydrate for every hour of exercise), making sure to also consume ½ to ¾ cup of water during every 15 to 20 minutes. (The water helps replace fluid lost through sweat and helps you digest the bar.) Following a workout, high-carbohydrate bars make a convenient choice along with some fresh fruit and a cup of milk, soy milk, or yogurt for added carbohydrate and protein.

SPORTS DRINKS

In workouts lasting an hour or more, you need carbohydrate replenishment as well as water. Sports drinks provide both.

Do they help you exercise longer? In a word, yes. In one study, researchers at Georgia State University asked men and women to run on a treadmill for 90 minutes at about 70 percent of their maximum effort. Then they ran a 10-K time trial. During the entire session, runners drank either a sports drink or a placebo beverage, consuming about 6 ounces of fluid every 15 minutes.

Results showed that the sports-drink group ran the 10-K significantly faster than did the placebo group. Moreover, those who took the sports drink rated their effort as being easier than the placebo group did.

Most sports drinks offer a blend of water along with carbohydrates, usually sucrose, glucose, fructose, or maltodextrins. A new sports drink, G-Push, utilizes a different carbohydrate source—galactose. Found in milk, this sugar may offer an advantage over typical sugars in sports drinks as it does not require insulin to make its way to your cells.

Odwalla's Simple Sports Drink blends carbohydrate from fruit juice and honey. The makers of the first carbohydrate gel, GU, have released GU_2O, a low-acid sports drink that is light tasting and may be easier on the stomach during exercise.

Pop Goes Your Workout

Many athletes ask me whether they can substitute soda for sports drinks during their workouts. I tell them to go right ahead if they want to feel sick during their workout. Sodas have 12 to 15 percent carbohydrate by weight, much more than the suggested range of 5 to 9 percent. If you quaff a drink with too much carbohydrate, you'll slow water absorption, which creates that sloshing feeling in your stomach.

Many sports drinks also contain sodium, potassium, and other electrolytes that help promote body-fluid balance. You don't need a lot, but a small amount of sodium serves three important functions. It makes you thirsty, which encourages you to drink more. It retains water, preventing dehydration and annoying potty stops. And it replaces some of the sodium you lose through sweat. But don't worry about increasing your risk of high blood pressure—sports drinks contain the same amount of sodium as found in a cup of 2 percent milk, only a tenth of your daily requirement.

Best For Endurance enthusiasts who exercise for more than an hour at a time.

What to Look For During exercise, you want a drink with between 6 and 9 percent carbohydrate. Anything above 9 percent slows digestion and promotes cramping, nausea, and diarrhea. Anything below 5 percent won't get enough fuel to your muscles.

To figure out the percentage of carbohydrate in a drink, divide the grams of carbohydrate per serving by the milliliters of drink per serving and then multiply by 100. For example, if a sports drink has

Comparing Sports Drinks
(per 8-ounce serving)

	Calories	Protein (g)	Carbohydrates (g)	Fat (g)
Accelerade	94	6.5	17	0
Cytomax	50	0	13	0
G-Push (G2)	70	0	18	0
Gatorade	50	0	14	0
GU_2O	50	0	14	0
Powerade	72	0	19	0
Simple Sports Drink	80	0	21	0

14 grams of carbohydrate per 240-milliliter serving, you would divide 14 by 240. Then multiply that answer (0.058) by 100. You end up with 5.8, which means the drink is nearly 6 percent carbohydrate.

Some research shows that your digestive tract better tolerates a blend of carbohydrates than it does just one type. Look on the ingredient label for different sugars, such as sucrose, fructose, glucose, and maltodextrin.

Also, look for a drink with 100 to 110 milligrams of sodium and 30 milligrams of potassium per 8-ounce serving.

Finally, buy the flavor you like. Studies show that you'll drink more if you like the taste of the drink. Experiment with different flavors and brands. And try them both when sitting around the house and while exercising. Studies also show that people rate the taste of a drink differently depending on whether they are drinking during a workout or after one.

Good Food Sources Sports drinks are scientific marvels, and few natural foods or beverages can match their formulations. If you want to try to make your own, however, mix 9 teaspoons of sugar, ⅛ teaspoon salt, and the juice of one lemon into 3 cups of water.

How to Use It Aim for 5 to 12 ounces every 15 to 20 minutes for workouts lasting more than 60 minutes.

CARBOHYDRATE GELS

Puddinglike in texture, carbohydrate gels generally come in small, individual serving packets. You simply rip off the top of a packet and squeeze the gel into your mouth.

Consisting of simple sugars and long-chain carbohydrates, these gels are fairly easy to eat and digest. But their two biggest pluses include size and portability. They typically weigh about an ounce per packet, so you can easily tuck a few into the waistband of your shorts for quick refueling.

Research shows that they work just as well as sports drinks and other performance foods. In one study, runners took either GU (one of the original energy gels) and water or an artificially sweetened placebo drink during a 2-hour treadmill run. The gel users downed a packet of GU every 30 minutes, along with adequate water. Compared to the placebo group, GU users maintained higher blood sugar levels, suggesting the GU had been digested and was available for the muscles as an energy source.

Some gels provide a simple mixture of carbohydrate and water, whereas others offer some electrolytes such as sodium, making them a better choice for longer endurance efforts on a hot day. A few gels contain nonessential extras such as amino acids, herbs, and even caffeine in amounts equal to that of about half a cup of coffee. While some fitness enthusiasts experience a boost of energy with this caffeine, others experience GI distress, so experiment with caffeinated gels on low-key training days, not during races.

Taste Matters

Whether you opt for a gel, a sports drink, fitness water, or an energy bar, it all comes down to a matter of taste—literally. That is, as long as you cover the physiological bases.

For workouts lasting less than an hour: Water is adequate. (Just be sure to get a good dose of digestible carbohydrate within an hour of your workout.)

For workouts lasting longer than an hour: You'll need fluid and energy replacement. Sports drinks, energy gels, and energy bars are all effective energizers. Regardless of your choice, aim for 30 to 60 grams of carbohydrate an hour, which comes to about 24 ounces of sports drink, two standard-size packets of energy gel, or one energy bar.

Best For Endurance fitness enthusiasts who exercise for more than an hour and who have little space to carry larger food items with them. Gels, bars, and sports drinks are all good sources of energy. However, sucking down a gel is easier for many people than gnawing on a bar. Sports drinks work well, too, but they are tough to carry with you during some types of exercise.

What to Look For You want a gel packet that contains 70 to 100 calories and 17 to 25 grams of carbohydrate.

Test out different brands and different flavors to see what you like best. Look for packaging that is easy to open. Remember, you'll be consuming the gels while moving; the ease with which you can rip open the pouch and squeeze out the gel (without dribbling half of it down your chin) is key.

Since some gels contain caffeine, be careful. Many fitness enthusiasts have complained of a laxative effect when they take these gels.

Comparing Carbohydrate Gels					
	Calories	Protein (g)	Carbohydrates (g)	Fat (g)	Caffeine (mg)
Carb-BOOM	107	0	27	0	0
Clif Shot	100	0	23	0	40
GU	100	0	25	0	20
Hammer Gel	100	0	23	0	50
PowerGel	120	0	28	0	50
Squeezy	100	0	25	0	0
Ultra Gel	133	0	24	0	0

My suggestion: If you want to give caffeinated gels a try, consume them during a low-key exercise session where you have easy access to a bathroom.

Good Food Sources If the price of gels (at $1 or more per pack) keeps you from using these refueling gems, try honey, a natural energy gel. Research shows that honey taken during endurance cycling efforts works as well as other carbohydrate gels. Available in packets or sticks that contain about 1 teaspoon and 25 calories, you'll need two to three honey sticks per ½ hour.

How to Use It When using gels, consume between 30 and 60 grams of carbohydrate per hour of exercise. That amounts to one to two gels an hour. Swallow them along with 8 ounces of water to help them move through your stomach and into your intestine quickly.

TAP AND BOTTLED WATERS

Whether bottled or from the tap, water is a sure bet for meeting your fluid needs. Most waters, depending on their source (such as an underground spring or lake), contain small amounts of calcium and magnesium and a handful of other minerals from the surrounding rocks and soil that contribute to your daily need. A few waters now on the market, such as Smart Water, are "enhanced" with added minerals.

Bottled waters can serve as a convenient way to rehydrate during a long day at work in a dry office. Just bring in a large water container and drink from it all day. Also, store some in your gym bag for use at the gym or to sip while in your car.

Best For Office workers and exercisers of all types, as most of us walk around in a state of chronic dehydration.

What to Look For No one brand is better than another, so simply choose the type that tastes the best to you.

Food Sources Thanks to strict government safety regulations on tap water, you can be assured that your local water supply is safe. While bottled waters on the market tout themselves as better tasting than what flows from the kitchen sink, research doesn't support any difference when it comes to hydration—tap water and bottled varieties work alike. Besides plain tap water, you also get water from fruit juice, sodas, coffee and tea, and other beverages.

Comparing Tap and Bottled Waters
(per 8-ounce serving)

	Calories	Protein (g)	Carbohydrates (g)	Fat (g)
Tap Water	0	0	0	0
Aquafina	0	0	0	0
Dasani	0	0	0	0
Fiji	0	0	0	0

How to Use It Throughout the day, drink at least 8 to 10 cups of water (either bottled or from the tap) as the foundation of your daily fluid intake. During exercise sessions lasting less than 1 hour, drink 5 to10 ounces of water every 15 to 20 minutes to stay hydrated. Check your urine color (urinate into a clear cup) as a gauge of hydration; pale yellow (lemonade-like color) equals good hydration, whereas dark or amber color (like apple juice) equals dehydration.

FITNESS WATERS

Until recently, people who exercised for an hour or less had few hydration options. They didn't need the calories of a sports drink. Yet some of the fitness enthusiasts I know didn't want to drink tasteless water.

Now, thankfully, we have fitness waters. Gatorade's Propel and Reebok Fitness Water both offer a mere handful of calories, plus a dash of vitamins and minerals, in great-tasting flavors. Other versions, like ChampionLyte, come sweetened with sucralose, along with a dash of electrolytes, and offer great taste with zero calories.

A blend of sugar substitute and electrolytes, these beverages offer tasty flavors to encourage drinking. Fitness waters make a great choice

Liquid Oxygen?

A newcomer to the fitness water scene, super-oxygenated water claims performance benefits through the addition of oxygen. Manufacturers of these super O_2 waters claim the extra oxygen gets into the body, giving a boost to both performance and recovery.

However, research from the University of Wisconsin showed that student athletes performed equally on a multistage treadmill test while drinking either plain water or the oxygen-juiced variety. Check the Nutrition Facts food label on these beverages, as some come sweetened with corn syrup and as many calories as soda.

Comparing Fitness Waters (per 8-ounce serving)				
	Calories	Protein (g)	Carbohydrates (g)	Fat (g)
ChampionLyte	0	0	0	0
Life 02	0	0	0	0
Propel	10	0	3	0
Reebok	12	0	3	0

when drinking plain water during a workout seems boring. If you like the taste, according to all the research, you will drink more. A few fitness waters come "supercharged" with oxygen and claim to boost performance. While this is intriguing, studies fail to show any boost with oxygenated waters—your lungs do a great job as is.

However, as these drinks contain only a small amount of carbohydrate, you'll need to include solid carbohydrate sources, such as fruit or energy bars, or turn to a carbohydrate sports drink for workouts lasting longer than an hour.

Best For Fitness enthusiasts who exercise for less than an hour and who are watching their weight. The electrolytes will help you retain more fluid, and the flavor encourages you to drink more. It also makes a great low-calorie beverage to sip throughout the day.

What to Look For Your drink should contain 50 to 150 milligrams of sodium, 10 to 100 milligrams of potassium, and less than 10 calories per 8 ounces. Choose the flavor and brand you find the tastiest.

Good Food Sources Because of the precise blend of electrolytes, these performance beverages do outperform most drinks that you can concoct in your kitchen. However, if you'd like to create your own low-calorie, flavored water, make herbal iced tea with peppermint, vanilla, or other herbal, calorie-free tea bags. You can add a dash of fruit juice or a squeeze of lemon or lime for extra flavor.

How to Use It Consume 5 to 10 ounces every 15 to 20 minutes of exercise.

RECOVERY DRINKS

To recover quickly and perform your best at tomorrow's workout, you must pay careful attention to what you eat and drink after today's session. Your muscles need carbohydrate, some protein, and plenty of fluids during the first 30 minutes after your workout in order to efficiently hydrate and fuel up. Miss that 30-minute window, and you may not have as much pep in your step tomorrow.

Yet many of us do miss that 30-minute window. Sometimes after a hot, long workout, solid food is the last thing your stomach wants. Also, sometimes other tasks—such as showering, packing up your gear, and traveling from your workout location to home—take precedence over eating.

That's where recovery products come in.

These products, such as Gatorade Energy, Endurox R_4, and Distance, deliver a hefty dose of carbohydrate, to the tune of 40 grams

Cooking 101

Pour about ½ cup of sports drink into a paper cup and put it in your freezer. After about 45 minutes, when the liquid becomes slushy, place a Popsicle stick in the center and continue freezing. Then after a workout—or anytime—peel away the paper and enjoy.

Comparing Recovery Drinks (per 8-ounce serving)				
	Calories	Protein (g)	Carbohydrates (g)	Fat (g)
Distance	190	7	38	1
Endurox R_4	180	8.5	35	0
Gatorade Energy	207	0	41	0
G-Push (G4)	110	0	27	0
Pro Performance	109	0	25	0

per 8 ounces. Some of these drinks also offer protein, which, according to several studies, may help your muscles restock glycogen (stored fuel) faster, speeding your recovery. Just don't drink them during exercise—they'll sit in your stomach.

Best For Endurance fitness enthusiasts who exercise aerobically for more than an hour and who either feel too hot or are too busy to eat real food within 30 minutes of a workout.

What to Look For You want a replacement product that does *not* contain stimulants, such as caffeine. These lead to fluid loss after exercise. Your beverage should contain 30 to 50 grams of carbohydrate for each 8 to 12 fluid ounces. (Aim for 50 to 100 grams of carbohydrate within 1 hour after your workout.) For protein, look for 8 to 13 grams for every 8 to 12 fluid ounces.

Good Food Sources Try a carbohydrate-and-protein-packed smoothie. Make it with fruit, a scoop of soy protein powder, and nonfat yogurt before your workout, and then stick it in the fridge. Drink it when you return from your workout. Frozen fruit juice pops also work well, particularly for those who feel too hot to eat.

How to Use It Aim for 50 to 100 grams of carbohydrate (200 to 400 calories) during the first 30 to 60 minutes after your workout. Beyond your replacement beverage, drink additional fluid (about 20 ounces for every pound lost due to sweating).

CAFFEINATED "ENERGY" DRINKS

Many fitness enthusiasts want a kick in the you-know-what to get them energized, both for their workouts as well as for their afternoons at the office. In response to that demand have come a cadre of engineered drinks with names such as Red Bull, Adrenaline Rush, Whoop Ass, KMX, and Berry Bomb.

These caffeinated drinks are rapidly becoming the beverage of choice over sodas, bottled iced teas, and even sports drinks for a quick energy fix.

Energy drinks consist of primarily water and sweetener, typically corn syrup, sucrose, or some other sugar. The amount of added sugar is on par with that of sodas and fruit drinks—about 25 to 40 grams (5 to 8 teaspoons of sugar) or 100 to 160 calories per 8-ounce serving. This is about twice the carbohydrate content of sports drinks, making energy drinks a poor choice to drink *during* a workout. The extra sugar hampers fluid absorption, giving you that sloshing feeling in your stomach.

The defining ingredient in these drinks, however, is a wallop of caffeine, sometimes in excess of 100 milligrams, which is more than twice that of a typical can of cola or cup of coffee.

Some of this caffeine may come hidden as guarana, an herbal source of caffeine. While manufacturers aren't required to list amounts of caffeine or guarana, be aware that these ingredients can boost heart rate, blood pressure, and feelings of anxiety as well as give you a greater sense of alertness and perhaps better reaction time. And since caffeine acts as a diuretic and ups urine production, you risk dehydration if you drink too many of these beverages.

Other common "energizing" ingredients include:

Taurine. The mystical ingredient that many Red Bull fans claim gives them a buzz is actually an amino acid, one of the 20 that make up protein. While taurine is vital for a variety of roles in the body such as aiding in fat digestion, no research shows taurine aids exercise performance. Since we make enough of this amino acid on our own, healthy adults don't need extra taurine from a beverage.

Vitamins and minerals. Energy drinks typically come with a dose of B vitamins, such as thiamin, riboflavin, niacin, and vitamin B_6. These vitamins play a big role in releasing energy from carbohydrates during exercise and in burning fats. And some studies have shown that serious exercise programs like daily running may slightly increase your need for these nutrients. But no science shows that drinking a beverage loaded with B vitamins results in any boosting powers.

Some beverages claim to enhance the body's immune system with added vitamin C and zinc. A few studies have shown that high doses of zinc taken in lozenge form (bathing the back of the throat) may lessen the duration of a cold virus. But no evidence shows that consuming extra zinc from a beverage bolsters immunity.

Some drinks contain chromium, a mineral intimately involved in the proper functioning of the hormone insulin. For the past several years, studies have shown that supplemental chromium doesn't aid in weight loss or muscle building. But many people may not consume enough of this mineral, especially those who eat a highly refined diet, which does not include beans, whole grains, and wheat germ (all good sources of chromium). So the chromium dose in a beverage could boost your intake into the healthy range if your diet is lacking.

Herbals. The list of herbals in many of the new energy drinks reads like an alternative medicine dispensary. These drinks contain a smattering of herbs—from astragalus (said to bolster immunity) to yohimbe (used to improve sexual function in men)—in varying amounts, often too small to cause an effect.

Drinks that suggest they enhance mood and revitalize the mind often contain a trio of herbs: *Ginkgo biloba,* kava kava, and St. John's wort. Several studies have shown that these herbs may have benefits in enhancing mood or memory. Ginkgo, for example, has been shown to improve memory in patients with Alzheimer's, but not so in healthy adults. Kava kava may be effective in reducing symptoms of mild anxiety, but like ginkgo, doses in these drinks are below therapeutic levels.

I actually view the suboptimal levels of herbs as a blessing, since potential side effects can occur from overdosing on many herbal products. Ginkgo, for example, acts also as a blood thinner at therapeutic doses of 120 to 240 milligrams daily. And if a person is also taking a daily dose of aspirin and vitamin E (which also thin blood), this may present a dangerous situation of excessive bleeding from a simple cut or scrape.

Creatine and other body shapers. Some of these energy drinks promise leaner and stronger bodies with the addition of creatine, L-carnitine, hydroxycitrate, and pyruvate. And some of these ingredients, such as creatine, do show promise as a strength aid. But there's a catch: The amount added to beverages is far below what is known to have any performance-enhancing benefits.

Best For Underweight college students planning to pull an all-nighter studying event. Because of the high sugar content in these drinks, they do not make ideal workout or diet beverages.

What to Look For Keep an eye on calorie counts, as downing a few "skinny" cans can add up to some unwanted calories. And check the ingredients list, noting the number of stimulants that may contribute to feelings of anxiousness and racing heart rate.

Good Food Sources Though it contains much less caffeine than some of these drinks, I suggest drinking hot or cold tea. Besides giving you some eye-opening caffeine, tea contains potent phytochemicals, which may bolster heart health.

Comparing Energy Drinks
(per 8-ounce serving)

	Calories	Protein (g)	Carbohydrates (g)	Fat (g)	Caffeine (mg)
Adrenaline Rush	135	0	35	0	120
Berry Bomb	120	0	30	0	na
KMX	114	0	30	0	38
Red Bull	109	0	27	0	120
Whoop Ass	105	0	27	0	na

How to Use It Don't drink caffeinated energy drinks before or during exercise. After exercise, along with yogurt or a tuna sandwich, energy drinks supply carbs for recovery.

HIGH-PROTEIN BARS

First developed for body builders in search of easy-to-eat gym food, high-protein bars have recently surged in popularity with the advent of high-protein weight loss diets. These bars have also become the bars of choice for vegetarians and other athletes in search of extra protein in their diets.

High-protein bars can provide as much protein as a tuna sandwich. The Daily Value for protein is 50 grams, but as a fitness enthusiast, you need more—about 75 to 100 grams daily. Some bars supply close to half of your needs.

Most bars use a lactose-free milk protein, which is a good source of essential amino acids. Another protein source, however, provides extra disease-fighting powers—soy. It's found in bars such as GeniSoy.

Comparing High-Protein Bars

	Calories	Protein (g)	Carbohydrates (g)	Fat (g)
Atkins Advantage	220	18	2.5	11
EAS Myoplex HP	240	20	29	5
GeniSoy	220	14	31	3.5
PowerBar Protein Plus	290	24	38	5
Promax Bar	270	20	39	5

Studies show that isoflavones in soy may reduce your risk for certain types of cancer and heart disease. They also may lower blood cholesterol levels and heart disease risk, slow the progression of osteoporosis, and more.

Be wary of bars labeled "low-carb." These bars typically rely on sugar alcohols such as mannitol and fillers like glycerin to sweeten and bulk up the bar size, and some manufacturers don't include these in the carbohydrate count. Your body processes these ingredients much like regular carbohydrates from fruits and grains. In fact, the FDA has recently warned some bar makers to revamp labels for an honest carbohydrate count.

Best For May be helpful for folks who fall short on meeting protein needs, such as vegetarian athletes and high-mileage runners who find it difficult to keep their weight steady.

What to Look For Most protein bars supply anywhere from 15 to more than 35 grams of protein. Check the source of protein on the ingredients label. Look for high-quality proteins such as soy, whey or casein (both from milk), and egg. These proteins supply your body with

Keep It Under Wraps

Use these tips when choosing an energy bar:

- Whether you're working out or sitting at your desk, drink at least 12 to 16 ounces of water with an energy bar.
- During exercise, you may find it difficult to chomp down a bar all at once. Simply take a bite at a time and rewrap your bar. Remember: Your goal is to eat one bar during an hour of exercise, not one bar in 5 minutes.
- If you've opened an energy bar and let it sit for a few hours (especially after taking a bite), toss it to avoid any trouble with contamination. When unopened, however, energy bars are ideal "traveling" fuel that don't require refrigeration.
- When the number of energy bar wrappers in your garbage can, on your car floor, or in your gym bag start outnumbering remnants from real food, you should get back in touch with fruits, vegetables, and other wholesome foods.

crucial amino acids for muscle repair. If the label lists hydrolyzed protein, the bar contains poorer-quality proteins made from connective tissue and animal hooves. Also take note of the fat count, as several high-protein bars enhance their flavor with artery-clogging saturated fat. Look for a protein bar with fewer than 5 to 7 grams of fat.

Good Food Sources You can easily meet protein needs from eating fish, soy, lean meats, beans, and eggs.

How to Use It An occasional high-protein bar may help make ends meet on those days your meal planning is off.

40-30-30 BARS

Based on the popular 1995 book *The Zone Diet,* which touts a 40-30-30 ratio of carbohydrate to protein to fat as optimal for weight loss and athletic performance, these bars are typically higher in fat and protein and lower in fiber than their high-carbohydrate counterparts.

The higher fat content makes many of these bars taste just like a candy bar, which some makers even state on the label. Most come fortified with an array of vitamins and minerals, with some bars offering well over 100 percent of the DV for certain nutrients. While some 40-30-30 bar manufacturers claim their products help burn body fat, the few studies performed with these bars fail to support such statements.

Best For Folks looking for more protein, but the higher fat and lower carbohydrate content makes these bars less desirable for use during exercise. But when combined with high-carbohydrate foods such as fresh fruit or whole grain bread, these bars can be used for a tasty recovery meal after a long exercise bout. Also, the extra fat may help stave off hunger, making these bars a snack option for days when real food isn't an option.

What to Look For If you are eating other fortified foods or taking a multivitamin, avoid bars with extra fortification. And check labels for total fat and saturated fat, as some bars pack as much as a candy bar.

Good Food Sources You can easily get enough protein and carbohydrates along with essential fats, vitamins, and minerals from soy burgers, fish tacos, or other wholesome foods.

How to Use It Eat these bars on occasion as a meal replacement with fresh fruit, but don't use them during exercise as their high fat and protein content may upset your stomach.

Comparing 40-30-30 Bars				
	Calories	Protein (g)	Carbohydrates (g)	Fat (g)
Balance	200	14	22	6
Ironman Hi Energy Bar	230	16	26	8
PR Bar	200	13	22	6
ZonePerfect	210	14	24	7

WOMEN-ONLY BARS

Bar makers must have heard women's complaints about many bars: "I want a bar that has what my body needs without all the calories." Voilà! Wildly successful Luna bars and EAS bars offer petite versions of their relatives, usually under 200 calories but packed with key nutrients for a woman.

Many bars, such as Luna, use heart-healthy soy protein and come fortified with calcium, folic acid, and iron, three nutrients often low in a woman's diet.

Best For Women who want a tasty snack when fresh fruit and other foods are out of reach. And men can enjoy them, too, as many of my male friends tell me they enjoy the less filling, smaller size of these bars.

What to Look For Look for a bar with 8 to 15 grams of protein and less than 5 grams of saturated fat.

Good Food Sources Real food such as a spinach salad, soy yogurt, and fresh fruit or fortified breakfast cereal provide great stand-ins for these bars.

Comparing Women-Only Bars				
	Calories	Protein (g)	Carbohydrates (g)	Fat (g)
Balance Oasis	180	8	28	3
EAS Results	200	11	28	6
Luna	180	10	24	4.5
PowerBar Pria	110	5	16	3

How to Use It Keep in mind that these bars have the same amount of protein as a glass of milk. If used to replace a meal (as some women tell me they do), eat them along with whole foods such as a cup of yogurt and fruit or a bowl of bean soup.

MEAL-REPLACEMENT BARS

Many bar eaters opt for these convenient packages rather than reaching for a real meal. Also, in an effort to trim waistlines, people are turning to bars for help in controlling calories and portion sizes.

Slim Fast meal bars, designed with the dieter in mind, may in fact assist in weight loss when used in place of a meal. A recent study showed that overweight women who replaced two of their three daily meals with a Slim Fast bar (or the drink) experienced greater success with weight loss and maintenance than women who didn't incorporate meal replacements. Weight loss experts note that many dieters do better with controlled eating regimens, helping to explain why eating a fixed meal bar (while monotonous) as opposed to real food may help people adhere to a weight loss regimen.

Best For Dieters who tend to experience difficulty with portion control.

Comparing Meal-Replacement Bars				
	Calories	Protein (g)	Carbohydrates (g)	Fat (g)
Balance Satisfaction	280	12	48	6
Ensure Energy Bar	230	9	35	6
Opti-Pro Meal	290	20	40	5
Slim Fast Meal On-The-Go	220	8	34	5

What to Look For Because you are using the bar as a meal replacement, look for one fortified with an array of vitamins and minerals. Make sure it has less than 5 grams of fat and contains 8 to 15 grams of protein.

Good Food Sources Any food that comes in an individual serving size such as a low-calorie frozen dinner or even a carton of yogurt can help control portions as well as a snack bar.

How to Use It Keep in mind that no single bar supplies the wealth of nutrients and health-boosting substances found in whole foods such as fresh vegetables, fruits, whole grains, nuts, and quality protein sources that should be a regular part of your daily fare.

Chapter 8

FUNCTIONAL FOODS

Some foods truly are as powerful as medicine. Some are not. Here's the information you need to sort through the hype.

For many years we've known that whole foods such as fruits and vegetables do much more than simply provide vitamins, minerals, and calories you need to keep your body healthy, energetic, and powered for both work and exercise. They also contain powerful substances called phytochemicals (translated "plant chemicals") that prevent numerous age-related diseases, from heart attack and cancer to blindness and memory loss.

Many of these same substances also act as powerful antioxidants that help to repair your muscles after a tough workout, allowing you to bounce back quickly with little soreness. As with vitamins and minerals, they keep your brain in top shape, give your skin a healthy glow, bolster your immunity, improve circulation, enhance blood flow, and generally help you to feel your best.

Over the years, as scientists have tried to isolate, name, and understand these powerful healing substances, different foods took their turn in the spotlight. Perhaps you remember the broccoli years. Then came the year of the carrot. Then garlic took center stage, then tomatoes—then too many other different fruits and vegetables to name.

As scientists isolated these substances with long-sounding names such as 3-n-butyl phthalide, resveratrol, and quercetin, the true confusion began.

Manufacturers began fortifying products such as orange juice, breakfast cereals, snack foods, juice drinks, and even potato chips with these phytochemicals, claiming that these new functional food products boosted memory, immunity, and energy. Consumers began spending billions of dollars each year on the functional food industry.

Let's take a look at some of these products to help sort the function from the fiction.

FUNCTION VERSUS FICTION

For a food to qualify as a "functional food," it must provide health benefits beyond that supplied by the basic nutrition of the food. Let's see how the following foods add up:

The Product Orange juice with calcium.

The Marketing Hook Orange juice makers were the first to capitalize on the functional food craze, adding the bone builder calcium to the drink. Other juice drinks soon followed, as well as a host of other products, from sports drinks to oatmeal. Manufacturers claim that even though calcium is easily available from many other foods—such as milk, yogurt, sardines, and leafy greens—many people still don't consume as much as they should to prevent bone loss. Calcium-fortified products are needed to help you meet the recommended 1,000 daily milligrams.

Function Versus Fiction Besides calcium, good old dairy products provide a good dose of quality protein, the B vitamin riboflavin, and vitamin D, which is needed for calcium to get to your bones. Even if dairy products are not on your list of foods due to allergies, lactose intolerance, or personal choice, other rich sources of calcium—tofu, greens, canned fish with bones, fish sauce, tortillas made with lime, sesame seeds, and figs—can help you to reach your daily dose.

Of course, calcium-fortified foods such as orange juice, cereal, or soy milk also help.

If you don't consume milk, fortified products can help you to meet your daily requirement and keep your bones strong.

The Product Omega eggs.

The Marketing Hook These eggs first appeared on grocery store shelves under the brand Eggland's Best. To make these designer eggs, farmers feed hens a mixture of flaxseed, fish oil, and algae. The omega-3 fatty acids in the hen feed make their way into the yolks of the eggs the hens lay.

Besides eggs, other foods—from cheese to milk to bread—are beginning to appear on supermarket shelves with added omega-3s. Researchers at Purdue University are currently looking for ways to change the fat profile of beef and game meat to include more omega-3 fats and less saturated fat.

Omega-3s are essential fats, typically lacking in most people's diets, that are crucial for a healthy immune system, vibrant-looking skin, and proper circulatory function. Studies show that omega-3 fats may help ward off cancer, heart disease, dementia, and other age-related declines in neurological function.

Each omega-rich egg generally contains about 300 milligrams of omega-3 fatty acids (the amount in a single 1-ounce serving of salmon) and about a gram less of saturated fat than a regular egg. They also contain slightly less cholesterol than regular eggs.

Function Versus Fiction It's true that most people consume much less of this healthy fat than needed. However, omega eggs are fairly expensive compared to regular eggs. If you don't want to fork over the extra money, you can get all the omega-3 fatty acids you need by eating fatty fish such as salmon two times a week.

The Product Margarine with sterols.

The Marketing Hook Two new margarines on the market—Benecol and Take Control—contain plant sterol esters, which act like fiber to cling to fat and cholesterol in your gut, preventing it from getting absorbed into your body.

Function Versus Fiction These margarines, when used as directed, truly do work as medicine. Research shows that they can reduce LDL cholesterol levels by up to 14 percent. However, these margarines are no excuse to follow an otherwise unhealthful diet.

If you have high blood cholesterol, give them a try, but know that they are not your only option. If you don't like the taste of these margarines, try using olive oil as a spread when possible. Otherwise, you can safely use butter sparingly, as long as you follow my heart-healthy food tips in "Heart Disease" in part IV.

The Product Juice drinks and other foods with ginseng and other herbs.

The Marketing Hook It seems like just about every juice drink on the shelves these days contains some sort of herb. For example, Arizona's Rx Elixirs come with guarana and ginseng for more energy, *Ginkgo biloba* for memory, and kava kava for stress reduction. Apple & Eve make Immune Boon Tribal Tonic with the herb echinacea. Robert's American Gourmet makes Kava Kava Corn Chips and Personality Puffs with St. John's wort and ginkgo. Finally, Snapple's Vitality contains grape seed extract and ginkgo for improved energy.

Function Versus Fiction Do these products really increase your energy, brain power, and mental calm? It's hard to say.

Some of the research on individual herbs, such as ginkgo, kava kava, and echinacea, is promising, showing that these herbs may boost memory, tranquility, and immunity, respectively. However, research also has failed to uncover energy-boosting powers for ginseng, the most common herb in all of these drinks.

And no research has been done on these particular products. For example, it's possible that these herbs may work in concert with other nutrients in the plants they come from to cause these beneficial effects. When you isolate the herb and put it in a drink, it may not continue to hold its power.

Also, the herbal content varies considerably. For most of these products, so little of the herb makes its way into the food or drink that it's doubtful the herb will do any good.

Also, some herbs interfere with absorption of drugs such as heart medication and even birth control pills. St. John's wort, for example, interferes with protease inhibitors used for HIV patients and decreases the effectiveness of heart medications and birth control pills.

THE TRUE FUNCTIONAL FOODS

Ever since the vitamin, mineral, and phytochemical supplement craze, experts have wondered: Once you remove lycopene from the tomato or the vitamin C from the orange, does it lose its health-boosting ability? What if the lycopene needs other substances, naturally found in tomatoes, to work?

Well, we simply don't know the answer to that question. However, many of us—myself included—believe that phytochemicals work in concert with other nutrients naturally found in food. Once you pick apart these nutrients and isolate them into a pill or product supplement, they probably lose some of their power.

Make Your Own Functional Food

Who needs products with added phytochemicals when you can make your own? These flaxseed buttermilk muffins not only taste great, they also supply a good dose of disease-fighting omega-3 fatty acids.

Flaxseed Meal Buttermilk Muffins

1 cup flour
½ cup whole wheat flour
½ cup flaxseed meal (use coffee grinder to process flaxseed)
½ cup quick oats
2 teaspoons baking powder
½ teaspoon baking soda
½ cup egg substitute (or 2 eggs)
1 cup buttermilk
4 tablespoons honey
⅔ cup raisins

Preheat the oven to 400 degrees. Mix all the dry ingredients together in a bowl. Combine the liquid ingredients in a separate bowl (keeping the raisins in reserve). Stir the liquid ingredients into the dry ingredients all at once, add raisins, and stir until thoroughly moistened but the batter still appears lumpy. Fill muffin tins lined with paper or foil cups about ⅔ full. Bake for 20 to 25 minutes. Serve topped with jam. Each muffin has 165 calories and a good dose of omega-3 fats.

Though some functional food products may help you stay healthy, I'm a true believer in reaping the goodness that Mother Nature has to offer. Many natural foods pack whopping doses not only of these important phytochemicals but also of health-boosting essential vitamins, minerals, and fiber.

To perform your best in this fast-paced, high-tech world, give Mother Nature's finest a try. Here are 15 of her best.

Soybeans

For centuries, soybeans and soybean products, such as tempeh and tofu, have been an integral part of Asian culture as both food and medicine—for good reason. Just 1 cup of cooked beans supplies 25 percent of your daily need for fiber and folate, along with about 50 percent of your daily protein needs. Soybeans are the only nonmeat source of complete protein, supplying all of the essential amino acids your body needs.

However, what truly makes soy a miracle food are its isoflavones, a type of phytochemical that has been shown to boost heart health as well as help ward off cancer and osteoporosis. These isoflavones, called *genistein* and *daidzein,* help keep the bad LDL cholesterol carrier from dumping cholesterol onto your artery lining. They also help to make your blood less sticky, preventing the sudden blood clots that can lead to heart attacks.

New research on rats shows that soy may also contain special substances that numb pain, possibly by hampering the way cells relay pain messages.

You need 25 grams of soy protein a day to do the job. You can get that amount by eating two soy foods a day, such as a soy sausage patty at breakfast and a soy burger or pasta with soy meatballs at dinner.

Tomatoes

Because I live in California, where tomatoes are grown, I eat tomatoes all summer long, as many as two tomatoes a day. My husband, Mark, whose family history puts him at high risk for heart disease, eats even more tomatoes and tomato products than I do—at my insistence . . . and his pleasure.

Tomatoes contain a phytochemical called *lycopene,* which acts like an antioxidant to prevent the bad LDL cholesterol carrier from initiating cholesterol buildup along your artery lining. It also shows promise as a cancer fighter.

This chemical comes from the carotenoid family—a powerful family of pigments that give fruit and vegetables their yellow, orange, and red colors. Lycopene is what makes a tomato red. (Ruby red grapefruit and watermelon also contain good amounts of lycopene.)

In addition to lycopene, tomatoes and tomato products such as pasta sauce and juice also supply plenty of vitamin C.

I love vine-ripened tomatoes because they taste as a tomato should—sweet and juicy. This extra juiciness is a direct result of lycopene. Tomatoes ripened on the vine often contain more of the phytochemical than those picked underripe and then ripened with special gases as they travel by truck while being shipped from one side of the country to the other. You can find vine-ripened tomatoes at farmer's markets during peak season throughout most of the country. You can also easily grow them in your garden.

Also, don't rule out processed tomato products such as juice and sauce. Because they are more concentrated, they actually contain more lycopene than fresh tomatoes.

Spinach

High in carotenes, calcium, and iron, spinach is a true power food. The carotenes help ward off age-related diseases as well as protect your exercising muscles from the damage of a harder-than-usual workout. The calcium keeps your bones strong, and the iron keeps your energy high.

A recent study suggests that regular servings of spinach and its cousin the collard green can lower the risk of age-related degeneration of the retina. Researchers surveyed more than 800 adults on their vegetable and vitamin intake and found that a weekly ½-cup serving of these greens cut risk for eye disease by a third, and a 1-cup serving reduced risk by half. Researchers believe that carotenoids, a family of pigments found in vegetables and fruits, protect the eye from cell-destroying free radicals. Beta-carotene, lutein, and zeaxanthin, the carotenoids in dark, leafy greens such as spinach and collards, appear to have the most benefit. (Though carotenoids are yellow, orange, and red pigments, the chlorophyll in spinach and other greens overpowers the carotenoids to create a deep green color.)

Use spinach instead of iceberg lettuce to boost the nutritional punch of your salads. Also, sneak cooked spinach into lasagna and other casseroles. Make sure to eat something acidic or high in vitamin C, such as tomatoes or oranges, along with your spinach to increase iron absorption.

Oranges

Oranges along with grapefruits, lemons, limes, and other members of the citrus family all contain a special group of phytochemicals called *bioflavonoids*. The unique bioflavonoids found in citrus fruits have been shown to effectively ward off cancer, heart disease, and diabetes.

Oranges are also packed with vitamin C. This powerful antioxidant may help your muscles recover faster after exercise as well as keep your immune system running strong. Oranges and other types of citrus are also a great source of folic acid, which helps build healthy red blood cells vital for carrying oxygen. This B vitamin helps clear your blood of homocysteine, a protein metabolite that damages artery walls, leading to heart disease. Citrus fruits also pack a good dose of fiber and potassium, both great for heart health. Finally, studies show that citrus fiber helps control appetite and aids in weight loss.

Include a serving of citrus fruits daily—a whole orange for a snack, grapefruit wedges in a salad, or citrus juice for breakfast.

Salmon

Most seafood, particularly fatty fish such as salmon and mackerel, are excellent sources of omega-3 fats. These essential fats, typically lacking in most people's diets, are crucial for a healthy immune system, vibrant-looking skin, and proper circulatory function. Studies also show omega-3 fats may help ward off cancer, heart disease, dementia, and other age-related declines in neurological function.

Seafood also provides a good dose of quality protein and minerals including zinc and copper, along with various vitamins such as niacin and vitamin B_{12}. Aim for two 3- to 4-ounce servings a week.

Flaxseed

Flaxseed, a dark brown version of sesame seeds, contain about 9 grams of fat in a 1-ounce serving. But more than half of the fat is alpha-linolenic acid, which is the plant form of omega-3 fats. Flaxseed is used to make flaxseed oil, a standout oil source of omega-3s compared to its competitors canola and walnut oil. For vegetarians or people who don't eat fish, flaxseed and products made from it are your best bet in getting these essential fats.

In one study, people with risky blood cholesterol levels ate three slices of bread made with ground flaxseed daily for three months. Following "bread" therapy, the participants' cholesterol levels dropped dramatically, especially levels of the bad LDL cholesterol. Also, the patients' platelets were less sticky following flaxseed consumption.

Getting the health benefits of flax means using flaxseed or bottled oil, both sold at health food stores and some grocery stores. When adding whole flaxseed to your diet, you must either purchase ground flaxseed (called *flaxseed meal*) or grind them yourself in a coffee grinder. The outer covering of an unground flaxseed is pretty tough and will go right through your system undigested.

Make sure to store flaxseed (meal or whole seeds) and flax oil in the refrigerator as the fats easily go bad. Use flax oil in salad dressings, tossed with cooked pasta, or drizzled on pizza. It's important to note that flaxseed oil cannot be used in cooking because at high temperatures the beneficial oils break down.

You can use ground flaxseed meal in hot cereals, soups, and smoothies—or virtually any way you want. There are also a few ready-to-eat breakfast cereals that are made with flaxseed meal that will help boost your intake of omega-3s with ease.

Brussels Sprouts

Along with broccoli, cauliflower, cabbage, and other members of the cruciferous vegetable family, Brussels sprouts contain nitrogen compounds called *indoles,* which have been shown to powerfully fight off heart disease and cancer.

Brussels sprouts also contain a good amount of the antioxidants vitamin C and beta-carotene, known to fight off cancer and other diseases as well as bolster immunity.

However, the same phytochemical that makes this family of veggies incredible disease fighters is also the same phytochemical responsible for their bitter taste. For best results, choose fresh, small Brussels sprouts and cook them until they are al dente, not until they are soft all the way through.

Garlic and Onions

Though garlic has received much of the headline attention, both garlic and onions contain important phytochemicals called *thioallyls,* which have been shown to lower blood cholesterol as well as help prevent the formation of blood clots.

These phytochemicals may also work to keep cancer-causing agents from latching on to cells. Garlic has been shown to lower the risk of colon and stomach cancer, and ongoing research suggests it may even lessen the chances of breast cancer.

These thioallyls come in different forms. For example, when you crush garlic, you release a thioallyl called *allicin,* which is what makes your breath stink after eating garlic as well as what may help unclog arteries. When you cook garlic, you release a thioallyl called *ajoene,* which acts like aspirin to keep blood from clotting.

You need about a clove a day to do the job. Use garlic and onions to spice up any dish.

Wine

Hippocrates, the father of medicine, referred to wine's healing powers hundreds of years ago. Yet we only recently proved him right.

Research now shows that one to two glasses of wine a day with meals lowers death rates from heart disease and stroke. The alcohol in wine—as well as in other alcoholic drinks—may protect the heart by raising the levels of HDLs. These cholesterol carriers scavenge the loose cholesterol in your blood vessels and carry it to your liver for disposal.

Also, special phytochemicals from the skins of grapes that end up in wine—particularly red wine—provide additional protection. Called *flavonoids,* these phytochemicals add flavor and color to wine. They prevent LDLs from dumping cholesterol on your artery lining as well as prevent dangerous blood clots.

But there's an important caveat. Moderation is key. People who reap the healing benefits of wine tend to have only one to two drinks with dinner. Drinking any more than that—or on an empty stomach—can leave you open to an array of health problems, including breast cancer. Additionally, too much alcohol hampers your recovery from exercise as it interferes with glycogen storage.

Variety Is Best

For optimal health, our bodies need some 40-plus essential nutrients. No one food has it all. Instead, eating a variety of whole foods—whole grains, fruits, vegetables, dairy, and meat—ensures that you get needed protein, fiber, fats, carbohydrates, vitamins, and minerals along with other substances called *phytochemicals,* which have disease-fighting abilities. For example, it's much healthier to eat a variety of different fruits and vegetables—even if some of them don't top the list of power foods—than to focus on eating only broccoli or tomatoes each day.

Chocolate

Chocolate happens to be my indulgent food that I typically eat every day.

Much to my chagrin, nutritionists have long vilified chocolate because of its heavy dose of saturated fat (not to mention sugar and overall calories). Yet research has shown that the type of saturated fat found in chocolate isn't the same type of artery-clogging saturated fat found in butter and bacon. Chocolate's fat (called *stearic acid*) doesn't seem to clog arteries like these other saturated fats do (thank goodness!).

Also, new evidence suggests that chocolate may prevent other foods from clogging up your blood vessels. Cocoa powder, dark chocolate, and milk chocolate all contain respectable amounts of phenols, chemicals that prevent cholesterol-carrying LDL from oxidizing and damaging your arteries. In fact, a 1½-ounce square of dark chocolate has the same amount of phenols as a 5-ounce glass of red wine. And a cup of hot chocolate made with nonDutched (not treated with alkali) cocoa powder has about 75 percent the level of a glass of red wine, according to the research done by Andrew Waterhouse, Ph.D., and his coworkers from the Enology Department of the University of California at Davis.

Though chocolate is definitely not as bad for you as was once thought, this treat will still pack in the calories. To avoid weight gain and satisfy your cravings, keep serving sizes small. Hold yourself to no more than 1 to 2 ounces of chocolate a day and make it dark, since dark chocolate has more polyphenols than milk chocolate (and white chocolate isn't real chocolate, so it has no polyphenols).

Barley

Barley and other whole grains contain a wealth of fiber and small amounts of healthy fats. Because barley and other grains come from plants, we know that they contain important phytochemicals, but researchers have only just begun to isolate and name them. Recent research shows that whole wheat, for example, contains natural antioxidants called *orthophenols,* which inhibit cancer. But only future research will uncover the powerful substances in barley, millet, and other grains.

We do know, however, that 1 cup of cooked pearled barley contains almost 10 grams of fiber, a third of your daily needs. This fiber is a mix of the soluble type known to lower blood cholesterol levels as well as the insoluble type known to keep your intestines working regularly.

Use barley and other whole grains as often as you can, particularly as substitutes for refined grains made from white flour. For example, use barley in soups, as an extender for meat loaf, or mixed with veggies as a pilaf.

Nuts

As with chocolate, nuts were once vilified for their fat and calorie content. But thanks to new research, we now know better.

Almonds have stolen much of the spotlight when it comes to the healing power of nuts, but just about every type of nut is good for you. Nuts are packed with heart-friendly monounsaturated fat. They are all loaded with antioxidant vitamin E, which may help reduce muscle damage as well as fend off age-related diseases.

Almonds in particular come with a healthy dose of important minerals, such as magnesium, iron, calcium, and potassium. In each ounce, you get 10 percent of your fiber and zinc needs, 25 percent of your magnesium needs, and a good dose of vitamin E.

Beans

Beans are a powerhouse food supplying a wealth of goodies. A 1-cup serving of beans packs almost half your fiber needs. And the fiber type in beans helps keep cholesterol levels in check, good news for your heart. Beans also supply a plentiful array of vitamins and minerals.

If you're a vegetarian, black beans, lentils, chickpeas, and other beans are your best source of protein, iron, and soluble fiber. High in carbohydrate, beans are also loaded with folate (folic acid), which may prevent birth defects during pregnancy and fight heart disease. Buy canned black beans, chickpeas, kidney beans, or any other type. Throw them in a blender with some spices to make a tasty sandwich spread or add them to soups and salads.

Berries

Strawberries—and many other berries—are low in fat and high in vitamins, especially beta-carotene, vitamin C, and folate. One cup of fresh berries offers more than 6 grams of cholesterol-lowering fiber. The type of fiber in berries is called *pectin,* which helps soak up cholesterol by-products in the intestine and carry them out of the body.

All berries contain health-promoting phytochemicals called *catechins,* which are also found in green tea (see below). Strawberries, in particular, contain an important phytochemical called *ellagic acid,* a powerful antioxidant that can inhibit tumor growth.

Thanks to hothouse farming and imported produce, you can find fresh berries year-round.

Tea

Tea—both green and black—has long been thought to have health-promoting properties, and research is beginning to bear that out. One study showed that green-tea drinkers have a lower risk of cancer of the esophagus than nondrinkers. Another shows that it may protect against skin cancer. The protective agent in tea looks to be a flavonoid catechin called *epigallocatechin gallate* (EGCG). It acts as an antioxidant, protecting cells from the damaging work of free radicals.

Black tea, made from the same leaves as green tea but blackened during the fermentation process, also contains EGCG. Though most research has focused on green tea, researchers suspect that black tea provides similar benefits. You can find both teas at any grocery store. Try to drink 1 to 2 cups a day.

Part III

EATING ACCORDING TO YOUR LIFE STAGE

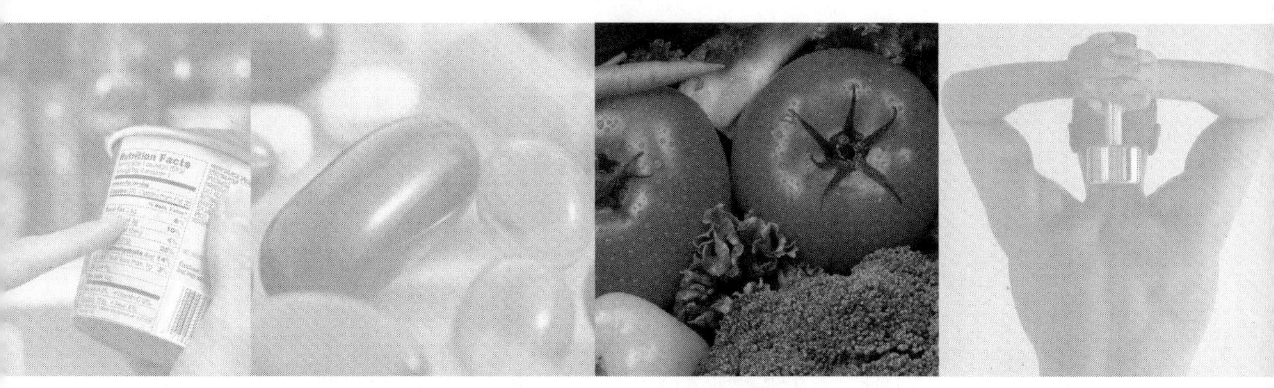

Chapter 9

EATING FOR FITNESS

Boost your performance, health, and motivation by following an individualized food plan based on your age and fitness level.

For years, people have used the U.S. Department of Agriculture's (USDA) Food Guide Pyramid to direct their eating choices. The pyramid, found on the side of cereal boxes and other food products, suggests a range of servings for grains, vegetables, fruits, meats, dairy, and fats.

No matter your age, no matter your fitness level, the pyramid suggests you make grains the cornerstone of your diet, followed by vegetables and fruit, then dairy and meat and topped with a small amount of fat and sweets.

It just doesn't work, particularly for people who exercise on a regular basis. Though the simple design of the pyramid creates an easy-to-follow food plan, the system is seriously flawed in numerous other ways, a problem that even the USDA, which designed the pyramid, now acknowledges.

Developed way back in 1992 during the relative dark ages of nutritional science, the USDA's Food Guide Pyramid desperately needs an overhaul.

But What About Those Other Diets?

All of my customized daily food and activity pyramids in chapter 10 will give you roughly 30 percent of your calories from fat, 15 percent from protein, and 55 percent from carbohydrate. Some other diets—such as the Dean Ornish program or the Atkins diet—recommend different amounts of macronutrients.

But such diets are not optimal for fitness. Here's why:

Super Lowfat Diets

Cardiologist Dean Ornish, M.D., says a 10 percent fat diet protects his patients from artery damage and helps heal already-clogged arteries. However, Dr. Ornish and others who promote very lowfat diets require you to accept a total package, which includes regular exercise, stress reduction, meditation, and yoga.

The combination of all those factors, not just the very lowfat diet by itself, probably unclogs blocked arteries. Also, for some individuals, a lowfat, high-carbohydrate diet tends to increase levels of circulating fats called *triglycerides,* while lowering healthy (HDL) cholesterol.

The Zone or "40-30-30" Diet

Promoters claim that following a 40 percent carbohydrate, 30 percent fat, and 30 percent protein diet speeds fat burning by better regulating and lowering the levels of insulin, the hormone that helps process carbohydrates. The science behind this reasoning is still unproven. Many of those who report success do in fact lose body fat, but mainly from calorie counting and cutting back on total calorie intake.

For example, the pyramid places all fats at the tippy top, cautioning us to eat them sparingly. Yet since 1992, we've learned that not all fats are bad. Some fats, such as the monounsaturated fats found in olive oil, promote health and can and should be eaten more often.

But What About Those Other Diets? *(continued)*

High Protein Diets

Several popular diet books, such as *Dr. Atkin's New Diet Revolution* and *Protein Power,* advocate cutting back or eliminating carbohydrates. This means eating no bread, pasta, potatoes, fruits, and vegetables, as well as very few dairy products. Instead, you eat more protein from tuna, meats, and eggs.

Following this carbohydrate-free eating plan will result in weight loss. As your body reacts to a very low-carbohydrate diet, it begins a metabolic state called *ketosis.* Rather than burning the standard mix of carbohydrate and fats for energy, your body now burns fats and fatlike compounds called *ketones* for fuel.

To fuel your brain, however, your body breaks down protein—not fat. It cannibalizes muscle, breaking it into amino acid building blocks and then converting these to sugar. Less muscle equals a slower metabolism, which is why people tend to gain weight as soon as they stray from the diet.

This type of diet is nutritionally unbalanced. You miss out on key vitamins and minerals, such as calcium, folic acid, and vitamin C, along with fiber. Additionally, the high-protein foods you are eating on this plan may be high in fat and cholesterol, which boost heart disease risk in susceptible individuals.

Others, such as the artery-clogging saturated fats found in animal products, should be minimized.

More important, we've also learned that not all people benefit from the same eating plan. For example, a man in his 60s needs more B_{12} and vitamin D than a man in his 20s. A woman in her 30s needs more folic acid than a woman in her 50s. A teenager needs more calcium than a child or even a pregnant adult woman.

Besides your age, your lifestyle also influences your optimal food choices. For example, those who walk, swim, run, or do some other type of physical exercise on a regular basis need more calories, protein, and nutrients than those who don't exercise.

In short, no single food guide pyramid fits all people.

Rather than have you follow the USDA's one-size-fits-all plan, I've developed seven new pyramids, found in chapter 10, each tailor-made to fit people at the following life stages:

- Children ages 4 to 8
- Children ages 9 to 12
- Teens
- 20s
- 30s
- 40s and 50s
- 60-plus

Follow the customized daily food and activity pyramid designed for your age, but don't stop there. You can further tailor your pyramid to your unique lifestyle habits, goals, and health background. (See sidebar, "Make Sure Your Genes Fit.") Each rung of each customized pyramid contains a range of servings for that particular food group. If you're fighting off weight gain, opt for the lower end of those servings, particularly for grains, protein-rich foods, calcium-rich foods, and fats. On the other hand, if you log 2 or more hours a day at the gym, you can probably opt for more servings.

I've also listed tips under each food category to help you use your pyramid to maximize your health. Each customized daily food and activity pyramid contains the following categories:

Fluids. The more you exercise, the more you sweat. A typical 165-pound person loses about 8 cups of fluid during the day. The same person sheds an additional 6 or more cups during a 45-minute run in the July heat. If you don't replace those lost fluids, you'll become dehydrated. Besides hurting your performance, chronic dehydration also increases your risk for kidney stones and bladder cancer.

Tip: Each of my customized pyramids provides a fluid range for your age. If you live in a hot environment and exercise outdoors, gravitate toward the higher end. Check your hydration by gauging your urine color—a darker color (like apple juice) equals dehydration, whereas pale yellow (dilute lemonade appearance) equals optimal hydration.

Grains. When you exercise, your muscles burn a type of carbohydrate, called glycogen, for fuel. To keep these important fuel levels optimal, you must eat a diet rich in grains, potatoes, and other types of high-carbohydrate foods. Besides carbohydrate, grains contain important B vitamins, such as thiamine, riboflavin, and niacin, that your muscles need to convert the carbohydrate you eat into energy.

Tip: While enriched refined-grain products made from white flour (such as crackers, white rice, and pasta) do supply these B vitamins, focus on whole grains (such as whole wheat bread, quinoa, and brown rice), which also provide the fiber you need for a healthy heart and digestive tract, as well as other key nutrients such as magnesium, zinc, and vitamin E not found in refined grains.

Vegetables. Exercise makes you breathe hard. The harder you breathe, the more oxygen your lungs suck in. While you need oxygen to sustain life, this gas tends to be unstable inside the body. And unstable oxygen molecules can oxidize, which damages your muscle cells as well as sets the stage for heart disease and cancer. Damaged muscle cells bring on inflammation and soreness, which makes your next workout feel harder than it should.

Most vegetables counteract oxidation by offering up antioxidants, important molecules that neutralize and repair damaged cells. Vegetables also house a wealth of other disease-fighting substances that help prevent cancer, diabetes, heart attack, and stroke.

Tip: Choose fresh, frozen, or canned vegetables, as these all supply a wealth of nutrients. Vegetables are also the lowest-calorie foods on the planet, making them the best friend of anyone trying to lose weight.

Fruits. As with vegetables, brightly colored fruit, such as kiwi, berries, and oranges, contain a wealth of antioxidants and other phytochemicals.

Tip: Though 100 percent fruit juice counts as a serving, you'll get more cholesterol-lowering fiber and other nutrients from whole and dried fruit.

Calcium-rich foods. Consuming dairy products is the easiest way to ensure you're getting plenty of bone-strengthening calcium. Besides strengthening bones, calcium helps keep blood pressure low, and recent research suggests it may even help you burn fat faster.

Tip: If you don't eat dairy, select calcium-fortified soy products or other calcium-rich foods such as calcium-fortified orange juice or cereal.

Protein-rich foods. Fit people need more protein than flabby people, about 80 or more grams of protein a day. This macronutrient is especially important after your workouts, when your body repairs muscle damage and shuttles energy back to your muscles.

Tip: Include soy, fish, eggs, and lean meat (think sirloin, not prime rib) in your postworkout meal. Lean meat, especially beef, is loaded with zinc, a mineral that most people need to optimize. And soy, fish, and other types of meat provide iron and other trace minerals, such as copper and manganese, that your body needs, especially during heavy training. Try to eat fish one to two times a week for its healthful omega-3 fats, which are known to prevent heart disease and joint pain.

Healthful fats. The monounsaturated fats found in nuts, avocados, olives and olive oil, and canola oil as well as the omega-3 fatty acids found in fatty fish and flaxseed help bolster heart health, help prevent cancer, and may even fight inflammation, muscle soreness, and the common cold. On the other hand, the saturated fats found in animal

Make Sure Your Genes Fit

Your unique genetics influence your optimal food plan. For example, some people are able to lower their cholesterol levels and improve their heart health by following a lowfat, high-carbohydrate diet. Others on the very same diet experience higher cholesterol levels. Also, some pregnant women have a higher need for folic acid than other pregnant women. And some people, usually African Americans, tend to experience a rise in blood pressure when they eat salt, whereas others see no effect.

Throughout my customized daily food and activity pyramids in chapter 10, I offer numerous tips to help you customize your eating plan to your personal health needs. However, to truly ensure you're following the best diet for you, I suggest taking your pyramid with you to your next checkup. Talk to your doctor about your family health history and personal health problems to get an idea of how to properly tweak your pyramid.

products and the hydrogenated fats found in processed foods both increase your risk for heart disease. No matter your age, try to optimize your consumption of healthy fats and minimize your consumption of heart-clogging saturated and hydrogenated fats.

Tip: All types of fat contain more calories per gram than either carbohydrate or protein. So if you're watching your weight, you should opt for the lower recommendation on your pyramid.

Sweets. Chips, cake, soda, and doughnuts all offer zero nutrients and hundreds of excess calories. Also, many of these foods contain either saturated or hydrogenated fat, two of your biggest artery cloggers.

Tip: One of the reasons you exercise is so you can eat the foods you love. So munching on cookies or fatty snack foods is not a big deal as long as these foods don't become dietary staples.

FOLLOWING YOUR CUSTOMIZED PYRAMID BEFORE, DURING, AND AFTER EXERCISE

In order to fuel your muscles and motivation properly, you must also know *when* to eat your pyramid foods.

For example, fueling up with a high-carbohydrate meal (think grains) before a workout will give you the motivation to get out the door as well as the energy to lengthen your workout. Eating during certain types of exercise can boost your endurance, speed, and reaction time. Finally, eating the right foods after exercise can help you to recover more quickly, enabling you to exercise harder and longer tomorrow.

Follow these tips to use your customized daily food and activity pyramid to your advantage before, during, and after exercise.

Before Exercise

- Eat 2 to 4 hours before a workout. To accommodate your workout schedule, you may need to rearrange your mealtimes. For example, you may eat lunch at 2 P.M. so you can work out at 6 P.M.

- Choose high-carbohydrate, lowfat, low-protein foods. Carbohydrate digests quickly, whereas protein and fat may sit in your stomach, making you feel nauseous during your workout.

- Eat about 400 to 800 calories at your pre-exercise meal. This amount should fuel your exercise without making you feel sluggish or full. A whole grain bagel topped with tomato slices and reduced-fat cheese or breakfast cereal and fruit with milk (or soy milk) are excellent choices.

- Drink about 10 ounces of water or sports drink 2 hours before exercise. This helps offset sweat losses during your work-

Sample Preworkout Meals

Try one of the following preworkout snacks 2 hours before your next run, bike ride, or swim:

- 6 ounces vegetable juice and ½ cup dried apricots
- 1 piece whole grain pita bread topped with 3 tablespoons fruit spread
- 1 glass of sports drink and 1 cup ready-to-eat, whole grain breakfast cereal mixed with 1 tablespoon raisins
- 1 package of instant oatmeal made with ½ cup vanilla-flavored soy milk or skim milk with a dash of cinnamon and sugar
- 1 toasted plain bagel with 2 teaspoons jam, 1 banana, ½ cup cooked rice sprinkled with cinnamon, and 1 cup sports drink

out. Also, 2 hours gives your kidneys time to rid your body of any excess fluid before exercising.

During Exercise

- Consume 5 to 12 ounces of either water or sports drink every 15 to 20 minutes of exercise. If you work out for more than an hour, make it sports drink to fuel your muscles and help offset sodium losses.
- Exercise tends to blunt feelings of thirst, so don't wait to feel thirsty before you drink.
- Consume 30 to 60 grams of carbohydrate for every hour of exercise. That comes to about 120 to 300 calories per hour

for endurance sports lasting 90 minutes or more and for stop-and-go sports such as tennis, basketball, and soccer. The carbohydrate will replenish spent muscle and brain fuel, boosting your energy and helping you to think more clearly.

After Exercise

- To help shuttle energy to your muscles and remove waste products, you must rehydrate quickly. Drink 2 cups of water for every pound of sweat you lose. Weigh yourself before and after exercise or monitor your urine color. Drink plenty of fluids until your urine runs pale yellow to clear.
- Eat a 100- to 400-calorie snack that contains both carbohydrate and protein during the first hour after your workout.

Sample Postworkout Meals

Try one of the following postworkout snacks within ½ hour of your workout:

- ⅓ cup each of soy nuts, dried papaya, and dried peaches eaten with an 8-ounce serving of cranberry juice
- ½ cup frozen blueberries swirled into 1 cup lowfat lemon-flavored yogurt eaten with a package (a 1-ounce serving) of wheat crackers
- 8-ounce carton of lowfat milk or soy milk with a nutrient-fortified energy bar that contains 8 to 10 grams of protein
- 1 small, microwavable bean burrito with 4 tablespoons packaged salsa and 1 small can (6 ounces) of orange juice
- 2 mozzarella cheese sticks, 1 toasted whole grain English muffin, and 1 orange

Carbohydrate goes straight to the glycogen stores in your muscles, which speeds recovery from exercise. Protein helps to repair muscle damage, boost immunity, and escort carbohydrate to your muscles. Your muscles are most receptive to carbohydrate replenishment during the first hour after activity.

- Stay away from caffeinated beverages such as cola, which tend to increase urine output, and carbonated beverages, which simply take longer to drink. On a hot summer day, consider having a Popsicle or cold smoothie, especially if you're overheated and don't feel hungry.

SERVING SENSE

Though my customized pyramids in chapter 10 contain differing amounts of food for various food groups depending on your age, I've

Size It Up

Food Group	Serving Size
Grains	½ cup cooked pasta, beans, couscous, or other grains (about the size of a computer mouse); 1 slice bread; ½ bagel; 1 ounce cereal (see box for serving size)
Vegetables	1 cup raw leafy greens (a little less than the size of a softball); ½ cup cooked or chopped vegetables
Fruits	1 medium piece of fruit (about the size of a tennis ball); ½ cup juice; ½ cup chopped fruit
Calcium-rich	1 cup milk, soy milk, or yogurt; 1½ ounces cheese (about the size of three dice)
Protein-rich	1 cup soybeans; 2 soy burgers; 2 to 3 ounces fish or lean meat (about the size of a deck of cards); 2 eggs
Healthful fats	1 ounce nuts (about 18 almonds); ⅛ avocado; 2 teaspoons oil
Sweets	Check labels for serving size and calorie count (refer to your pyramid for sweets allotment)

kept the serving sizes consistent (see table, "Size It Up," on page 175). For example, one serving of pasta is the same amount for a four-year-old as it is for a 60-year-old.

During the first few weeks of your new food plan, you may need to carefully measure foods to ensure you stay within the right number of servings for the day, especially if you have become accustomed to "supersize" portions. With time, however, you'll develop your serving sense and automatically eyeball the correct portion sizes.

Chapter 10

FIT EATING AT EVERY AGE

Use the customized daily food and activity pyramid designed with your fitness in mind.

Within this chapter, you'll find seven eating plans for the seven major stages of life: children ages 4 to 8, children ages 9 to 12, teens, 20s, 30s, 40s and 50s, and 60-plus. Each eating plan not only optimizes the nutrients most important for that life stage (for example, by including more calcium for teens and more folic acid for women in their 30s) but also factors in common lifestyle barriers to fit eating.

For example, those in their teens and 20s often survive by eating on the go from vending machines, minimarts, and restaurants. Rather than tell you all to start cooking, I instead offer ways to get the nutrients you need from "fast" food. Another example: We all know that children need to eat more vegetables. Rather than beating you over the head with that fact, I offer simple yet effective strategies to optimize your child's nutrition, even for the pickiest eaters.

Because nutritional needs change quickly and dramatically from birth to age 4, I have not included a food plan for this age group. If your child is younger than age 4, consult your pediatrician about the best food plan for him or her.

FIT EATING FOR AGES 4 TO 8

Children need relatively few calories but a lot of nutrients to fuel their active growing bodies. As a result, children must eat foods that give them a big bang for their caloric buck in order to fit all the nutrients they need into a small amount of calories.

Few children eat enough of the right foods. Foods such as Goldfish crackers, cupcakes, hot dogs, Cheez Whiz, and soda provide little in the way of nutrition but a lot in the way of calories. It's not uncommon for children to be deficient in numerous vitamins and minerals, fiber, and even protein at this age, as the vast majority of what they eat doesn't contribute to their nutritional needs.

But fear not—you *can* get your child to eat healthful foods. I know, because I raised two children.

Start your child's diet metamorphosis by quitting your job as a short-order cook. Most picky eaters come from families with moms or dads who offer to cook something special for the kids. As mom and dad eat their fish with steamed broccoli, the kids eat hot dogs or pizza.

Prepare just one dinner every night for the entire family, not one dinner for you and one for your children. Don't force your children to eat everything on their plates, but serve up a little of everything and encourage them to try a bite of everything. If they pick at their food, fine. But don't offer to cook a separate "kiddie" meal.

Besides dinner, breakfast is also an important meal, particularly for school-aged children. Studies show that children who head to school on an empty stomach tend to perform worse on math, reading, and memory tests. They also tend to consume fewer vitamins and minerals and less fiber and protein than their breakfast-eating peers.

Breakfast doesn't have to take a lot of time. Cereal with milk provides a quick-and-easy way to start the day and a great way to sneak in 5 or more grams of fiber. If your child doesn't like high-fiber cereals such as Wheat Chex or Raisin Bran, mix those cereals with a sweeter kid cereal such as Lucky Charms.

Besides cereal, good quick breakfast options include a peanut butter and jelly sandwich for your child to eat on the way to school, leftover macaroni and cheese with a piece of fruit, leftover pizza with a can of vegetable or fruit juice, or a smoothie made with soy or regular milk or a carton of yogurt and two types of fruit.

Customized Pyramid for 4- to 8-Year-Olds

Stick to the following food groups, number of servings, and exercise prescription daily to optimize your child's health and physical development.

Physical Activity: 60+ Minutes Few schools offer physical education classes these days, so encourage movement as much as you can. Resist the urge to "baby-sit" your kids with the VCR or computer games. Exercise at this age doesn't have to be structured, but kids need to move. Otherwise, they will become more and more sedentary as they age and more likely to gain weight. Take them to a playground and let them run around with friends or tackle the swing set or seesaw. Play tag and other active games with your kids. You will boost not only their health but yours as well.

Fluids: 2 to 3 (8-Ounce) Glasses Take steps to ensure your child meets quota here, as children's bodies don't sweat as efficiently as an adult's does, making them more prone to heat illness during exercise. Don't compound matters by allowing your children to exercise while dehydrated.

Fortunately, your child needs a relatively small amount of fluid compared to an adult, so meeting these fluid needs should not be hard. Encourage your child to drink healthful fluids with meals, such as milk with dinner and fruit juice with lunch. Many children this age love sports drinks, probably because of the wild assortment of colors and names. As most sports drinks contain a lot fewer calories than soda, they provide a great hydration option for children, particularly active ones.

Grains: 6 Servings Children need their age plus 5 in grams of fiber. That means a 4-year-old should be eating 9 grams, a 5-year-old 10 grams, and so on.

Few kids pull it off.

Try to break your child out of the refined-carbohydrate trap. Sure, boxed foods such as macaroni and cheese and snack crackers offer quick-and-easy meals and snacks, but they also provide little fiber and few vitamins and minerals. Experiment with whole grains. If your child is already strongly attached to foods made from white flour, slowly add these whole grains to refined ones by mixing whole wheat noodles in with refined ones or brown rice in with white.

Vegetables: 3 Servings Many parents complain that their children don't eat vegetables. Here's a little trick: Involve them in vegetable preparation from an early age. What children select, grow, or prepare, they will often eat.

Take your children with you to the grocery store. While in the produce section, ask your child to choose a vegetable for dinner. For example, you might ask your child to find a red vegetable for the salad or a green or a purple vegetable for a side dish.

Then, when preparing the meal, allow your child to help by pulling the vegetables out of the fridge, washing them, and assembling them on a plate.

Certain vegetables will be a harder sell than others. Children do have more sensitive taste buds at this age, so what tastes bitter to you will taste extremely bitter to them. The bitterness from Brussels sprouts and broccoli comes from the indoles, the healing substances that prevent disease. Don't give up, though. You can hide some of the bitterness with sauces. Get creative and keep offering these foods, setting the stage for a lifetime of healthful eating.

Fruits: 2 Servings Buy fruit and offer it as a snack. Younger children may not be able to eat a whole piece of fruit, so make it fun by

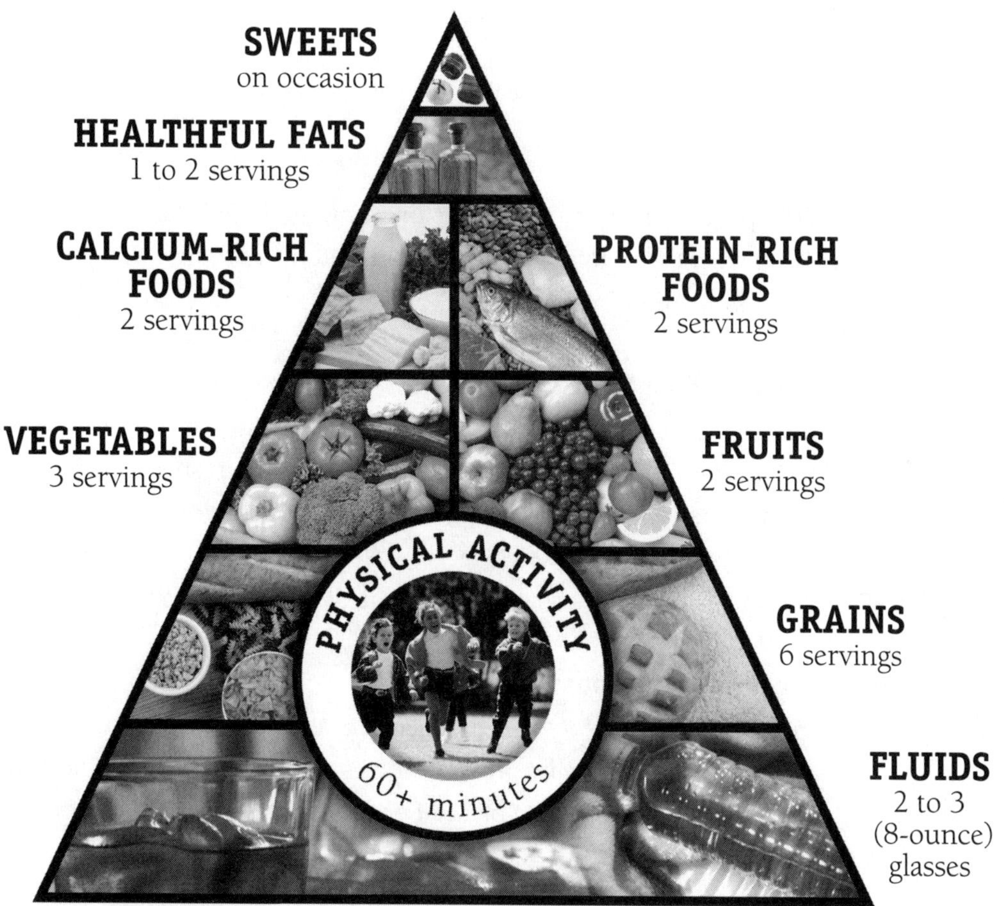

CUSTOMIZED DAILY FOOD AND ACTIVITY PYRAMID
FOR CHILDREN 4 to 8

Let Them Snack

I've raised two children, so I know it can be tough to get them to sit down to a meal and eat everything on their plates. So don't force them. Children by nature are distracted. They probably won't be able to only eat three meals a day. Allow them to snack, eating as often as every 2 hours. Just make sure you serve quality snacks such as chopped carrots, dried or fresh fruit, nuts, or fruit juice.

chopping apples and other fruits into unique shapes. Also, offer them 100 percent fruit juice or vegetable juice to drink rather than soda or other nonfruit juices.

Calcium-Rich Foods: 2 Servings Children need quite a bit of calcium compared to the amount of calories they eat—to the tune of 800 milligrams. If your kids won't drink milk, you can sneak in calcium by putting milk or yogurt into soups for a creamy texture, offering nonfat pudding for dessert, serving cereal with milk for breakfast, or making a lowfat milk shake or smoothie with milk or yogurt and fruit.

Protein-Rich Foods: 2 Servings Wean your child off processed meats such as hot dogs and luncheon meat as a way of life, and begin serving healthful, quality protein sources such as eggs, beans, and fish. Many children won't eat a piece of grilled or broiled fish, but they will often eat fish if you include it in another dish such as a tuna noodle casserole or salmon salad sandwich. Also, try adding fish such as clams to pasta sauce.

Healthful Fats: 1 to 2 Servings By age 2, children don't need as much fat as they did during infancy, and research shows many kids eat too much of it. Focus on healthful fats as much as possible from olives, olive oil, avocado, nuts, and nut butters. Nuts can provide a great healthful snack that you won't have to force your kids to eat.

Sweets: On Occasion Kids eat more sweets than you think. Don't feel obligated to serve dessert every night of the week or include a cupcake in their lunch bag. Also, remember that soda falls into this category.

FIT EATING FOR AGES 9 TO 12

As many as 20 percent of children in this age group are now considered overweight. Lack of physical activity at home and at school means kids burn few calories. Yet these same kids tend to eat a lot of food.

With the fast-paced American lifestyle, parents often have little time to cook, resorting to taking kids out to eat, often to family-style restaurants such as TGI Friday's or to fast-food restaurants such as McDonald's. Such places offer little in the way of portion control, serving up dinners that contain 1,000 calories or more. Buffet-style family restaurants pose the greatest weight-watching challenge because kids pile their plates with unhealthful, high-calorie, high-fat choices such as fried chicken and french fries and then head to the dessert counter for one, two, or three servings.

Besides eating huge portions, kids also eat a lot of empty calorie foods such as snack chips and soda. Junk foods often make up as much as three-fourths of the calories that kids eat. It's nearly impossible to fit all the vitamins, minerals, fiber, protein, and other nutrients into the remaining fourth. In fact, research has found some children aged 9 to 12 to be deficient in key vitamins and minerals, fiber, and protein.

In short, most kids need a diet overhaul.

Start this overhaul by teaching your kids about portion control. Go over my customized daily food and activity pyramid with them, allowing your children to check off and measure their servings each day. Also, try to wean them off fatty high-calorie foods and introduce more healthful, lower-calorie foods in their place. Include a high-fiber food such as brown rice, whole grain cereal, vegetables, fruit, or beans at every single meal to help kids feel full longer and improve intestinal function.

Customized Pyramid for 9- to 12-Year-Olds

Follow this pyramid to raise a trim, fit child.

Physical Activity: 60+ Minutes Encourage your kids to move by setting a good example. If you're currently sedentary, get off your rear and move. Start a walking program and take your kids along with you. On the weekends, do something active as a family, such as going for a family bike ride or hike. Allow your child to try numerous sports, as research shows concentrating on just one sport may cause exercise burnout.

Fluids: 5 to 8 (8-Ounce) Glasses Gravitate toward low-calorie or noncalorie fluids, saving the soda for special occasions. Preteens and teens drink as much as 55 gallons of soda a year, a huge source of empty calories that tends to displace more nutritious beverages such as milk or fruit or vegetable juice—and sometimes even meals. Offer water as often as possible, jazzing it up with a shot of fruit juice or lemon.

Grains: 6 to 11 Servings Begin to teach your child that snack chips and crackers don't count as grains. Try to make at least half of these grains "whole" by choosing brown rice over white, high-fiber cereal over sugary cereal, and whole wheat bread over white.

Vegetables: 2 to 5 Servings Kids aged 9 to 12 will turn their noses up at vegetables just as younger children will. However, research done at schools in California shows that kids who *grow* their vegetables tend to eat them. Many California schools now offer gardens for kids to plant seeds and grow vegetables. The schools serve up the fruits of the students' labor at the cafeteria salad bar. More kids at these schools now dish up salad than before the garden experiments.

If you live in a climate that precludes gardening, include your children in meal planning, shopping, and preparation. This is a great

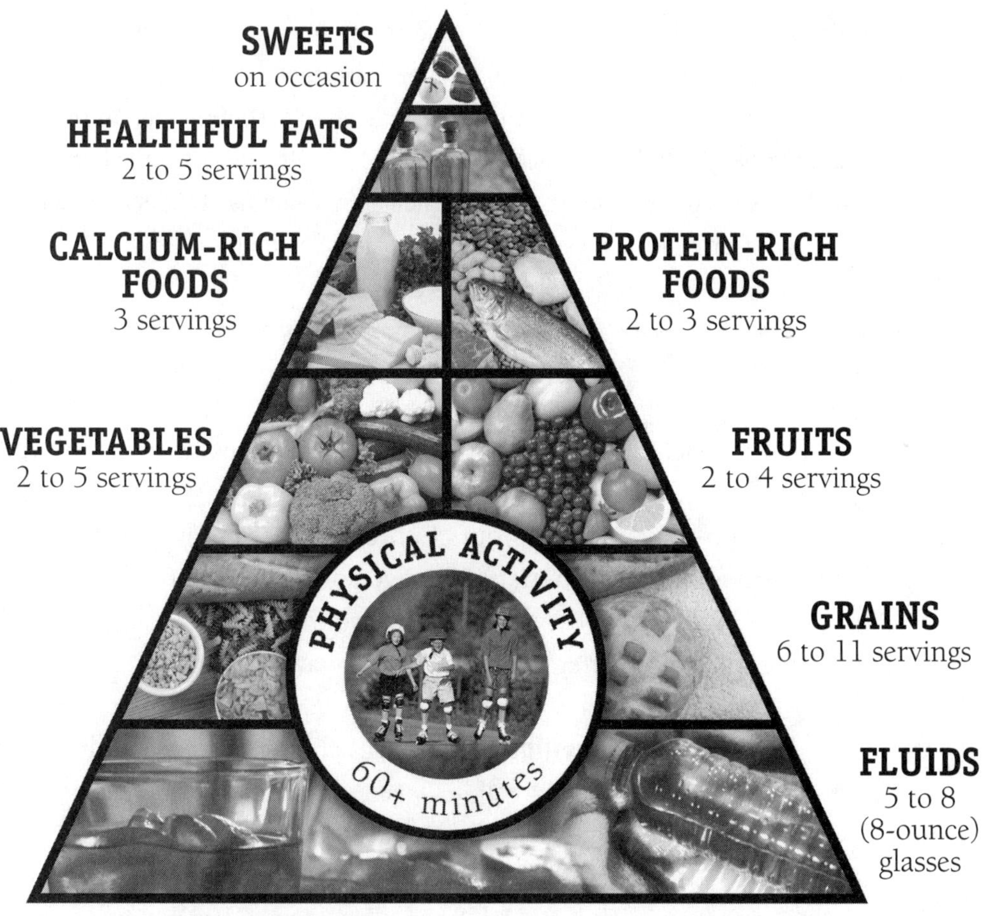

CUSTOMIZED DAILY FOOD AND ACTIVITY PYRAMID
FOR CHILDREN 9 to 12

Supersized Portions, Supersized Children

A 12-ounce soda contains roughly 150 empty calories, but few kids stop at 12 ounces.

Convenience stores and fast-food restaurants now offer up huge sodas of 20 ounces or more. Just one of these drinks contains nearly as many calories as your child eats for breakfast. The sheer magnitude of these empty calories often displaces healthful foods, particularly milk, and contributes to weight gain.

Besides out-of-control super sodas, snack foods also tend to displace healthful foods. Kids snack a lot at this age, with snack foods often accounting for 16 to 20 percent of their daily calories. You may not be able to control what your kid eats at school, but you can control what you offer at home. Serve up healthful snacks such as dried or fresh fruit, chopped vegetables, bean salads, and nuts.

age to teach kids how to cook, a skill that will come in handy when they become adults!

You can also guide your children's choices simply by talking to them about the importance of vegetables and healthful eating. The more knowledge they have about healthful eating, the more likely they'll make smarter food choices when away from home.

Fruits: 2 to 4 Servings Offer your children whole and dried fruit as snacks as often as possible. Give them berries for their cereal, apples in their lunch bags, and bananas to eat as a snack after school. Most kids can operate a blender, so whipping up a fruit smoothie (½ cup fruit juice, ½ cup lowfat vanilla yogurt, ½ banana, ½ cup frozen berries, and 3 ice cubes) makes a tasty treat.

Calcium-Rich Foods: 3 Servings Kids aged 9 to 12 rarely get as much calcium as they need, often because they tend to drink soda instead of milk. Try to get your child to drink milk during at least one meal. It's okay to flavor the milk with chocolate, as long as they drink it. Follow up with calcium-rich snacks such as flavored yogurt and string cheese.

Protein-Rich Foods: 2 to 3 Servings Begin to teach your child about saturated fat, a type of artery-clogging fat found in animal products. Shop together and pick out the leanest cuts of meat and poultry. Try to eat fish one to two times a week.

Healthful Fats: 2 to 5 Servings Stay closer to two servings if your child carries extra fat. Focus on healthful fats such as olives, olive oil, avocado, nuts, and nut butters. Nuts provide a great healthful snack your kids will eat without giving you any lip. Serve them at least once a week.

Sweets: On Occasion Your kids will find sweets to eat at school, so you don't need to offer them at home. At home, try to come up with more healthful desserts, such as chocolate-covered strawberries or nuts, or strawberry shortcake.

FIT EATING FOR TEENS

Between the pages of teen magazines, on billboard advertisements, in music videos, and on the movie screen, unnaturally skinny models, actors, and actresses paint an unrealistic picture of the ideal body—and plenty of teens are buying into the image.

Because the actors and actresses that appear on television, in movies, and in the pages of magazines are unhealthfully thin, with body sizes well below what's considered normal, teens are faced with a nearly unachievable ideal. For example, research from Brigham Young University in Provo, Utah, has found that excessive dieting and use of diet pills increase in direct correlation with the amount of time teenage girls spend reading women's beauty and fashion magazines.

Parents often unconsciously contribute to poor body image. In fact, eating disorders generally start at home, in children as young as age five. If you spent their childhood dieting and asking if certain clothes made you "look fat," you probably conditioned your teen to follow in your footsteps.

Body image used to be only a problem for teen girls. But more and more boys now exhibit signs of disordered eating. I recently counseled the parents of a rail-thin soccer player. The boy burned hundreds of calories out on the field but often refused to eat dinner when he arrived home from practice. He told them that he was dieting so he could develop a "six-pack." Yet his postpractice fast hampered his muscle recovery, and his performance on the field was slipping as a result.

To counteract poor body image and eating disorders, put the focus on healthful eating rather than on dieting and calories. Talk to your teen about the difference between healthful and unhealthful fats, for example, rather than labeling them all as "fattening." Keep your own calorie counting and dieting to yourself and refrain from any "Do I look fat?" comments.

Besides poor body image, many teens also suffer from poor food choices. Rather than eating true meals, they snack and graze all day long. They tend to receive the vast majority of their calories in the form of fast-food and minimart meals and vending machine snacks. These empty calorie foods crowd out more nutritious foods, causing mineral and vitamin deficiencies in many teens.

To encourage healthful snacking, keep ready-made snacks at home for teens to grab on their way out the door. For example, I keep sealable plastic bags filled with dried fruit, trail mix, and even a breakfast or energy bar for my teenage daughter, Natalie. She'll swipe a bag on her way out the door and snack from it between school and swim practice rather than buying cookies from a vending machine. Whole fruit left in plain view out on the counter offers a great snack option for teens to grab in the afternoon after school.

Customized Pyramid for Teens

Encourage your teen to stick to the following food groups, number of servings, and exercise prescription daily for optimal health and physical performance.

Physical Activity: 60+ Minutes If your teen plays a school sport, he or she probably gets 60 minutes a day plus a dose of bone-and-muscle-building strength training. However, if your teen doesn't play a sport, take him or her to the gym with you and explore the weight room together. Strength training will help teens, particularly girls, build and preserve strong bones that will help prevent osteoporosis later in life.

Fluids: 6 to 11 (8-Ounce) Glasses Your teen will drink soda when you're not around. It's a given. So don't put the focus on it at home, as the typical minimart large soda contains 500 calories! Instead, stock the fridge with bottled water and seltzer and encourage your teen to drink milk, even if it's chocolate flavored. Though chocolate milk contains more calories than plain milk, it contains the same amount of calcium, an extremely important mineral for this age group.

Grains: 6 to 14 Servings If your teen plays sports, he or she will need plenty of grains to fuel those active muscles. Yet most teens have trouble meeting their requirement for this food group primarily because of their sleep schedule. If you have a teenager, then you know they can sleep for as many as 12 hours at a time. Your teen may wake in the morning with just enough time to dress and race out the door to catch the bus, missing breakfast and two grain servings. Then, if your teen plays a school sport, he or she might arrive home from practice at 7 P.M. so tired that he or she heads straight to bed, skipping dinner and even more grain servings.

Encourage your teen to start the day right with grains at breakfast. Stock easy-to-grab options such as breakfast bars and whole grain bagels. Then encourage your teen to snack throughout the day on grains, trying to eat whole grain options, such as a sandwich made with whole grain bread, five to seven times during the day.

Vegetables: 3 to 6 Servings Offer these at dinner as your teen probably won't eat much in the way of vegetables during the day. Ask

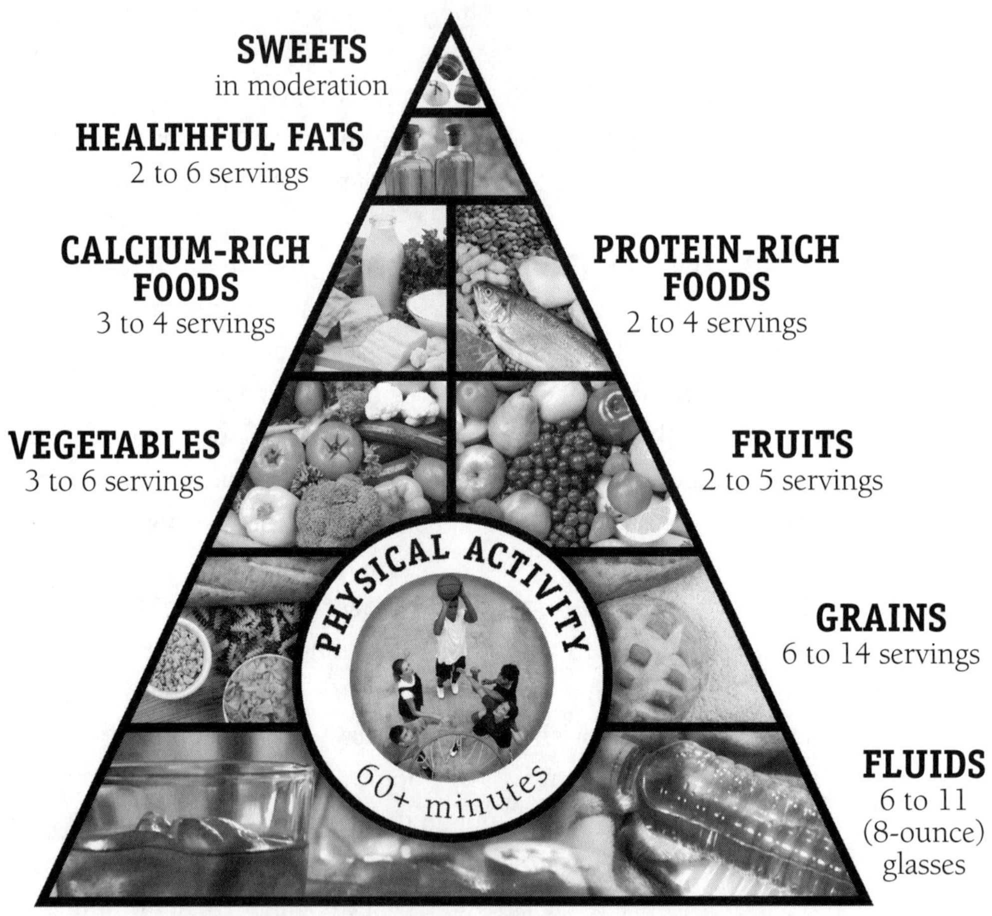

CUSTOMIZED DAILY FOOD AND ACTIVITY PYRAMID FOR TEENS

your teen to prepare the salad for dinner or to steam some broccoli or asparagus in the microwave.

Fruits: 2 to 5 Servings Put dried fruit in sealable plastic bags and offer it as a quick snack. Also, keep whole fruit, such as apples, peaches, or pears, out on the counter for easy grabbing. Fruit smoothies made with a scoop (10 to 15 grams) of soy protein powder makes a great postpractice recovery meal and a great, simple, and tasty treat.

Calcium-Rich Foods: 3 to 4 Servings Teens need more calcium than at any other time in their lives to help build strong bones. Try to get your teens to fit in as much calcium as possible by serving milk with dinner, encouraging them to drink chocolate milk instead of soda, and offering other high-calcium options such as calcium-fortified juice.

Protein-Rich Foods: 2 to 4 Servings Active teenage boys need the higher end of the protein requirement, whereas girls can usually get away with just two servings. It's hard to fit four protein servings in a day, especially if your teen equates lunch with chips and a soda. Encourage your teen to choose high-protein options at the minimart or fast-food restaurant, such as a bean burrito at Taco Bell, a plain hamburger at McDonald's, or beef jerky with chocolate milk at the 7-Eleven. When making dinner at home, try to serve up fish one to two times a week.

Healthful Fats: 2 to 6 Servings If your teen is on the chunky side, hold fats to just two servings. Emphasize healthful fats such as olives, olive oil, nuts, nut butters, and avocado. Teach your teen about artery-clogging saturated fats, found in animal products such as whole milk and fatty cuts of meat, as well as unhealthful hydrogenated fats, found in fried and processed foods.

Sweets: In Moderation For other age groups, I recommend only eating sweets "on occasion," yet teens, particularly teenage girls, will often eat sweets every day. It's a given. For optimal health, however, sweets should account for no more than 10 percent of their daily calories (about 200 calories). But for most teens, sweets make up 20 percent or more of their diets. Rein them in by offering sweets only rarely at home, but don't expect them to give up sweets for Lent.

FIT EATING FOR YOUR 20s

My son, Grant, recently left for college at California State University in Chico, 2 hours away. Two days after settling in to apartment life, Grant called me. He asked, "Mom, when I go grocery shopping, what am I supposed to do?"

I told him somewhat incredulously, "When you go to the grocery store, you buy food to eat." After talking a few more minutes, I understood his predicament. He didn't know what foods he should be eating or how to pick them out.

Perhaps you are facing the same challenges.

During your 20s you move out of your childhood home or college dorm and begin to fend for yourself, often for the first time. Suddenly you begin to appreciate mom and dad more than ever, missing that magical thing called "cooking" that they used to do for you. When faced with this sink-or-swim time period, many of those in their 20s sink like a dead weight. Rather than learn the basic strokes of healthful eating by planning meals, shopping for ingredients, and cooking, many people in their 20s instead survive on restaurant meals, snack foods, and frozen dinners.

This eating-out lifestyle tends to pile on extra calories, calories that generally don't get burned off during the typical 8-hour-a-day desk job.

To fight off first-job "seat-itis" (extra fat accumulated from sitting down all day long), you must practice portion control when eating out. For example, ask the waiter to put half of your order in a to-go box before even bringing it to the table. Then eat your leftovers the next day for lunch.

Also teach yourself the basics of food shopping and cooking in baby steps. You might aim for one at-home dinner a week and then eventually work your way up to two or three. To help pick out the best foods for those dinners, you'll find tips under each rung of your customized pyramid.

Customized Pyramid for Your 20s

Stick to the following food groups, recommended servings, and exercise prescription for optimal weight, health, and physical performance.

Physical Activity: 30 to 60 Minutes During high school and college, you naturally accumulated activity simply from walking from one class to another. But once you take on your first desk job, your calorie burning plummets. So work in 30 to 60 minutes of some form of aerobic exercise most days of the week.

Also, starting at age 20, most people begin to lose muscle mass, at the rate of ½ to up to 2 pounds of muscle for each decade of life. This loss of muscle slows your metabolism, causing you to gain even more weight. However, you can easily reverse muscle loss by strength training two to three times a week.

Fluids: 6 to 10 (8-Ounce) Glasses Stock your refrigerator with bottled waters, sports drinks, and 100 percent fruit or vegetable juice, such as orange, tangerine, grapefruit, prune, or tomato juice. Look for real fruit juice boosted with added calcium or antioxidants if you're falling short on meeting calcium needs or skimping on your fruits and veggies.

Grains: 6 to 11 Servings Grains supply the energy that fuels your workouts and, if you choose the right types, can also help you prevent disease. Opt for whole grain breads and bagels made from sourdough, wheat, rye, and oats. Use these for quick sandwiches for lunch or even for dinner. But be careful, as many breads claim to be "whole wheat" but really aren't. Always check the Nutrition Facts label to make sure the bread contains 3 grams of fiber per serving.

For breakfast, buy whole grain cereals that provide 5 grams or more of fiber per serving (such as Raisin Bran or 9-grain hot cereal). For dinner, opt for instant, boil-in-a-bag brown rice rather than those packaged pasta concoctions, most of which contain more than 5 grams of fat per serving.

Vegetables: 3 to 5 Servings Vegetables are naturally low in calories, so they'll help you keep off creeping weight. Spinach provides a wonderfully versatile and healthful option as you can purchase a resealable package and pull out a handful to stick on pizzas, add to sandwiches, and even mix into scrambled eggs. In addition to spinach, also purchase resealable packaged spring salad mix for fast-fix salads. It will last more than a week in the fridge.

Fruits: 2 to 4 Servings Dried and fresh fruits provide great healthful snacks. Go for variety and color. Buy Fuji apples to grab on your way to work. Buy red grapes for easy snacking at home. And always stock up on berries—blueberries, raspberries, strawberries—for easy healthful additions to breakfast cereal and yogurt.

Calcium-Rich Foods: 2 to 3 Servings To meet your requirement, look for fat-free or reduced-fat milk, yogurt, buttermilk, and, my favorite, chocolate milk. Try single-serve drinkable yogurt, which makes a great "take-along" snack that packs a good dose of protein, calcium, vitamin B_{12}, and riboflavin. Just steer clear of full-fat cheeses like cheddar and Monterey Jack, which are loaded with artery-clogging saturated fat.

Protein-Rich Foods: 3 Servings Try to eat fish one to two times a week. It's the easiest meal you'll ever make and couldn't be better for your health. Just stick a fillet in a frying pan and cook for 3 minutes on each side, or broil a fillet or steak in the oven for 7 to 10 minutes per inch of thickness. Microwaving a salmon fillet topped with olives and marinara sauce also makes a quick fish meal. Look for premarinated

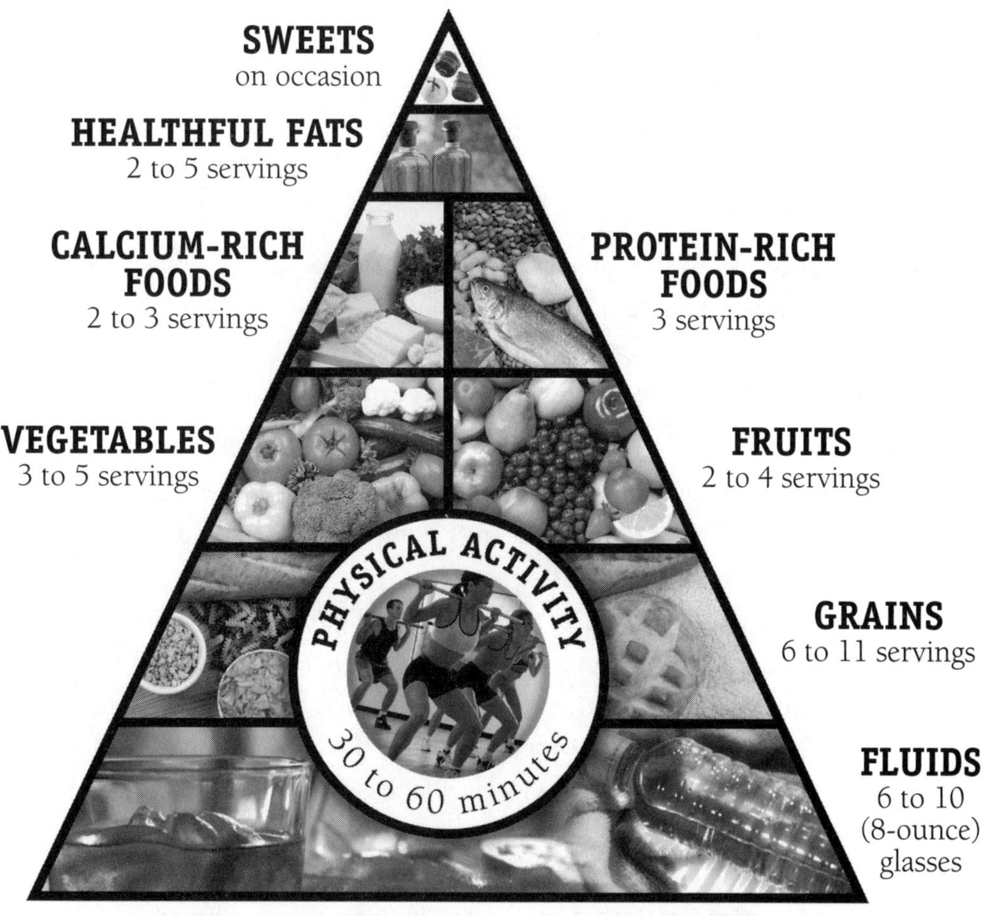

CUSTOMIZED DAILY FOOD AND ACTIVITY PYRAMID
FOR YOUR 20s

Pile Up Your Frozen Assets

Many of those in their 20s equate frozen food with TV dinners. Yet the frozen food aisle at your local supermarket offers many quick-and-easy meal choices that are also easy on your waistline and heavy on solid nutrition. Good options include:

- Frozen dinner entrées with less than 8 grams of fat per 300 calories, such as stuffed peppers, three-bean chili, herb-roasted chicken, beef portobello, and chicken in peanut sauce.
- Veggie burgers made with soy.
- Rice bowls such as Szechuan style with edamame (whole soybean).
- Frozen meal starters that contain an assortment of vegetables for you to stir-fry with chicken, tofu, lean ground beef, or fish.

fish such as salmon or catfish, along with chicken or other meats, that make a quick meal on the grill along with veggies and grains.

Healthful Fats: 2 to 5 Servings Optimize your consumption of monounsaturated fats from olive oil, olives, avocado, nuts, and nut butters, and minimize your consumption of saturated fats from animal products (butter, full-fat dairy, fatty meats) as well as hydrogenated fats from processed foods (fried foods, snack crackers and chips, most bakery treats).

Sweets: On Occasion If you have a sweet tooth and find that you can't stop at just one, buy prepackaged sweets that provide automatic portion control. For example, rather than eat ice cream out of the container, try a mini ice cream sandwich. Instead of an entire chocolate bar, try a small truffle or a Hershey or Dove miniature.

FIT EATING FOR YOUR 30s

On your 13th birthday, you celebrate becoming an official teenager. On your 16th birthday, you celebrate turning your legal driving age. At 18, you become a voter, and at 21, a legal drinker.

Though age 30 certainly pales in comparison to these other milestones, it marks the day when most people leave behind the irreverent, carefree days of youth. For example, financial planners encourage you at age 30 to start putting the maximum into your 401(k) to save for retirement. I'd like to add another milestone to turning 30. The end of your 20s and the beginning of your 30s marks a time when you should begin investing in your health.

During our teens and 20s, many of us felt invincible, often too invincible to focus on getting enough calcium or vegetables. Yet during our 30s, most of us realize that invincibility is just a cruel myth.

In order to live healthy, strong, and happy into old age, you must maximize your consumption of healthful foods—starting now. It's time to wave good-bye to those carefree days of your 20s when you ate out every night. You need to plan nutritious meals and figure out that thing called "cooking."

Take one of your days off from work and turn it into your meal-planning day. Flip through magazines and cookbooks. You might even treat yourself to an hour with the Food Network. Do anything that will inspire you to cook. Then figure out five meals for the week. You don't have to create five time-intensive gourmet meals, but you should include a source of protein, one to two servings of fruits or vegetables, and a whole grain. For example, a red pepper and spinach omelet served with whole grain toast and sliced fruit for dessert counts as a quick-and-easy, nutritious dinner.

If you have kids, take some of the stress off yourself by planning just one dinner a night—not two. You already have enough on your plate—literally and figuratively—without having to also serve as a short-order cook. Expecting your children to eat the same foods you eat will not only save time, it will also help you raise less picky eaters. An added bonus: You'll eliminate some weight gain because you'll no longer swallow the remnants of your kids' hot dogs or macaroni and cheese.

Customized Pyramid for Your 30s

Stick to the following food groups, recommended servings, and exercise prescription for optimal weight, health, and physical performance.

Physical Activity: 30 to 60 Minutes Try to move for at least 30 to 60 minutes on most days, including strength training two to three times a week. If you have kids, you can multitask by including them in your fitness routine. Push your kids in a jog stroller as you walk or jog. Or play tag with them for at least ½ hour or more.

Fluids: 4 to 10 (8-Ounce) Glasses Choose low-calorie beverages such as iced tea and bottled water and drink up. The extra fluid will help to delay feelings of hunger. Monitor your consumption of alcohol, as these beverages contain a lot of calories and tend to lower your willpower. Your original plan of meeting a coworker for one beer after quitting time can easily turn into two or three drinks over a plate of nachos or cheese fries.

Grains: 6 to 12 Servings When planning meals, think of grains as the vehicle that transports vegetable and protein servings into your body. Mix spinach, peas, and corn into brown rice, for example, or make whole wheat pizza dough and top it with peppers, spinach, onions, garlic, broccoli, tomato sauce, and soy pepperoni. Or cook up some whole wheat pasta and toss it with a red sauce packed with eggplant, onions, garlic, and peppers.

Vegetables: 3 to 5 Servings Vegetables provide your best defense against aging. Also, should you decide to have a baby, the high amounts of folate in most vegetables will help prevent birth defects. Snack on raw veggies, such as cauliflower or carrots. Sneak leafy greens into sandwiches or add them into stir-fries, soup, or scrambled eggs. Keep frozen vegetables on hand at all times and add them to just about every dish. Use bagged lettuce for quick-and-easy salads.

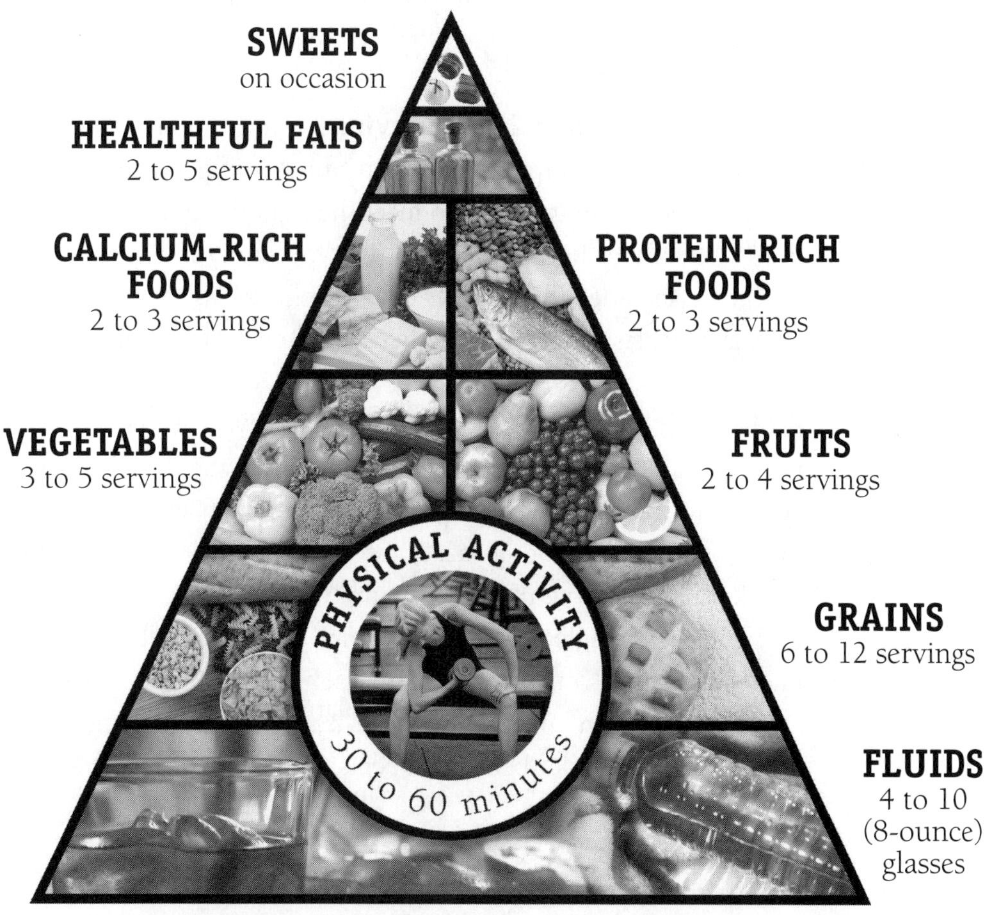

CUSTOMIZED DAILY FOOD AND ACTIVITY PYRAMID
FOR YOUR 30s

Fruits: 2 to 4 Servings In addition to fighting disease, fruits like strawberries, apricots, and cantaloupe ooze with a bounty of vitamins, especially vitamin C, and an array of antioxidants including flavonoids and carotenes, which help protect your muscles from oxidative damage caused by heavy workouts. Preliminary research also shows that certain flavonoids found in fruit like oranges and berries help protect the skin from the damaging impact of UV light. Reach for variety—the more colorful your selection, the greater the array of antioxidants.

Calcium-Rich Foods: 2 to 3 Servings Your number of calcium servings pales in comparison to your number of grain servings. Yet many people are more likely to meet their grain requirement. If you don't like milk or have discovered that your body can't easily digest its lactose, include other sources of calcium, such as calcium-fortified juice at breakfast or even a Viactiv calcium chew as a midday snack.

Protein-Rich Foods: 2 to 3 Servings If you're pregnant, you need an additional protein serving to help fuel the development of your child. Focus on quality protein sources such as soy, eggs, lean meats, fish, poultry, and beans. Though meats such as beef and poultry offer quality protein as well as important vitamins and minerals for your exercising body, they also come with artery-clogging saturated fat. Cut back on as much of this fat as possible by removing the skin from chicken and buying extra-lean ground beef and sirloin steak instead of fattier beef cuts such as T-bone and regular ground beef or chuck.

Healthful Fats: 2 to 5 Servings Stick to two servings if you are watching your weight and go up to five if you're very active and lean. Choose healthful fats such as olives, olive oil, avocado, nuts, and nut butters over saturated fats found in butter and animal products and trans fats found in processed foods.

Eating for Pregnancy and Lactation

Your nutrient needs go up when you get pregnant and during breast-feeding. Theoretically, you can probably get all of these nutrients from food, but few women do.

Let's face it—few of us eat perfectly all the time. That's where prenatal vitamins come in.

The three most important nutrients for pregnancy are iron, folate, and vitamin B_{12}. Folate and B_{12} are both used in gene replication, which goes on at a very high rate during the first few months of pregnancy, when you might not even know you're pregnant. Also, doctors are now learning that some women may have a higher need for folate than once thought, putting their babies at a higher risk of neural birth defects.

When you start trying to conceive, begin taking a prenatal vitamin that contains 400 to 600 milligrams of folate and 100 percent of the DV for B_{12} and iron.

Despite popular belief, your calcium needs won't increase during pregnancy, because your body absorbs more of it automatically from your diet. Just make sure to drink a vitamin D–fortified product such as milk to ensure your body absorbs plenty of this mineral.

Finally, both pregnancy and breast-feeding increase your need for fluids. During pregnancy, your kidneys are working overtime to filter not only your wastes but also the wastes of your growing fetus. You need plenty of fluids to dilute those wastes and ease the job on your kidneys. During lactation, you can lose up to 1 quart of fluid in breast milk production each day. Drink at least 8 to 15 glasses of water a day to ensure proper hydration during breast-feeding.

Sweets: On Occasion Many supermoms and superdads feel they need to make dessert every night in order to be "good" parents. You don't. In fact, you shouldn't. Not only will this strategy create undue stress for you, it will pad the waistlines of everyone in the family. Hold dessert to just once or twice a week, and offer more healthful options such as berries with frozen yogurt.

FIT EATING FOR YOUR 40s AND 50s

I'm living proof that your metabolism doesn't *have* to come to a screeching halt at midlife.

The average person experiences a 2 to 3 percent drop in metabolic rate for every decade after age 20. Each 1 percent drop roughly equals 15 fewer burned calories per day. You must either cut those calories from your diet or add them to your exercise regimen if you want to keep off creeping weight.

For many years, scientists had thought that this metabolism drop was largely beyond our control. They knew that most people lost an average of 1 to 2 pounds of muscle during each decade of life. Because every pound of muscle burns between 35 and 50 calories a day, researchers thought some of this metabolism slowdown could be reversed with strength training. However, they also thought that part of the drop was simply that—a drop that you could do little about.

I went right along with this theory until recently when I toured the exhibitors area at an international sports medicine conference. One of the exhibitors was showcasing a new, fairly simple device that measured resting metabolic rate.

Both my good friend Kris Clark, age 48, and I, age 45, decided to give it a try. Kris sat down in the chair, put the mask over her face, and a few minutes later learned that she burned 1,470 calories a day just by breathing, digesting, and living. That was 14 percent above the norm for her age and roughly what's considered normal for a woman in her 20s.

I sat down in the chair, put the mask over my face, and amazed everyone in the room when the machine calculated that my *resting* rate was 2,100 calories, 70 percent above my norm and the amount that a 16-year-old boy probably burns during his sleep.

Both Kris and I exercise regularly. I strength train a bit more consistently than Kris, and the efforts showed up in my metabolic rate. Kris and I are living proof that your metabolism doesn't have to slow with age, providing you feed it with enough exercise to keep it running.

Most people, however, don't. Our sedentary lifestyles tend to cause a large drop in muscle mass over time. The more muscle you lose, the more your metabolism slows. If exercise isn't a priority for you, you'll need to cut back on what you eat in order to hold off excess fat.

If you exercise less than an hour a day, pay close attention to portion control during meals. For a week, use measuring cups and spoons to dole out your foods. This will help provide an accurate picture of what ½ cup of pasta or a serving of cereal looks like. You'll probably be surprised to learn that you generally eat much more than a recommended serving—eating much more than the number of grain, protein, or fat servings you're supposed to consume in a day.

Customized Pyramid for Your 40s and 50s

Stick to the following food groups, recommended servings, and exercise prescription for optimal weight, health, and physical performance.

Physical Activity: 30 to 60 Minutes Thirty daily minutes of cardiovascular exercise will boost your health and prevent disease. However, if you want to keep off creeping weight, increase your exercise duration to 60 to 90 minutes. You can accumulate some of that time by incorporating more walking into your day. Try walking to work, taking frequent walk breaks while at work, and so on. In addition to aerobic exercise, build metabolism-boosting muscle by strength training two to three times a week.

Fluids: 4 to 10 (8-Ounce) Glasses If you're highly active and live in a hot climate (and therefore sweat a lot), you'll need closer to 10 glasses a day. If you live in a cold climate, sweat little, and weigh little, you probably only need four glasses. Monitor your urine to make sure you are well hydrated. You should empty four full bladders of pale yellow urine a day.

To help prevent weight gain, cut back on your consumption of liquid calories. Alcohol is a big gut buster. So are sodas. Opt for lower- or no-calorie beverages such as club soda with a hint of fruit juice instead.

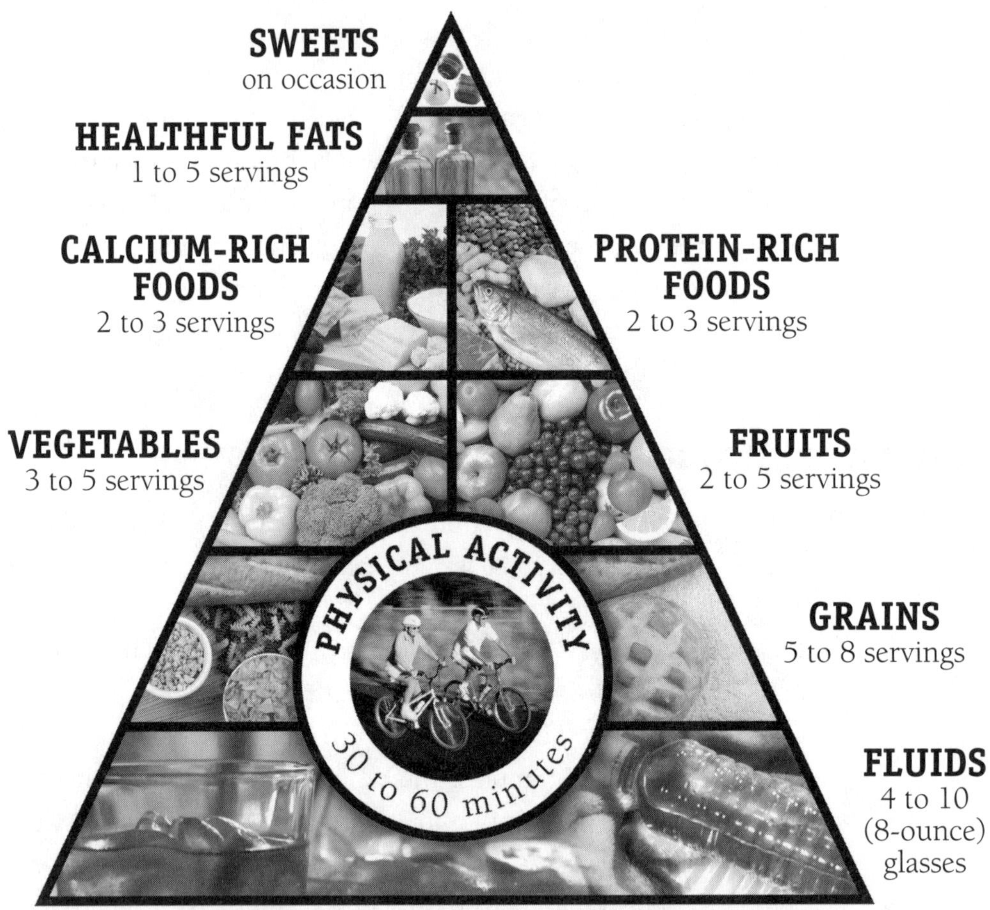

CUSTOMIZED DAILY FOOD AND ACTIVITY PYRAMID
FOR YOUR 40s AND 50s

Grains: 5 to 8 Servings Until your 40s, grains provide the bulk of your diet, followed by fruits and vegetables. But to cut calories and maximize nutrients for disease prevention, that changes during your 40s and 50s.

Try to make most of your grain servings come from whole grains such as whole wheat bread or brown rice. Avoid processed "grains" such as crackers, as these usually contain small amounts of hydrogenated fats, a dangerous type of fat thought to clog arteries and increase cancer risk. These snack foods also offer little in the way of fiber or nutrients.

Finally, carefully measure your grains, as many people eat much more than they realize.

Vegetables: 3 to 5 Servings Not only are vegetables low in calories and packed with appetite-suppressing fiber, they also provide your best weapon against age-related disease. If you're a woman, your estrogen levels will begin to drop during your 40s and 50s, putting you at a greater risk for weakened bones, heart disease, high blood pressure, and diabetes. Men commonly gain their guts during these years, which puts them at a greater risk for high blood pressure, diabetes, heart disease, and some cancers.

Boosting your vegetable intake will help prevent all of those diseases as well as provide the potassium your body needs to combat a jump in blood pressure from the typical American high-sodium diet.

Fruits: 2 to 5 Servings Like vegetables, brightly colored fruits contain a wealth of nutrients that will help prevent disease. Yet each type of fruit offers different types of disease-fighting nutrients, so variety is key. Try to expand beyond your fruit staples of apples and bananas. Try a new brightly colored fruit every week for optimal disease protection.

Calcium-Rich Foods: 2 to 3 Servings Calcium will help keep blood pressure low and bones strong. Calcium may even help to prevent middle-aged spread, as recent research shows that it boosts

Gut Control

You don't gain a gut overnight—although it may seem like it when you suddenly notice that it's there. Overeating by a mere 10 calories a day will add a pound of fat to your body over a year's time. Many people overeat by much more than that, to the tune of 100 extra calories, padding their frames by 10 pounds a year. Heaping servings of grains, sweets, and other foods easily add on 100 or more calories daily, so know how much you put on your plate!

fat burning and hinders fat storage. Opt for lowfat or nonfat options, such as 1 percent or fat-free milk or nonfat yogurt, to cut back on artery-clogging saturated fat.

Protein-Rich Foods: 2 to 3 Servings Put the focus on beans and fish for optimal heart disease and cancer prevention. Fish contains an important fat called *omega-3 fatty acid,* which has been shown to help prevent heart disease, cancer, and even joint pain, so try to eat fish at least two times a week. Beans—a great source of soluble fiber—will also help keep cholesterol levels in check as well as keep you regular, important in preventing colon cancer.

Healthful Fats: 1 to 5 Servings Aim for the low end of this recommendation if you're watching your weight. Focus on healthful fats from nuts, olives, olive oil, and avocado. Try to eat nuts five times a week to maximize heart disease and cancer prevention.

Sweets: On Occasion If your exercise habits coupled with portion control are keeping you slim and trim, go ahead and splurge on 200 or fewer dessert calories a day. If you're watching your weight, eat these only on occasion.

FIT EATING AT 60-PLUS

By the time you enter your 60s, your calorie needs have come full circle.

You began life requiring few calories but a high amount of nutrients to fuel your growing body. As your body grew into your teens and 20s, you needed comparatively more calories and fewer nutrients. However, the sedentary nature of American life coupled with a natural drop in metabolic rate means that you'll need fewer and fewer calories for every coming decade after age 20 if you want to fend off weight gain.

By the time you enter your 60s, your metabolism may be running 10 to 15 percent slower than it did during your 20s, and with sagging activity levels, this translates roughly into 500 to more than 1,000 fewer burned calories a day. The end result: You may need to cut back to a meager 1,000 daily calories to hold off creeping weight.

At the same time, you must maximize your consumption of disease-fighting vitamins, minerals, fiber, and phytochemicals to strengthen your chances of living to a ripe old age with vigor and maximum quality of life. To fit all the vitamins, minerals, fiber, phytonutrients, carbohydrate, protein, and healthful fats you need into 1,000 to 1,400 calories, you must make every meal count by eating the most nutritious foods from each category on your customized pyramid.

Customized Pyramid for Your 60s and Beyond

Stick to the following food groups, recommended servings, and exercise prescription for optimal weight, health, and physical performance.

Physical Activity: 30 to 60 Minutes Include strength training two to three times a week. Strength training will help preserve bone mass and muscle mass. Studies show that 70- and 80-year-olds who start a strength training program can rebuild lost muscle, trading in their spindly chicken legs for the shapelier legs of their youth—so it's never too late! This extra muscle will help to boost your metabolism, allowing you to consume more food without gaining weight.

Fluids: 4 to 10 (8-Ounce) Glasses As you age, your thirst mechanism falters, neglecting to trigger you to drink when you're dehydrated. That's one reason why older people experience more health problems in the heat—they're usually dehydrated, which hinders the body's ability to cool itself. So count off your fluid servings each day and monitor your urine. You should empty four full bladders a day of pale yellow urine.

Start your morning with a glass of water. After 8 hours of sleep, you're dehydrated. You need the water. Then follow up with a water break every 45 minutes to an hour.

Because you need so few calories, opt for low-calorie beverages such as water, herbal or regular iced teas, or even diluted sports drinks. To jazz up water, try sparkling water with a small shot of lemon or lime juice.

Grains: 4 to 6 Servings Make every single one of your grain servings count. Try to eliminate refined grains such as white rice or pasta or bread made from white flour as well as sugary, fiberless breakfast cereals. Processing removes the outer shell of these grains, refining away the fiber, vitamins, protein, and overall goodness.

Instead, opt for whole grains all the time. Besides an array of disease-fighting phytonutrients, whole grains contain healthful fats, protein, and fiber. The fiber in particular helps move waste through your intestines, preventing colon cancer. Start your day with a fortified breakfast cereal that contains at least 5 grams of fiber, such as Multibran Chex or Kashi Go Lean. Follow up with whole grains at lunch and dinner, such as brown rice, barley, whole wheat berries (kernel), quinoa, millet, wild rice, and amaranth.

Vegetables: 3 to 5 Servings This is the only food group on your pyramid where you can go beyond the upper limit and not see the effects on your waistline, as most vegetables contain a mere 25 calories per serving. Though vegetables offer very few calories, they contain a wealth of disease-fighting nutrients. For example, you can get your entire day's worth of vitamin C in just one serving of chopped red pepper. Gravitate toward brightly colored vegetables such as dark leafy greens, as these tend to contain the most nutrients.

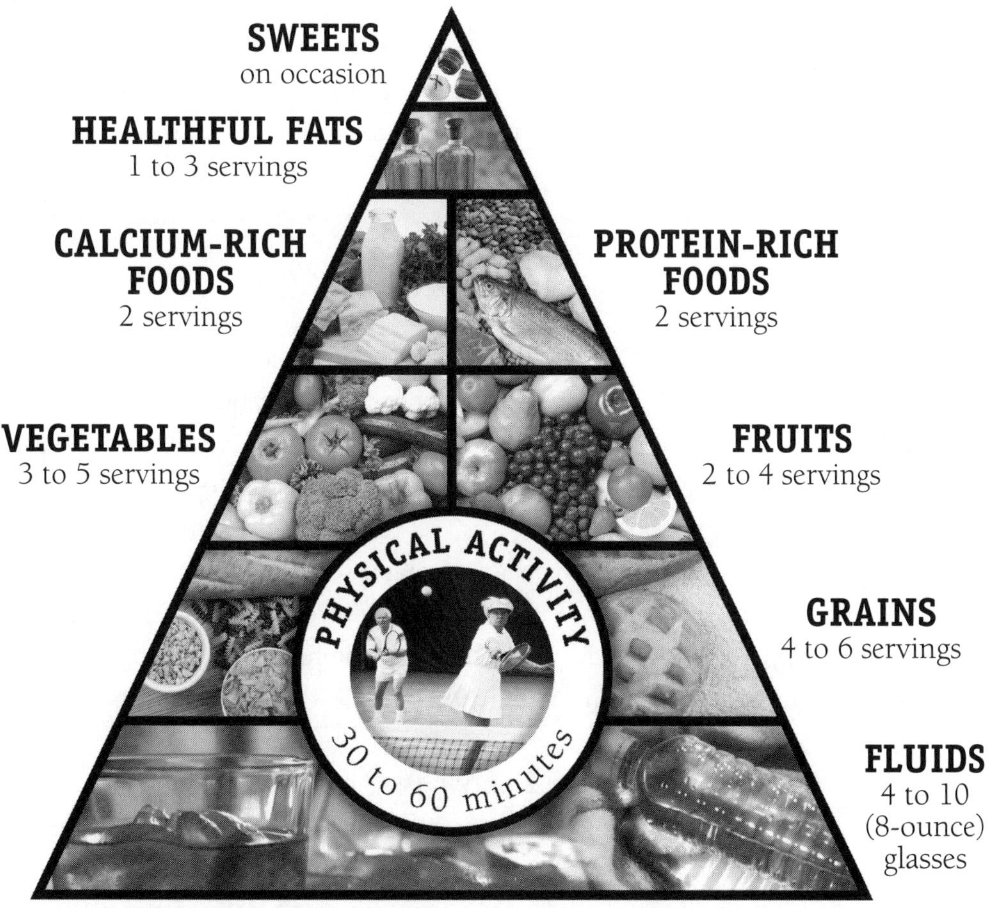

CUSTOMIZED DAILY FOOD AND ACTIVITY PYRAMID
FOR YOUR 60s AND BEYOND

Supplemental Insurance

As you age, you need more calcium, vitamin D, and vitamin B_{12}, and few of those aged 60-plus receive all they need from food. Lower-calorie diets often don't leave enough room for 1,200 to 1,500 milligrams of calcium (the equivalent of four to five glasses of milk), and your body absorbs less B_{12} and manufactures less vitamin D with age.

Try to get at least half of your calcium requirement from food, allowing a separate 500 to 1,000 milligram supplement to make up any shortfall. Follow up with a multivitamin that contains 100 percent of the DV for vitamins D and B_{12}.

Fruits: 2 to 4 Servings Along with vegetables, brightly colored fruits such as blueberries, strawberries, mango, pineapple, and apples help to prevent heart disease, cancer, and other age-related diseases.

Though fruit is certainly not a high-calorie food, many are not low-calorie foods either.

For example, one banana contains roughly 100 calories. Compare that to an entire red pepper at 20 calories, and you can easily see which is the true diet food. If you're watching your weight, stick with just two servings from this food group.

Calcium-Rich Foods: 2 Servings You need calcium for your aging bones, but you don't need the saturated fat or calories that come with it. Opt for fat-free milk, nonfat yogurt, or nonfat, calcium-fortified soy or rice milk. Be careful with cheese, as even the lower-fat varieties generally add quite a big calorie wallop.

Protein-Rich Foods: 2 Servings Opt for broiled fish at least twice a week, as it contains healing fats and generally fewer calories than meat. Beans, soy foods, and eggs also offer high-quality protein for few calories. When you opt for red meat, watch your portion size and choose lean cuts. Your 3-ounce serving (the size of a deck of cards) is much smaller than the typical steak or burger. Opt for sirloin and chop it up for fajitas or other dishes to make the small amount seem larger.

Healthful Fats: 1 to 3 Servings Hold yourself to the low end if you're watching your weight. Try to make all of your fats come from the healthful end of the fat spectrum, focusing on nuts, nut butters, olives, olive oil, avocado, canola oil, and flaxseed meal or oil. Try to eat nuts three to five times a week, as this fat source is extremely good for your heart.

Sweets: On Occasion Opt for the lowest-fat, lowest-calorie options, such as fruit Popsicles or sorbet. Consider combining your "sweet" with a healthful food. For example, try drizzling chocolate syrup on top of fruit.

Part IV

PERFORMING AT YOUR PEAK

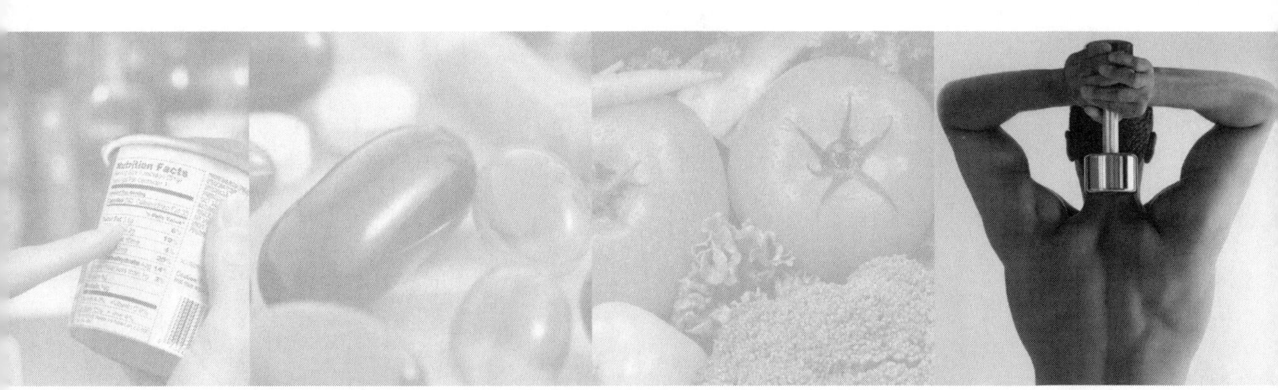

AEROBICS

Tips to help you dance, kick, punch, and march with more pep.

Aerobics classes have come a long way since the days of the Jane Fonda leg lifts. Today numerous different types of classes exist, opening up aerobics classes to women and men of all shapes, ages, sizes, and fitness backgrounds.

If you lack the coordination for the choreographed moves of a dance aerobics class, you might enjoy a kickboxing class with its standard series of kicks and punches. If you need something fun to motivate you to work out, you might enjoy African dance and other contemporary-themed classes. If you feel as if only a drill sergeant could get you to give it your all, you can enroll in a boot-camp-style class.

Whether you do step aerobics, take kickboxing classes, do organized African dance, or take some other recent incarnation of the original Jane Fonda type aerobics class, you can increase your calorie burning and class enjoyment by paying careful attention to performance nutrition.

I've found that many women who take these classes, however, somehow don't consider them an athletic workout. Yes, they look to these classes as a way to burn calories, as a way to condition their heart and lungs, and as a way to tone their muscles. But they also see them as a social outing, and they rarely watch what they eat before and after class.

I've done just about all the different types of aerobics style workouts at one time or another, and I've seen what happens firsthand when people don't eat the right type of foods before class. They merely go through the motions.

The instructor yells for them to kick, and they barely lift their leg. The instructor says to march in place, and they look as if they are trudging through mud. The instructor says to shimmy their hips, and they respond with a halfhearted twist. The instructor says to drop and give him 10 push-ups, and they go in slow motion, completing about two when the rest of the class has banged out 10.

Yet these very same people are the ones who will congratulate the instructor for creating such a great workout. Even though they burned so few calories during their halfhearted attempt at working out, they feel just as fatigued as if they had given their all.

So my very first tip for better aerobics performance is this: Take eating seriously. You can burn a heck of a lot of calories during your class—or hardly any—depending on your energy level when you show up. Here are some ways to keep energy levels high:

Snack. Two to three hours before your class, eat a small snack that contains about 50 to 75 grams of carbohydrate, particularly if you will head to class straight from work. This snack will top off the fuel tanks in your muscles and stabilize blood sugar levels, helping to energize your muscles and brain for your workout. Good midafternoon snacks include a handful of dried apricots and a cup of sports drink, four whole grain crackers spread with 2 tablespoons of jam, or one energy bar and ½ cup cranberry juice.

Bring a water bottle to class. The room may not feel hot when you first show up, but start bouncing around and you'll begin to lose a lot of fluids through sweat. If you do your workout early in the morning or just after work, you're probably already dehydrated when you show up. After your nighttime fluid fast, you wake up dehydrated. After a long day of breathing in dry office air, you're probably also dehydrated.

During class, this dehydration will make your head feel like an expanding, hot balloon. It can also lead to an exercise-induced headache, particularly with all of the jumping around. Dehydration allows your blood to thicken, preventing it from transporting nutrients as easily to your brain and muscles. End result: fatigue.

Try to drink a glass of water ½ hour before class and then follow up by taking sporadic sips from your water bottle during class. Not all instructors will give you a water break, allowing you to run to a nearby fountain for a sip. If your instructor tends to go all-out for the entire time, you may have to insert your own water breaks. Dance over to your water bottle and march in place as you drink. Try to take frequent breaks with small sips. The consistent smaller sips will also help you to jump without feeling a splashing sensation in your stomach.

Consider a sports drink. If you head to aerobics class just after rolling out of bed (or do an aerobics video first thing in the morning), you won't have time to fuel up with a snack. So do the next best thing: Consume calories as you work out. Rather than water, consume a sports drink during your workout. And don't worry about the calories from the sports drink counteracting your calorie burn. An entire 16-ounce sports drink contains only 120 calories. Those calories will add spunk to your workout, helping you to work off many more extra calories as a result.

Know the safety considerations. Some types of aerobics classes such as kickboxing can easily lead to injury if done incorrectly because these classes involve quick movements. If you're taking a new class and don't know the moves, do them slowly with care. Don't hold hand weights, and listen carefully to the teacher's instructions about proper form. In general, you should never lock or snap your joints when punching, kicking, or otherwise extending your limbs. You may need to exercise at a lower intensity during your first couple classes before you'll get the hang of proper form. However, a couple classes with a lower-than-usual calorie burn will be well worth it down the road when you can continue to exercise at a high intensity without discomfort.

Gravitate toward an instructor with similar musical tastes. Researchers have long searched for the ideal workout music to fuel motivation. However, they've found that no one type of music motivates every fitness enthusiast to work out at a higher intensity. Rather, the best type of music for you is the music that you personally find inspiring. If you feel the urge to move when you hear hip-hop, you may not perform at your best at a class that blasts oldies tunes. If you love eighties music, then you may trudge through a workout with New Age

Your Preseason Program

You can take aerobics classes year-round, so there's truly no "off-season." However, you can still train your body to perform better during these classes and reduce your injury risk with the following drill. Because many of these classes, particularly kick-boxing and boot-camp-style ones involve a series of quick movements, you'll benefit from a training program that helps you to hone your reaction time. The faster your reaction time, the faster you'll drop and give the instructor 10 push-ups when prompted.

You can boost your reaction time by trying this drill with a partner. Stand and hold a large fitness ball in front of your body at torso level. Ask your partner to stand facing you and to whack your fitness ball with an open palm from various directions. This sounds simple, but you'll find that you must work numerous abdominal muscles—as well as your brain—to continue to hold on to the ball as your partner comes at it from all directions.

Once you get the hang of this drill, increase the difficulty by trying it with your eyes closed. You can also try other drills by asking a partner or two to toss large fitness balls or small heavy balls at you from all directions. Make sure to do this in a large room or outside—you don't want to break anything.

punk. If you exercise at a gym, make a habit of asking the instructors about the type of music they tend to play during their workouts. Then choose the teacher who plays the music you like the most.

AMENORRHEA

When you lose your period, your bones and your heart weaken.

When many female athletes stop menstruating, they smile and happily say good-bye to their periods. The lack of menstruation allows them to train harder without the distraction of cramps and other menstrual symptoms.

Yet lack of menstruation is nothing to smile about. When menstruation stops, it means that a host of hormones, including the female hormone estrogen, are low. Besides stopping your period, depressed levels of estrogen also results in bone mineral loss or premature osteoporosis. You also need estrogen to help prevent cholesterol from building up along the lining of your arteries.

Studies show that young women with amenorrhea experience the weakened bones and diseased arteries of women two to three times their age. This results in serious and chronic stress fractures, including fractures of vertebrae similar to those seen in 80-year-old women.

Worse, if amenorrhea lasts long enough, these changes become irreversible. Some studies show that as many as four years after regular periods return, bone mass continues to be low in women who once had amenorrhea.

Menstruation 101

An estimated 25 to 40 percent of female endurance athletes report trouble with menstruation. An even larger percentage of athletes experience problems with ovulation. In other words, they menstruate regularly but don't release eggs.

In almost all cases, amenorrhea is a result of misguided dieting, not a direct result of exercise. Often, women dramatically increase their amount of exercise without simultaneously increasing calorie intake. For example, a well-designed study on monkeys done at the University of Pittsburgh found that increasing the amount of exercise without increasing calorie intake encourages the body to slow the metabolism. In other words, the body goes into starvation mode, slowing the metabolism to hold on to fat stores. This causes an athlete to burn fewer calories during sleep than a sedentary person.

In the University of Pittsburgh study, thyroid hormone (responsible for regulating metabolism) dropped by 20 percent, enough to suppress ovulation. Another study, this one from Beth Israel Deaconess Medical Center in Boston, found that when calorie levels or stores are low, the body also responds with low blood leptin levels. Leptin is the hormone that became famous a number of years ago when researchers linked abnormal leptin levels to obesity. Leptin is responsible for telling your brain that fat stores are adequate or full. When calories are low, leptin may signal the brain to turn off the reproductive system. It acts like a safety mechanism. When fat stores and calories are low, your body may not be capable of carrying a baby to term.

Studies show that many high-mileage athletes can run on unusually low numbers of calories without losing weight. It's as if they take on the efficiency of a high-mileage car, getting more miles to the calorie than before.

In one study, female marathon runners who averaged more than 65 miles a week consumed a mere 1,400 calories a day. Since sedentary women of normal weight typically eat 1,500 to 2,000 calories a day, it doesn't seem possible that the women runners could maintain their weight on so few calories, but they did. Running 65 miles a week should have boosted calorie needs by 800 calories a day.

This creates a nasty catch-22 for many women as extra pounds stubbornly cling to their bodies. In an attempt to lose weight, they may ramp up their exercise even more as well as cut even more calories. In response, thyroid, estrogen, and leptin levels drop yet again, slowing the metabolism even more. End result: You lose little to no weight, but you do lose your period.

Throw a full-blown eating disorder, such as anorexia, into the equation and periods stop even faster.

Healthy eating taken to an extreme can also cause menstruation problems. High amounts of fiber, about twice the DV of 25 grams, and low intakes of protein (such as a vegetarian diet) can result in amenorrhea. Research shows that athletes who consumed more fiber experienced more trouble with irregular menstruation compared to other athletes who ate less fiber. High-fiber diets may lower levels of circulating estrogen, already lowered by a low amount of body fat and high amount of exercise.

Fortunately, research shows that menstruation can easily be restored—and so can your metabolism—if you simply eat a little more. Here are some tips:

Eat a snack every day. If you've been cutting calories and increasing exercise in an effort to lose stubborn weight, adding calories back into your diet may seem counterproductive. However, simply adding a 100-calorie snack a day may be enough to fix metabolism and menstruation problems. This extra snack will signal your metabolism that food is plentiful, flipping the switch to allow it to burn calories faster. You also burn calories simply to digest food, so eating a midafternoon snack will boost calorie burning during that time of the day.

Good 100-calorie snacks include a banana, a cheese stick and a handful of baby carrots, half an energy bar, or a slice of whole grain bread spread with 1 tablespoon of apple butter.

Take a calcium supplement. Your bones need all the help you can give them. You need 1,500 milligrams of calcium a day, every day. Increase your consumption of calcium-rich foods such as dairy products and deep green leafy vegetables. Also, take a 500-milligram calcium supplement twice a day with meals.

Don't use estrogen as a fallback. Medical doctors often prescribe birth control pills to women with amenorrhea to help restore menstruation by boosting the amount of circulating estrogen. However, though these pills may make your symptoms disappear, they may not protect your bones.

Researchers in Spain studied the bone mineral density of those with severe anorexia and amenorrhea after these women began taking birth control pills. After an entire year of therapy, bone mineral

Are Athletes at Risk?

No one knows for sure exactly what conditions may bring on an eating disorder, but most likely it's a lot of things going on at once: personality type, genetics, type of sport (those sports that demand thinner bodies for either performance reasons or appearance), and other environmental factors.

Dr. Jorunn Sundgot-Borgen, from the Norwegian University of Sport and Physical Education, studies factors that may trigger or exacerbate eating disorders in female athletes. In one study, Dr. Sundgot-Borgen evaluated athletes, including middle- and long-distance runners.

She found that anorexia, bulimia, and a subclinical eating disorder called *anorexia athletica* were likely to take hold when an athlete began dieting or had frequent weight fluctuations. Also, those athletes who started dieting at a younger age were more likely to develop an eating disorder. A traumatic event such as an injury also appeared as a trigger for eating disorders, perhaps because of forced inactivity, which, in turn, may have caused unwanted weight gain.

Other researchers have noted that eating disorders may be connected to your genes. In fact, substance abuse problems and clinical depression, both inheritable conditions, are common in bulimics and anorexics. And while exercise typically is viewed as good for the mind, some susceptible individuals may develop disordered eating habits under certain exercise conditions.

density remained low, even though the women were menstruating. Other factors, beyond estrogen, may keep bone mineral density low, particularly if dietary factors are not addressed.

Get help. If amenorrhea accompanies other factors such as eating disorders and osteoporosis (known as the *female athlete triad*), you'll need professional help to overcome the problem. You'll need to see a dietitian, psychologist, psychiatrist, or medical doctor. Your family and coaches should also be involved in your treatment. See "Disordered Eating" for more information.

ASTHMA

Eating strategies coupled with the right medication may ease this growing epidemic.

When you suffer an asthma attack, the muscles in your bronchial tubes—the gateway to your lungs—tighten and your bronchial lining swells, creating less space for air to pass through. This inflammation can produce mucus, which also restricts breathing. The result is labored breathing, chest tightness, and coughing.

Besides making exercise difficult, asthma inflicts its tolls in many other ways, including 10 million missed school days each year. Asthma is the third most common reason for hospitalization in those age 15 or younger.

Doctors diagnose an increasing number of children and adults with asthma each year, with asthma prevalence jumping a startling 75 percent between 1980 and 1994, according to statistics from the Centers for Disease Control. Many scientists blame increases in air pollution and global warming, which may increase allergens such as grass pollen, for the dramatic rise in asthma cases.

Besides pollen and air pollution, other irritants such as germs, cold air, smoke, fumes, and dust can also trigger an asthma attack. So can exercise. Those with one type of asthma, called *allergic asthma,* may suffer an attack after exercise ends, in response to drier airways caused by mouth breathing. Another type of asthma, called *exercise-induced asthma,* may strike within a few minutes after exercise begins as a direct result of faster, more forceful breathing.

Neither type of asthma, however, should spell an end to your fitness efforts. Regular exercise helps improve lung function and lung capacity. The better your fitness level, the fewer asthma attacks you experience.

Swimming provides an ideal form of exercise for people with asthma because the warm, humid environment tends to prevent an attack. Yoga offers another beneficial form of exercise, as one study found that two-thirds of asthma patients who practiced yoga were able to reduce or stop taking their medication.

In addition to exercise, various nutritional strategies may help ease symptoms. We need more research before we'll know for sure whether or not the following strategies truly help ease symptoms. However, as all of these strategies are also good for your overall health, it doesn't hurt to try them:

Stay well hydrated. Hydration is important for everyone, but particularly for those with asthma. Fluids help to keep your airways moist, helping to prevent an attack. Make sure to drink 5 to 12 ounces of fluid for every 15 minutes that you exercise.

Eat the right fats. And avoid the wrong ones. Though research has yet to prove the connection, many experts suspect that an imbalance of omega-3 fats to omega-6 fats causes many inflammatory diseases, including asthma. Omega-3 fats, found in fatty fish such as salmon, tend to prevent inflammation, whereas omega-6 fats, found in many cooking oils, tend to promote it. Most of us eat too many omega-6 fats and too few omega-3s.

Increase your consumption of omega-3 fats by eating fish twice a week and using ground flaxseed in baking recipes. Eating more fish and seafood will also help you consume another important asthma-fighting nutrient: selenium. This mineral aids an antioxidant enzyme that works at the surface on the cells in your lungs to help prevent inflammation. Besides seafood, other foods rich in selenium include grains and beans.

Lower your consumption of omega 6-fats and other undesirable fats by cutting back on butter, margarine, processed foods that con-

Quick Tip

If you have asthma or suspect you have asthma, talk to your doctor about prescription medication that can prevent and stop asthma attacks. These medications often include using an inhaled bronchodilator. You'll be able to take a couple puffs from your inhaler 15 minutes before you exercise to prevent an attack during exercise, or take a puff during or after exercise, when you feel symptoms coming on.

Also, because pollution such as ozone, carbon monoxide, and sulfur dioxide can trigger an asthma attack, monitor air pollution levels and choose indoor exercise on days when the smog count is high. That also goes for days when the pollen count is high or on cold, dry days.

tain hydrogenated fats, fried foods, and full-fat animal products. Also, cook with olive or canola oils rather than other vegetable oils (corn, safflower).

Wean yourself off the painkillers. If you regularly take ibuprofen or aspirin to soothe the muscle aches inflicted during intense or longer-than-usual exercise bouts, you may be contributing to your asthma. Though these medicines are known for their anti-inflammatory effects on your muscles, some research suggests that they may actually *cause* inflammation in the lungs.

Examine your diet. A very small amount of asthma sufferers—about 5 percent—may have food allergies that contribute to their asthma. (Many more people *think* they have food allergies than actually do.) The most common suspects are MSG (the salt substitute found in Chinese and canned food) and sulfites (found in wine and processed foods). To cut back on both additives, focus your diet on whole foods—fruits, vegetables, and whole grains—and away from foods that come out of a bag, box, or can.

Load up on fruits and vegetables. Children who eat diets low in fruits and vegetables tend to wheeze and experience other asthma symptoms more often than children who eat more produce, finds a recent study. Fruits and vegetables are rich in antioxidant nutrients that may help protect the cells in the bronchial tubes and lungs from damage and inflammation.

Many fruits and vegetables are also high in vitamin C, which several studies have shown may help minimize allergic and exercise-induced asthma by lowering airway reactivity.

Finally, people who eat a high amount of fruits and vegetables tend to consume lower amounts of sodium (because they eat less high-sodium processed food). High consumption of sodium has also been associated with asthma, though no one has proven the connection.

Fruits and vegetables are also good for your overall health. Try to eat more than five servings a day, closer to 10 or 11 if you can. Make several of those servings vitamin C–rich sources, such as citrus fruits, bell and hot peppers, spinach, tomatoes, berries, kiwi, and melons.

Eat a tomato a day. Tomatoes and other pink and red produce contain a substance called *lycopene.* In one study published in the journal *Allergy,* people with exercise-induced asthma were able to reduce their symptoms by taking supplements that contained this nutrient.

However, you don't need to go the supplement route to get enough lycopene. Pink grapefruit, watermelon, and tomatoes all qualify as rich sources. Try to eat a tomato product every day, such as red sauce on your pasta one day, tomato juice the next, and tomato slices in your salad another time. In addition to fighting asthma, you'll also help prevent heart disease and cancer.

Pile on the beans. Black, pinto, kidney, and other beans are all rich in the mineral magnesium, which may help ease asthma symptoms. Though research is too preliminary to suggest taking magnesium supplements for asthma, eating more beans can't hurt, as beans are also rich in heart-healthy fiber. Try to eat several servings of beans a week. Other magnesium-rich foods include whole grains and green leafy vegetables.

BASKETBALL

Improve your dribbling, shooting, and running with these foods.

As a nutrition consultant for the Sacramento Kings, I've dealt with just about every basketball-related nutrition question you can ask. Kings players have asked me what foods they can eat to improve their reaction time, hand-eye coordination, sprint speed from one end of the court to the other, and staying power.

Even if you're not a professional basketball player, the same eating strategies apply. Whether you want more stamina for an afternoon of pickup at the gym or a better reaction time for a big high school tournament, follow these Kings-tested tips:

Eat familiar foods before a game. Because I consult and root for the Kings, I actively root *against* the L.A. Lakers. When the two teams came head to head in 2002, I wasn't unhappy to read in the newspaper that Lakers star player Kobe Bryant wouldn't be playing because of a bad case of food poisoning. According to the news report, he thought his intestinal problems were a direct result of the bacon double cheeseburger and cheesecake he had eaten the night before at his hotel.

I'll get to why that's not exactly the best before-game dinner in a bit, but it goes without saying—don't experiment with your GI tract before a game. Eat only foods that you know will digest well. If you are traveling, stick to foods that are less likely to harbor harmful bacteria and other organisms.

Pay attention to your timing. If you play in a league or for a school where you must travel to games, pay attention to the amount of time that elapses between your last meal and the game. I've found that many players do fuel up with an energizing high-carbohydrate meal. But during the time it takes to pack up gear, drive to the game, unpack, and then warm up, hours can elapse. By the game's start, you've got an empty stomach and low blood sugar.

Try to eat a high-carbohydrate meal or snack within 2 hours of your game or practice. Bring food along with you to eat in the car during the trip, such as a resealable bag full of your favorite breakfast cereal, an energy bar, a sports drink, dried fruit, or a bagel.

Get acquainted with sports drinks. In the old days, we didn't encourage basketball players and other nonendurance athletes to consume sports drinks during a game or practice. We figured that they didn't burn enough calories during the game to result in muscle fuel depletion. Turns out that we were wrong.

Two recent studies now show that consuming a sports drink that contains 6 to 9 percent carbohydrate can increase running speed, reaction time, agility, and hand-eye coordination in those who play sports that involve sudden bursts of stop-and-go activity, such as basketball. In one of these studies, female basketball players drank either a sports drink or placebo beverage during a four-quarter game. During the last 10 minutes of the second half, researchers asked the women to perform a 15-meter sprint along with a dribbling-and-shooting drill. Those who had the sports drink were able to sprint faster and were more likely to score on the dribble-and-shoot than those who didn't have the drink.

Drinking a carbohydrate beverage during practice or a game improves reaction time by directly acting on the brain. Your brain burns glucose for fuel. Keeping blood sugar levels stable by drinking a sports drink helps supply your brain with consistent fuel, allowing you to think more clearly and make better decisions on the court.

Your Preseason Program

If you play on a team during one part of the year, you can improve your game by working on your agility and jumping skills during your off-season. Try the following exercises:

Shuttle run. Set up a series of cones or objects about 20 yards apart. Run through them, up and back, weaving in and out. You can also try it while dribbling a basketball. As your skills improve, set the cones up closer and closer together.

Jumping squats. With your feet a shoulder's width apart, squat down and then spring up, landing on a diagonal with your left foot a few feet in front of your right, as if you were jumping up to catch a rebound shot. Continue switching legs back and forth, trying to spring as high as you can and land as fluidly as you can, repeating 10 to 20 times.

Second, sudden sprinting from one end of the court to the other burns carbohydrate almost exclusively for fuel, whereas other less intense activities such as running and walking burn a mix of carbohydrate and fat. This high amount of carbohydrate burning can deplete stores in localized sections of your lower leg muscles, causing you to slow your sprinting speed.

Take a sports drink to your next game or practice, aiming to drink about 4 to 8 ounces during every 15 to 20 minutes of play.

Drink more. You'll sweat *a lot* during a basketball game or practice in a hot gym. Your sweat rate depends on your genetics, as well as how vigorously you play and how much you sit on the bench. To make sure you drink enough fluid to replace what you lose, weigh yourself without clothes before and after your games and practices. Every pound you lose during a game or practice equals a pint of sweat. To avoid dehydration and the accompanying lethargy and headache, replace every pound you lose with 16 to 20 ounces of fluid, preferably 20.

Eat during halftime or between games. You might be able to make it through one game on a sports drink or water. But if you are planning a long afternoon of numerous pickup games at the gym or a daylong tournament, you'll need to eat real food during your rest breaks to keep your blood sugar levels up and your muscles fully stocked with fuel. During your break between games, eat a high-carbohydrate light meal of about 500 to 800 calories, such as a light sandwich with fruit or an energy bar with some trail mix made primarily of dried fruit.

Recover well. The Kings tend to reserve the best restaurant in Sacramento after their games. They pile in around 11 P.M. and order up filet mignon, shrimp cocktail, and lobster. I often suggest that they try to eat some bread and a salad along with these high-protein choices. There's nothing wrong with celebrating with tasty protein options after a game, but make sure to eat some carbohydrate along with it. You'll need the carbohydrate to help restock your muscle fuel stores for tomorrow's game or practice—or just for a long day at the office.

If you play on a high school team, you may find your food options limited late at night, which is probably why most of you hit the local fast-food establishments. Whether you find yourself at the local McDonald's, Burger King, or Wendy's, stick with one or two plain burgers, a lowfat milk shake, and a side salad. Stay away from the fries and burgers piled high with fatty toppings such as cheese, bacon, and special sauce.

CANCER

Foods that protect your cells from damage.

Cancer ranks as our number two killer, behind heart disease. Yet many more people worry about cancer than heart disease, possibly because cancer is harder to understand. So before we talk about ways to prevent or slow cancer's progression, let's first take a look at how the disease develops.

Usually, the cells in your body grow, divide, and die. However, each day, your body confronts a host of carcinogens, substances that can damage your cells.

These carcinogens enter your body through the air you breathe, the food you eat, the water you drink, and the sunlight that penetrates your skin. Once inside your body, they may damage cells, altering the cell's DNA, the genetic list of instructions that guides the cell's activities.

Your body will try to repair damaged DNA but can sometimes fall behind. In the unrepaired cells, the set of instructions that tells the cell to "stop dividing" remains deleted, and the cell divides out of control, creating more cells with defective DNA. These abnormal cells divide more rapidly. Left to multiply, these abnormal cells begin to squeeze out normal tissue, making it tough for the affected organ to do its job.

Cancerous cells also grow and live for a longer-than-usual period of time, sometimes entering your bloodstream or lymph system and then traveling to other parts of the body—a process called *metastasis*.

What You Can Do

You can take many steps to reduce cancer risk, as up to 60 percent of all cancers are directly linked to lifestyle habits such as diet and exercise. You're already doing your part to prevent cancer by staying fit. Exercise may help prevent some cancers by improving glucose control, which in turn lowers the demand on many organs, including your pancreas. Exercise also speeds bowel transit, which means toxins in your waste move through your intestines faster, reducing their chances of damaging cells in your colon and rectum. Exercise also keeps levels of estrogen steady, which may help prevent estrogen-related cancers such as breast cancer.

For the minimum in cancer protection, work out for at least 30 minutes five or more days of the week. For optimal protection, push your workout time up to 45 minutes.

In addition to exercise, nutrition can help to dramatically reduce your risk of developing cancer. Numerous different types of foods contain important substances called *antioxidants,* which help to neutralize carcinogens in your body as well as repair damaged cells. Research now shows that optimizing your intake of antioxidant foods works better than taking antioxidant supplements, possibly because food presents these important nutrients to us in the right amounts and combinations.

Boosting your consumption of these foods as well as lowering your consumption of cancer-causing foods will help you to keep your cells healthy. Here's how:

Use olive oil liberally. People in Mediterranean countries develop less cancer than those in the United States. Researchers suspect the Mediterranean focus on olive oil may partly explain the protection. (People in these countries also tend to eat more fish and fruits and vegetables than we do.)

Olive oil contains high amounts of monounsaturated fat, a heart-protective fat type that shows promise as a cancer fighter, particularly for breast, skin, and colon cancers. Olive oil also contains phenols, the same type of phytochemical found in red wine, as well as substances called *lignans.* Both lignans and phenols possess potent antioxidant properties, helping to protect your cells from the damage that can set the stage for cancer. Because extra-virgin olive oil contains the most phenols, choose this type over nonvirgin varieties. Dip your bread in it, use it as a salad dressing, mix it into marinades, toss it with pasta, and cook with it.

Cut back on refined foods. A study of more than 2,000 people in Italy found that those who consumed more fruit, vegetables, fish, poultry, and olive oil—and fewer starches such as bread, cakes, and desserts—

Your Anticancer Menu

Breakfast

9-grain cereal topped with 2 tablespoons chopped almonds

¾ cup fresh blueberries and a drizzle of honey

¾ cup soy milk

Snack

6 ounces veggie juice

2 dried peach halves

Lunch

1½ cups hearty bean soup (lentil, onion, greens)

3-inch square whole grain corn bread spread with 1 tablespoon fruit spread

1 cup fresh fruit salad

12 ounces iced herb tea with lemon

Snack

1 cup nonfat yogurt topped with 3 tablespoons dried cranberries

Dinner

3 ounces lean beef stir-fry with bok choy, garlic, and snow peas (1 cup total) served over 1 cup brown rice

1 cup spinach tossed with 2 tablespoons olive oil dressing

1 ounce dark chocolate

Nutritional analysis—calories: 1,800; protein: 80 grams; carbohydrate: 290 grams; calories from fat: 19%.

Cooking 101

Take your favorite chili, stew, or meat loaf recipe, cut back on the meat and add onions, diced peppers (green or red), carrots, leeks, corn, or any other vegetable you can think of. To quick breads, muffins, and cakes, add cranberries, raisins, crushed pineapple, grated carrots, pureed prunes, or chopped dates or figs. It's surprising how you can transform an old favorite into a more delicious and nutritious treat.

were less likely to develop colon cancer. Cut back on refined foods as much as possible, substituting whole foods in their place. Switch from white bread to whole grain as well as pasta made from white flour to pasta made from whole wheat or quinoa. Instead of snack crackers, eat crunchy raw vegetables. Instead of cake, try fruit with whipped topping.

Experiment with soy. The little soybean may help prevent just about every age-related disease, including cancer. Soybeans contain substances called *isoflavones* that act like medicine to lower the incidence of both breast and prostate cancers, not to mention heart disease and osteoporosis. These isoflavones may weakly act like the hormone estrogen, helping to prevent this hormone from promoting bad cell growth. Isoflavones may also inhibit different proteins involved in cancer formation as well protect your cells from the DNA damage that leads to cancer. Aim for 25 milligrams of soy protein a day by eating more soy-rich foods such as veggie burgers and other meat substitutes.

Load up on produce. Fruits and vegetables contain important antioxidants useful in preventing just about every type of cancer in your body. They are also high in fiber, which helps to speed waste transit through your bowel, preventing the toxin buildup that can lead to colon cancer. A diet high in fruits and vegetables also tends to be low in salt, which may contribute to stomach cancers, as well as low in saturated fat, which may contribute to breast cancer.

Most of us claim we are eating plenty of fruits and veggies, but, when it comes down to it, most of us are not getting enough. A recent survey of American adults in 16 states revealed that just 23 percent consumed the recommended five servings a day of fruits and vegetables. To sneak more in, keep convenient fruits and veggies on hand, whether they are fresh, frozen, or canned. Stock your freezer with frozen berries or peaches, for example.

Add veggies to almost anything. Slip some slices of cucumber, tomato, or dark leafy lettuce into your sandwich. Add chopped greens, such as kale or spinach, to a can of soup. Grate carrots, jicama, or radishes into your dinner salad. Serve yourself two cooked or raw servings of vegetables at dinner or your main meal. If you're steaming broccoli, simply add in beans or cauliflower for an extra serving.

Cut back on alcohol. Though alcohol may aid heart health, it has also been linked to mouth, throat, larynx, esophagus, liver, and breast cancers. Limit your consumption to two daily drinks for men and one for women. A drink equals 12 ounces of beer, 5 ounces of wine, or 1.5 ounces of 80-proof distilled spirits.

Monitor your red meat intake. No one is exactly sure why red meat may increase risk for some types of cancer. Many of the studies that found this link were retrospective, looking back on the eating habits of people. Though we don't know for sure, red meat may not be as much to blame as what people tend to eat with it—potato chips, French fries, twice-baked potatoes, and so on. As long as you cut back on saturated fat and bump up your vegetable consumption, there's no reason not to make red meat a part of your diet. Just make sure to choose the leanest cuts (sirloin over prime rib, ground sirloin over ground chuck).

CHRONIC FATIGUE

If you feel as if you've been hit by a truck—even when you first wake up—these tips will help.

Are you dragging through your workouts? Are you unable to concentrate? Do you generally feel compelled to lie on the couch rather than do much of anything else?

Such chronic fatigue can be frustrating because the cause and solution to your fatigue can be elusive. For example, if your fatigue is accompanied by flulike symptoms that persist along with the inability to sleep soundly, you may have chronic fatigue syndrome (CFS), which may have roots in a muscle disease or virus. However, if your sluggishness comes with weight gain and a feeling of cold intolerance, you may have a thyroid disorder, one that may require medication. Then again, a general feeling of malaise and tiredness along with an intolerance to cold may signal a completely different condition called anemia.

To find out precisely which fatigue-causing condition you have requires a trip to your family physician. You and your doctor will have to do some careful sleuthing, looking at your diet, blood test results, symptoms, and lifestyle habits.

If your doctor has diagnosed you with anemia, chronic fatigue syndrome, or fibromyalgia (the most common causes of chronic fatigue as well as ones that respond well to dietary changes), follow your doctor's advice, along with the tips in this section.

Anemia

Your red blood cells serve as oxygen delivery carts for working muscles and other cells in need of this precious gas for energy metabolism. Poor red blood cell production results in compromised oxygen delivery. End result: You feel lethargic.

A host of nutrients are vital for healthy red blood cell production, including iron, folic acid, vitamins B_6 and B_{12}, and protein. (See sidebar, "Are You Deficient?") A physician-ordered blood test is the only way to determine if you have anemia, as well as which nutrient may be causing the deficiency. Once you know for sure you have anemia, follow these tips to keep red blood cell production strong:

Beef up your diet. You need iron to pull oxygen into your red blood cells. To keep levels optimal, eat readily absorbed forms of iron such as lean meats and fish at least twice a week. Also choose iron-fortified breakfast cereals and include vitamin C–rich fruits such as citrus fruits, which boost iron absorption from nonmeat foods such as cereals and beans. Avoid taking an iron supplement (unless prescribed by your physician), as these lead to constipation and block the absorption of the mineral zinc.

Start your day with cereal. You need vitamin B_6 to make hemoglobin, a protein inside your red blood cells. One of the easiest ways to ensure you're eating enough is simply to start your day with a fortified breakfast cereal. You can also sprinkle wheat germ over foods or eat a daily banana (one of the best fruit sources).

Eat your veggies. Fruits and vegetables are great sources of folic acid, an important B vitamin that helps build red blood cells. Reach for at least two daily servings of citrus fruits, including oranges and grapefruit, and green leafy vegetables, such as broccoli, asparagus, and kale. Fortified grains (cereals, bread, pasta, and rice) are also a good source of this vitamin.

Take a B_{12} supplement. You need B_{12} to make red blood cells, and the ability to absorb this important vitamin declines with age. If you're over 50, take a multivitamin with 100 percent of the RDA for B_{12}, as the body absorbs the pill form more readily than from food. Since B_{12} is only found in meats, milk, and other animal products, look to fortified food sources (soy milk, breakfast cereals) if you are a vegetarian.

Sleep More, Sleep Better

People often "burn the candle at both ends" by getting up early for a workout and then staying up late due to time demands, but this chronic sleep deprivation can make you feel chronically tired. Make sure you're getting a good 8 hours on a regular basis. To get a better night's sleep, eliminate caffeine after 2 P.M. and forgo alcohol after 6 P.M., as both can hinder sleep.

Focus on quality protein. You need protein to make hemoglobin and red blood cells. To make sure you are getting all of the amino acids (the building blocks of protein) that you need, focus on complete protein sources such as fish, lean beef, poultry, low-fat dairy, eggs, and soy, which all supply a complete set of all of the essential amino acids. Eat two to four servings of protein-rich foods a day.

Chronic Fatigue Syndrome and Fibromyalgia

Chronic fatigue syndrome and fibromyalgia are two related conditions that can make you feel as if you've been run over by a truck—from the moment you get out of bed. In addition to fatigue, fibromyalgia is accompanied by muscle soreness, and chronic fatigue syndrome with swollen glands.

Both conditions are tough to diagnose and even tougher to treat. Here's what research shows may help:

Take a B-complex supplement. A study published in the *Journal of the Royal Society of Medicine* found that people with chronic fatigue syndrome are usually deficient in the B vitamins pyridoxine, riboflavin, and thiamin. More research is needed to find out if a deficiency causes the condition or if people with chronic fatigue syndrome somehow

Are You Deficient?

If you have anemia, too little of any of five important nutrients may be to blame. Following are descriptions of what each of these nutrients does, as well as information on how your doctor can tell if you're running low.

Iron

What it does: This mineral sits within the red blood cell and latches on to oxygen, making it indispensable for energy metabolism.

How your doctor can tell if you're deficient: When your doctor takes a look at a sample of your blood, your iron levels will be low and your blood cells will appear weak in color and size.

Vitamin B_6

What it does: This B vitamin helps assemble the protein in red blood cells, called *hemoglobin*.

How your doctor can tell if you're deficient: Your hemoglobin count will be below 12 in women and 14 in men.

Vitamin B_{12}

What it does: Too little B_{12} hampers red blood cell production and creates a form of anemia that may also lead to nerve damage.

How your doctor can tell if you're deficient: Your red blood cells will appear larger than normal and irregular in shape. Also, a B_{12} absorption test may show hampered absorption.

Folic Acid

What it does: Another B vitamin, folic acid works alongside vitamin B_{12} to make copies of your red blood cells, replenishing the supply that dwindles daily.

How your doctor can tell if you're deficient: Your red blood cells will look abnormally large and oval shaped. Also, your urine sample will reveal a low level of folic acid excretion product.

(continues)

Are You Deficient? *(continued)*

Protein

What it does: A must for making fresh hemoglobin and blood cells, protein in insufficient amounts in your diet may bring on both anemia and a weak immune system.

How your doctor can tell if you're deficient: Your blood test will reveal low circulating levels of liver proteins. Also, a review of your dietary patterns will show a low protein intake.

have trouble absorbing or processing these vitamins. Either way, a B-complex multivitamin can't hurt. Find a B-complex vitamin that provides 100 to 200 percent of the RDA.

Stick with your exercise program. When you're dead tired, exercise may be the last thing you feel like attempting. However, research shows that regular aerobic activity lasting for 30 minutes three times a week can help alleviate symptoms of both conditions. Attempt exercise during the afternoon, as that will help you sleep better at night. Also, go easy on yourself. If you're just starting an exercise program, build up very gradually, starting with just 5 minutes of a light activity such as leisurely walking and adding 1 to 2 minutes each week, until you build up to ½ hour.

Consider therapy. Numerous studies show that behavioral therapy can dramatically lower symptoms of chronic fatigue syndrome, possibly because those with CFS tend to be chronic overachievers. Ask your family physician for a referral to a therapist who specializes in cognitive behavioral therapy.

CYCLING

Surviving long rides often means experimenting with unusual foods.

There's nothing quite like a long ride through wine country. I sometimes spend as many as 4 or 5 hours in the saddle, as my riding buddies and I enjoy the lush rolling hills. Inevitably, however, on every ride, one of my riding partners looks askance at my ride grub and questions, "You're eating that?"

Cyclists, as with many other endurance athletes, tend to focus on three main food groups when they ride: energy bars, energy gels, and sports drinks. Those foods all supply convenient and easily digestible muscle-fueling carbohydrate. However, when I'm in the saddle for 4 or more hours, the sweet taste of those foods tends to get to me.

Among my riding buddies, I'm famous for introducing seemingly untraditional foods into the ride menu. For example, I often beg for the group to stop at my favorite deli so I can order my midride tomato sandwich. In addition to an energy bar or two, I pack many other foods into my cycling jersey, including baked potatoes, dried fruit, and even leftover rice.

Right about now, you're probably also thinking, "She's eating what?" However, as you'll soon see, these foods and many others provide great, easily digestible carbohydrate to help you maneuver your ride. So whether you're planning on spending hours in the saddle or only your lunch break on the local mountain bike trail, use these tips to boost your performance:

Eat early and often. Many cyclists wait until they feel hungry or tired before they reach into their back pocket for food. However, if you wait until you feel fatigued, your blood sugar has already dropped, and you'll never fully catch up.

To stay energized during your ride, start consuming calories in the first half hour, aiming for 100 calories for every half hour of riding.

Quick Tip

Many cyclists experience trouble opening prepackaged foods while in the saddle. You can make this easier by opening them before the ride or tearing a small portion of the packaging so you can easily rip off the rest with your teeth. For example, open your energy bars before you get on the bike. Simply open the package seams, put the bars in your jersey pocket with the open side facing away from your sweaty back, and then get on your bike.

Don't gorge. Some cyclists see long rides as an excuse for an eating event, eating way too much food and feeling sick and sluggish as a result. If you tend to feel stuffed on your rides, try splitting up your food into separate servings. Place 100 calories (the amount in one banana, one large Fig Newton, or one gel pack) at one end of your jersey pocket. Then place a different type of food, perhaps a handful of animal crackers, into a little plastic bag to serve as your second snack. That way you'll work your way through your snacks at the right times, eating enough calories without eating too much.

Make drinking easy. Cycling ranks as one of the easiest sports for transporting food. Special jerseys allow cyclists to store energy bars and the like in no-bounce pockets. The bike itself is equipped to carry water bottles. However, many cyclists fail to drink enough fluids because they lack the balancing skills needed to grab and drink from a water bottle while in motion. Also, some types of cycling, such as navigating an extremely curvy road or climbing on a mountain bike, make one-handed cycling difficult.

You need to finish off two water bottles an hour. If you find that your bottles remain partially full at the end of your rides, invest in a water carrier such as the type made by CamelBak that allows you to fill as many as 100 ounces of fluid into a soft, light bladder that you wear on your back. These backpack water carriers contain convenient drinking nozzles that you clip to your jersey, allowing you to sip water without moving your hands off the handlebars or slowing your pedaling cadence.

For road riding, fill your water pack with water, as your food will supply the carbohydrate you need. If you're mountain biking, however, fill it with a sports drink. Many mountain bikers fail to take the breaks needed to nibble on food, so the calories from your sports drink will help fuel your muscles to climb and allow you to stay on your bike longer. Just make sure to wash out your water bottle with warm soapy water after each ride to prevent bacterial growth. (If you'll be filling the bladder of a CamelBack unit with sports drink, look for one with an end wide enough to insert your hand for easy scrubbing and drying.)

Experiment with taking breaks. If you ride for longer periods of time, and particularly if you plan to ride a century (a one-hundred-mile ride) or an endurance bike race such as a 24-hour mountain bike team event, you need to know what you can eat during your downtime that won't interfere with your riding time.

During longer practice rides, break at least once an hour. You can make these breaks fun. Take them at a local coffee shop, bakery, or deli. Experiment with what amount of food you can comfortably digest during that break and still get back on your bike to ride. Besides eating, use your breaks to stretch out your neck, shoulders, arms, and legs.

Perfect your eating form. To safely steer while grabbing for food in your back pocket, move one hand to the center of your handlebars. Even better, try no-handed drills to get used to balancing the bike with just your feet and legs. (For safety reasons, stick with one-handed riding when in a group of riders.) When you grab your water bottle, don't look down. Instead, keep your eyes on the road and simply use one hand to swat around until you feel the bottle. If you have trouble pulling and pushing the bottle back into the carrier, adjust the carrier.

Branch out. Food boredom ranks as one of the biggest contributors to "bonking" (running low on blood sugar, giving you a light-headed, that's-all-I-can-ride feeling). After a while, the sports drink, energy gels, and energy bars all taste the same. You get sick of eating sweet foods and begin to eat less and less. Eventually, the fatigue, dizziness, and telltale signs of low blood sugar set in. To avoid food boredom on long rides, experiment. Any high-carbohydrate, low-fat food will do. Try the following, all available from your kitchen cabinet or convenience store along your ride route:

- **Dried pears.** These high-carbohydrate, low-fiber treats remain intact and free from "pocket junk" (bits of food or crumbs) when stored in your back pocket, even without a protective bag. They also come in fairly large pieces, making them easy to grab.
- **Guava paste.** Available at Spanish grocery stores, this carbohydrate-packed paste made from guava fruit comes in cellophane-wrapped cubes the size of three sugar cubes. This paste gets to your head and muscles faster than any other food I've tried, providing extremely quick energy.
- **Leftover rice.** Most cyclists don't think of rice as a perennial ride food. Try it. I often stick leftover rice sprinkled with a little sugar in a sealable plastic bag and then suck some out when I need it. The neutral taste of the rice helps overcome the monotony of eating typically sweet ride foods.
- **Leftover baked potatoes.** Baked potatoes are another great food to help you overcome sugar mouth. Eat these during the first part of your ride before they "overbake" in your back pocket.

Your Century-Ride Menu

If you're planning on competing in an endurance race or a charity ride, use the following sample menu to keep your eating on track.

Before the Ride

3 6-inch pancakes
2 tablespoons jam or syrup
6 ounces orange juice
1 banana
Coffee

During the Ride

At 20 miles: 1 banana, 1 cup sports drink
At 35 miles: 1 energy gel
At 52 miles: Lunch stop—2 fig bars, 2 slices bread with light filling (turkey or cheese slices or jam), 1 apple, 1 cup sports drink
At 75 miles: 2 cups sports drink, 3 dried pear halves
At 90 miles: 1 cup sports drink, 2 fig bars

After the Ride

2 cups pasta with ¾ cup meat sauce
1 cup wild rice salad
2 cups green salad with garbanzo beans, cucumbers, 1 tablespoon oil-vinegar dressing
1 slice sourdough bread
12 ounces iced tea

Nutritional analysis—calories: 3,086; protein: 91 grams; carbohydrate: 552 grams; calories from fat: 19%.

- **Animal crackers.** Just stick them in a plastic bag and eat them throughout the ride.
- **Fig bars.** Like dried pears, these cookies don't collect a lot of pocket junk or lose their shape.
- **Pretzels and chips.** I like to bring along something salty for long rides. The salt helps replace sweat losses and encourages drinking. More important, it helps counteract the sweetness of energy bars and energy gels. Try salted pretzels or salted fat-free potato chips.
- **Sour candy.** SweeTarts, Jelly Bellies, and other types of sour candy provide muscle-fueling carbohydrate without the sweetness of energy bars or gels.
- **Beef jerky.** Okay, so this one's higher in protein than carbohydrate, but if you really hate sweet foods, it's not a bad alternative.

Recover with calories. When you end your ride, place recovery eating higher on your priority list than cleaning up and storing away your bike. During long rides, your muscles use up stores of glycogen, your reserve of carbohydrate energy. You must replenish this glycogen before your next ride in the bike saddle. Eating within the first half hour after your ride will more efficiently restock your muscle fuel stores than waiting until more than an hour has passed.

During that first half hour off your bike, try any of the following foods or meals:

- 1 cup sports drink, 1 banana, and 1 energy bar
- A tuna sandwich, 1 cup pasta salad, and 1 cup fruit salad
- 1½ cups pasta tossed with tomato sauce, 1 cup fat-free milk, and 1 fig bar

- 2 ounces of pretzels, 8 ounces of fruit juice, 2 oatmeal cookies, and 1 mozzarella cheese stick
- 1½ cups ready-to-eat cereal, 1 cup fat-free milk, 2 tablespoons raisins, and 1 apple
- 1 bean burrito, 1 cup tomato–garbanzo bean salad, and 1 orange

DIABETES

Food and exercise act like medicine to manage this epidemic.

Type 2 diabetes is becoming a national epidemic. Over the past decade, type 2 incidence has climbed a staggering 40 percent among 40-year-olds and 70 percent among people in their 30s. Once considered an adult disease, type 2 also afflicts many overweight and out-of-shape children and teens. In fact, those younger than age 20 have experienced a 10-fold increase in this deadly disease.

And since many people don't routinely get their blood sugar levels measured, an estimated 8 million people probably unknowingly have diabetes.

Many more people have what is referred to as insulin resistance, or syndrome X, a type of prediabetic condition that dramatically increases your heart disease risk.

To prevent or reverse these deadly disorders, you must first understand how your metabolism works.

When you eat, blood sugar or glucose levels rise. The hormone insulin, secreted from the pancreas, ushers the glucose into muscle and fat cells where it's either burned as fuel or stored.

In healthy people, blood glucose levels return to normal within a few hours, but in those with diabetes or insulin resistance, the body's cells resist insulin's action. It's as if someone is knocking at your door,

Quick Tip

High blood insulin and glucose levels often go unnoticed in the early stages because they don't make you feel any different. That's why everyone should have their blood sugar levels tested starting at age 35 or 40 (earlier if you have family history).

Ask your doctor for a blood glucose test especially if you:

- Have a direct relative (mother, father, sister, brother) with diabetes.
- Are sporting excess weight, especially in the belly region.
- Gave birth to a baby weighing more than 9 pounds or were diagnosed with gestational diabetes.
- Are Hispanic, black, or non-Caucasian (at greater risk).

Compare your results (two consistent readings taken on different days) to the values listed here:

Fasting Blood Glucose

Healthy	60 to 109 milligrams/deciliter
Insulin-resistant	110 to 125 milligrams/deciliter
Diabetic	126 milligrams/deciliter or higher

but no one answers. So the pancreas pumps out more insulin and knocks a bit louder.

In some people, most likely due to a genetic defect, the pancreas tires from its workload and can't keep pace with demand, and blood glucose levels climb into the diabetic range. (In type 1 diabetes, the pancreas completely fails and no insulin is produced, making replacement necessary for survival.)

With both diabetes and insulin resistance, blood sugar doesn't get to where it belongs, choking off the flow of nutrients to cells. Blood vessels become diseased, leading to an array of problems—infections (particularly urinary tract and in the feet), nerve damage (which can cause impotence), heart disease, blindness, and kidney failure. Researchers have found that children who have diabetes experience artery clogging at a young age. They are also more likely to experience early onset of puberty, with girls menstruating up to four and a half years too early.

Also, high insulin and blood glucose levels tend to bring on syndrome X health problems—high triglyceride and low HDL levels, high blood pressure, and sticky, clot-prone blood.

Dodging Diabetes

The good news: Diabetes and its ill effects can be controlled successfully through a healthful diet and regular physical activity. Here's how to turn the disease around:

Get physical. Exercise boosts the body's sensitivity to insulin. In other words, a softer knock opens a cell's door to glucose, which helps blood sugar levels remain in the healthy range.

For example, diabetes is virtually nonexistent in rural areas of Southeast Asian countries where life involves lots of physical labor. But when people move to the city and live more affluently, activity levels fall off, and diabetes incidence rises. When it comes to insulin sensitivity, however, the goodness of exercise is transitory. If you stop, you lose the benefit.

Make your days as physical as possible, by walking every chance you get, taking the stairs, and playing with your children or your dog. Include cycling, swimming, jogging, or other continuous, calorie-burning activity at least three but preferably five days a week.

Seek middle management. Many people want to blame eating too many sweets for their risky sugar levels. Instead, it's more likely

What Is Type 1?

About 5 to 10 percent of all people with diabetes in the United States have type 1, or insulin-dependent, diabetes. In this form, the pancreas fails altogether in producing insulin, usually by childhood or before age 20. The cause: a genetic predisposition that causes a "self-destruction" of the insulin-secreting cells of the pancreas.

People with type 1 diabetes must carefully time their insulin replacement (injections or use of an insulin pump) with the amount of carbohydrate they eat. Also, since exercising muscles use glucose for fuel, the timing, intensity, and duration of a workout must be monitored so that glucose levels don't plummet to dangerously low levels. Start slowly at fitness. Build up gradually to moderately intense exercise at least three times a week and five to seven times for best results. Consult your physician before starting an exercise program.

that too many calories plump up fat cells making them resistant to insulin.

More overweight people develop type 2 diabetes, especially those who carry their extra weight around the waist or abdomen. With excess fat, the likelihood of insulin resistance increases, which, in turn, pushes the pancreas to work harder. Fat storage around the middle appears to make matters worse as fat cells in this region appear more prone to developing insulin resistance. Losing as little as 10 to 15 pounds can improve insulin sensitivity. And if you keep the weight off, the benefit stays.

Eat smart. Eating a diet with plenty of water-soluble fiber, the type in beans, oats, and fruit, helps steady the release of sugar into the bloodstream. Include these foods frequently in your daily fare (see sidebar, "Dining with Diabetes in Mind"). Also, select whole grain versions of pasta, bread, and bagels.

Dining with Diabetes in Mind

This meal plan has added fiber and foods that help keep blood sugar levels in check.

Breakfast

1 cup oatmeal (with 2 tablespoons chopped almonds and ¾ cup vanilla soy milk)

1 whole orange

1 slice whole grain bread with 1 tablespoon apple butter

Lunch

1 bean burrito (whole wheat tortilla, 1 cup black beans, ½ cup brown rice, salsa, 1 ounce lowfat cheese, ⅙ sliced avocado)

1 cup fruit salad

Snack

½ cup fruit-nut trail mix (dried apricots, peaches, walnuts, soy nuts)

1 kiwi, sliced over ½ cup plain lowfat yogurt

Dinner

3 ounces grilled tuna over 1 cup couscous

2 cups green salad with 2 tablespoons olive oil dressing

1 cup steamed asparagus with 1 tablespoon grated Parmesan cheese

1 baked apple topped with cinnamon and 2 tablespoons chopped pecans

Nutritional analysis—calories: 2,090; protein: 100 grams; carbohydrate: 282 grams; calories from fat: 30%.

While not all health professionals agree on this one, some research suggests that more fat, rather than less, may be best for some people with diabetes. Eating a diet with 30 to 40 percent of the calories from heart-healthy fats, mostly monounsaturated (olive and canola oils) along with nuts and fish helps keep HDL levels up and triglyceride levels down.

For some people who are insulin-resistant or diabetic, a high-carbohydrate diet boosts triglyceride levels—more bad news for heart health. But backing off on refined carbs shouldn't put a dent in restocking your glycogen stores for your workouts. Just substitute several daily servings of fresh fruits, vegetables, and whole grains.

Don't smoke. It goes without saying that smoking brings with it a multitude of health problems. While researchers aren't clear how, smoking further aggravates insulin resistance. It's as if when smoke is around, the cells won't answer the door when insulin comes knocking.

Drink responsibly. A few studies show that moderate alcohol consumption—one to two drinks daily—may lower the risk of a heart attack in people with diabetes. Alcohol, whether from red wine, beer, or distilled spirits, boosts HDL levels ever so slightly, which in turn lowers heart disease risk. But don't start drinking, if you don't already, as there's no evidence that risk for developing diabetes is lowered with alcohol consumption.

DISORDERED EATING

When dieting and exercise become an obsession, you need professional help.

Many of us use exercise to help control our weight. We may find ourselves working off occasional indulgences, for example, by jogging or walking extra miles to make up for last night's fried chicken dinner.

Yet this eat-and-sweat-it-off behavior can easily mushroom into a compulsion that, at the very least, removes the joy of fitness and eating and, at the most, results in life-threatening malnourishment.

Several studies show that compared to nonathletes, athletic men and women, especially those in sports where body weight and shape is an issue, such as running and gymnastics, have a greater incidence

Is It Normal or Is It an Eating Disorder?

The answer to that question depends on your answers to the following questions:

- Are you preoccupied with food and your weight?
- Do you binge frequently and then exercise as a way to cope?
- Does the thought of gaining weight evoke so much fear that you regularly restrict or deprive yourself of food?
- Even though people tell you that you are thin, do you feel fat?
- Do you feel anxious if you can't exercise?
- Do you have a secret stash of food?
- Do you feel that you would like yourself more if you were thinner?
- Do you feel guilty when you eat?

If you answered yes to four or more questions, you have developed an unhealthy relationship with food and should seek counseling.

of abnormal eating behaviors and full-blown clinical eating disorders such as anorexia and bulimia.

Eating disorders often begin during adolescence. More than half of teenage girls report that they are dieting or think they should be dieting. Most are attempting to lose the 40 pounds that they typically gain between ages 8 and 14.

Dying to Be Thin

Eating disorders result in a myriad of health problems. Low calorie intake or sporadic eating, for example, results in poor exercise performance and endurance. Cheating the body of food doesn't allow you to eat enough protein, vitamins, and minerals like zinc. End result: a weakened immune system, chronic illnesses, and fatigue. You are prone to more injuries and take longer to recover from them.

But more threatening to your long-term health is a condition known as the female athlete triad: disordered eating, cessation of your menstrual cycle, and osteoporosis (the debilitating bone disease typically seen in elderly women). Too few calories and too much exercise can lower levels of the hormone estrogen, responsible for normal ovarian function. Too little estrogen will cause periods to cease. Estrogen plays a vital role in bone health and in preventing heart disease. Low estrogen levels in young women lead to brittle bones just like those seen in elderly women.

There are numerous types of eating disorders, but the most common among fitness enthusiasts include anorexia nervosa, bulimia, subclinical eating disorders, and the closely related condition, exercise addiction. Following are some hallmarks of each.

Anorexia Nervosa

Anorexia is characterized by a cluster of symptoms including self-induced starvation, an intense fear of becoming fat, a body weight that's 15 percent below normal for height, and, in women, the loss of a regular menstrual cycle or amenorrhea (see "Amenorrhea"). Fine facial and body hair may grow (called *lanugo*) on an anorexic, in the body's last-ditch effort to stay warm.

Anorexics view themselves as fat despite their frail appearance. Their distorted body image drives them to lose even more weight, usually through severe calorie cutting and excessive exercise, giving them a feeling of control. Often perfectionists and highly motivated, anorexics are typically college educated, single, and from middle- to upper-class families. Yet they also have low self-esteem believed to stem from an upbringing with overly protective or controlling parents.

Bulimia

By some reports, 15 to 25 percent of all female college athletes suffer from this eating disorder.

Bulimia is characterized by frequent episodes of binge eating, with as much as 2,000 to more than 10,000 calories in a single binge. This is typically followed by feelings of extreme guilt prompting purging (usually vomiting or the use of laxatives and diuretics) of the unwanted calories to prevent weight gain. For bulimia classification, bingeing and purging episodes occur at least two times a week for three months.

Bulimics may also purge by exercising excessively, such as jogging or stair stepping for hours. Bulimics often feel helpless and out of control during binges. Because bulimics are usually normal in body weight and appearance and often binge and purge in secrecy, family and friends may be unaware of their battle with food. Despite this normal appearance, bulimics often brush with death as severe vomiting causes loss of electrolytes such as potassium, which can result in heart failure.

Subclinical Eating Disorders

Since anorexia and bulimia don't develop overnight, many fitness enthusiasts may be suffering from what's called a subclinical eating disorder. This includes skipping meals, 24-hour fasts, calorie restriction, and occasional purging (maybe once a week instead of the two times or more per week seen in bulimia) as a means to lose weight. People with a subclinical eating disorder may also be obsessed with their weight and very fearful of becoming fat. These eating disorders are

Quick Tip

If you think you have an eating disorder or know someone who has one, contact the following organizations for more information:

National Eating Disorders Association
603 Stewart Street, Suite 803
Seattle, WA 98101
Phone: (206) 382-3587 or (800) 931-2237
Web site: www.nationaleatingdisorders.org

Anorexia Nervosa and Related Eating Disorders (ANRED)
Box 5102
Eugene, OR 97405
Web site: www.anred.com

believed to be rampant in such sports as gymnastics, crew, wrestling, volleyball, and running.

Exercise Addiction

When you feel obligated to exercise—either to burn calories or even to burn off stress—you're considered an exercise addict. Exercise begins to function as a drug, quickly becoming the top priority of your life, even though you probably no longer enjoy it. Rather, you feel compelled to exercise, doing more and more of it, even though the activity may make you sore or cause injuries. You may keep detailed records of your exercise duration and frequency. When you don't exercise, you feel guilty or anxious.

Getting Help

With treatment, 60 percent of those with eating disorders recover. Treatment requires the involvement of physicians, dietitians, and mental health professionals. In extreme situations, especially in women with prolonged cases, hospitalization may be required. As with other serious diseases, prevention is key. This requires vigilance on the part of parents, coaches, and friends to look for signs of abnormal eating and exercise behaviors.

If you think you have an eating disorder, get help. Your disorder is ruining both your emotional and physical health. If you think you know someone with an eating disorder, follow these tips:

Never manipulate someone who has an eating disorder. People with anorexia will resist efforts to get them to eat, even with your well-meaning encouragement. She or he may pretend to take the food to make you happy and may even eat it but later purge it through vomiting so as not to gain weight. Because the condition is often built around a flawed way to seek control, manipulating or bossing someone with an eating disorder will only make the problem worse. Rather than trying to force someone to gain weight or to eat, let your friend or loved one know you care about his or her health and you are there as support.

Gather information on treatment programs. People with eating disorders need professional help that involves not only nutritional support and medical care but also psychological treatment. Unfortunately, these programs can be expensive and are not always covered by insurance.

Look for community service agencies, since these are often not as expensive. Also, consider taking part in a clinical trial—you can then get free treatment. Go to the Anorexia Nervosa and Related Eating Disorders (ANRED) Web site (www.anred.com) for information about current research trials.

Encourage your friend or loved one to seek help. This is the hard part. Most people with eating disorders will deny that there's anything wrong. If you're a parent or legal guardian of someone 18 or younger with an eating disorder, sign your child up for a physical and psychological exam. If either doctor recommends hospitalization, listen.

If your loved one or friend is older than 18, you can't force him or her to seek treatment. Instead, express your concerns gently. Encourage treatment, but don't force it. You might provide information about the disorder, listen to his or her concerns, and offer to attend the first treatment session. Offer the best gift you can—your support and caring.

Never make remarks about weight. Someone with an eating disorder hears "You're too thin" as a compliment and "Good, you're finally gaining weight" as a call for more dieting.

ENERGY

Advice for those who give 110 percent—and then give a little more.

I know all about full schedules. I wake most mornings at 5 A.M., answer e-mail, and then head out for a swim or bike ride. Then I'm off to the university, where I lecture 550-plus students, meet with students during office hours, return phone calls, write articles for magazines and trade journals, read medical journals, and attend meetings.

At 4 P.M., I head home for a bike ride, a strength workout, or a power walk or a run with one of my dogs. Then there's dinner with the family followed by more work. When I hit the hay at 10 P.M., I fall asleep in less than a second.

If I didn't eat right, I'd probably curl up under my desk by midafternoon. If, like me, you squeeze the last drop out of every minute of your day, the following tips will help you navigate your jam-packed schedule with more vigor:

Eat a handful of raisins. Raisins are a great source of the mineral boron, which may help combat drowsiness. In a series of studies performed by the U.S. Department of Agriculture (USDA), healthy men and women who ate low-boron diets for several weeks suffered from slowed brain activity compared to those who took a boron supplement.

We don't yet know how much boron is needed for healthy brain function, but USDA researchers gave study subjects 3 to 4 milligrams of boron, a dosage equivalent to that found in about 3 ounces of raisins. You can also consume that much boron from 1 ounce of almonds.

Pack a tuna sandwich for lunch. Tuna is one of the best food sources of selenium, a mineral that may boost mood, lift spirits, and contribute to feelings of clearheadedness. (Brazil nuts are also high in this mineral.)

Researchers at the USDA tested the effects of selenium on mood by feeding half of the men in a study only 40 percent of the recommended daily selenium requirement, while the other half took in about 350 percent. When researchers tested the moods of both groups, the high-selenium group felt more elated than depressed, more energetic than tired, more clearheaded than confused, and more confident than unsure. Sounds like a fabulous "drug" to me, but be cautious about taking large amounts of selenium as this mineral can cause toxicity problems. (See "Word of Caution" sidebar.)

Tuna is also high in protein, which can help prevent the all-too-common midafternoon slump. A high-carbohydrate meal—pasta, bread, and fruit, for example—can alter levels of the brain neurotransmitter serotonin, causing feelings of drowsiness. But adding protein, such as tuna or tofu, to your lunchtime pasta can provide the right mix of nutrients in the blood, including amino acids that alter brain neurotransmitter levels to boost alertness.

Always eat breakfast. No matter how frenzied your day, don't skip breakfast, truly the most important meal of the day. Many studies on children have shown that reading, memory, and other cognitive skills falter when they miss breakfast. Going all night without food, followed

Cooking 101

Whenever you need a quick pick-me-up but don't have time to actually prepare a meal or a snack, try one of my favorite energizing snacks: a sorbet sandwich. Take 3 tablespoons of strawberry sorbet and wedge it between two caramel corn rice cakes. The coldness of the sorbet combined with the crunchiness of the rice cakes will give you the jolt you need to tackle your next task.

by a foodless morning, causes blood sugar levels to dip. Since sugar (in the form of glucose) is the brain's primary fuel source, it's no wonder memory and other thinking powers go downhill.

When I know my day will be anything but serene, I start the morning with a high-energy breakfast to fuel me with enough calories and nutrients to last me until lunch. I'll have a glass of 100 percent fruit juice along with 1½ cups of 9-grain hot cereal. I stir 1 tablespoon of isolated soy protein powder into the cereal before cooking and then add a little extra liquid. After cooking it, I stir in ¼ cup of golden raisins and 1 ounce of chopped pecans. Then I top the whole concoction with ¾ cup vanilla-flavored soy milk.

Drink coffee wisely. Drinking a cup or two of coffee can certainly improve feelings of alertness and clearheadedness and even bolster performance on monotonous tasks such as typing or filing. But too much of this pick-me-up can easily brew into a caffeine habit that can backfire, causing fatigue. Caffeine junkies—the people with a perpetual cup of coffee (or tea or cola)—have developed a dependency on caffeine. Without a steady allotment of the stimulant throughout the day, they go into caffeine withdrawal, feeling tired and irritable.

If you view coffee or other caffeinated beverages as a life source (and I'm speaking from personal experience here), try phasing caffeine

Word of Caution

If you're tempted to boost your brain power by taking a selenium supplement, beware. This mineral is highly toxic in large doses. Stick to dosages no greater than 400 micrograms, or about five to seven times the daily requirement (which is 55 micrograms). Better yet, concentrate on getting selenium from your diet. In addition to tuna, other good food sources include nuts, chicken, turkey, lean beef, and whole grain breads and cereals.

out a little at a time to regain your own natural feelings of energy. Start your "detox" by trimming one-fifth of your typical daily caffeine intake for a few weeks. You may experience some fatigue or headaches for a day or two as your body adjusts. Then, when you've gotten accustomed to this regimen, gradually continue cutting back a bit at a time. Once you're down to a cup or two in the morning, you can decide whether you want to eliminate caffeine altogether.

Perk up with water. Your brain is more than 70 percent water by weight, and if this percentage dips below a critical level when you become dehydrated, you'll feel listless, dull, and headachy.

According to the USDA, most Americans drink only one-fourth of their fluid needs as plain water; they get the rest from coffee, soda, and food. Keep yourself energized by starting your morning off with an 8-ounce glass of plain water (yes, even before your morning coffee). Then keep a bottle of water handy and drink about 1 to 2 quarts throughout the day. Every time you start to feel sluggish, reach for that bottle of water and take a big swig.

Freshen up with fiber. Besides keeping your intestinal tract healthy, relieving constipation, and lowering blood cholesterol, fiber may also help you feel energized. A recent study from the journal *Appetite* suggests that including a high-fiber breakfast cereal like Kellogg's All-Bran lowered self-assessed ratings of fatigue compared to eating a low-fiber cereal. Researchers suggest that the higher fiber intake, which prevents constipation, may in turn lessen feelings of sluggishness.

Boost your fiber intake by selecting breakfast cereals that supply at least 20 percent of the DV for fiber (5 grams per serving). Also include several servings of fruits and vegetables daily along with beans and whole grains.

Snack periodically. Whenever you feel as if you need a little jolt, eat a small snack. Reach for snacks that are crunchy and really hot or really cold to help wake up your senses. Keep these snacks high in nutrient-packed, carbohydrate-rich foods and light on calories (stay under 200) to avoid weight gain. Here are some examples:

- One frozen fruit bar.
- Drinkable fruit-flavored yogurt (sold in 8-ounce plastic bottles) mixed with ½ cup club soda.
- One ready-to-eat cereal bar like Kellogg's Nutri-Grain tossed in the microwave for less than a minute and then spread with 1 tablespoon fat-free cream cheese.
- One package of precut veggies with reduced-fat dip.

FATIGUE DURING OR AFTER EXERCISE

Remedies to help keep you energized to the finish line—and beyond.

Most people who start exercising on a regular basis say they feel more alert and vibrant compared to when they were sedentary. However, for some people, exercise can be a drag. They tell me that they feel tired halfway through a workout and end up calling it quits earlier than expected. Then, afterward, they feel bushed and struggle to stay awake while at work.

The good news: Midworkout and postworkout fatigue can almost always be remedied with proper nutrition. Here's what to do:

Eat the right foods before exercise. During a workout, your muscles burn a type of carbohydrate fuel called *glycogen*. Your liver also stores this carbohydrate energy to supply your blood with sugar for your brain to use throughout the day. Following your workout, your blood sugar levels may take a dip as you run low on this fuel, resulting in a postworkout slump.

You can turn this around by fully stocking those muscle and liver glycogen gas tanks before your workout. About 2 to 3 hours before a long workout, eat high-carbohydrate foods such as cereal, bread, low-fat muffins, or fruit. (Stay away from high-fat foods before your workouts. Doughnuts, fatty meats, or high-fat dairy products may cause early fatigue because they digest slowly and don't directly fuel the brain.)

The carbohydrates will be released into your bloodstream during your workout, serving as fuel for your exercising muscles and conserving your stored liver glycogen to later power your brain at work.

Snack during your workout. During a long exercise session of an hour or more, eat foods that have a high glycemic index (GI). The GI is a measure of how quickly a carbohydrate food is processed, releasing sugar into the bloodstream. High-glycemic foods are exactly what you need to fuel your muscles and keep fatigue-causing fatty acid levels from climbing. Aim for 30 to 60 grams of carbohydrate for every hour of exercise. That comes to about 120 to 300 calories per hour. Good high-glycemic choices include sports drinks, raisins, bread, potatoes, and cookies sweetened with molasses.

Eat again—after your workout. I know, I'm starting to sound like a broken record here, but eating a small amount of food before, during, and after exercise is the most effective way to eliminate fatigue.

Tips for the Night Shift

Like it or not, our bodies respond to sunlight, preferring to wake up with dawn and wind down at sunset. When you work at night, you keep the lights on when your body prefers to wind down for sleep. The lights may stimulate you to stay awake, but the darkness outside keeps signaling your body to sleep. Then when you go home in the morning, the sunlight signals your body to awaken, when you're ready to go to bed.

Inevitably, those who work the night shift report that they feel constantly sleep deprived, a situation that can wreak havoc on your health. Recent studies show that chronic sleep loss may play a part in age-related diseases such as hypertension and diabetes.

Here's how to help yourself stay more alert at work as well as sleep better by day:

Shift your meal patterns. Eating a large meal before you go to work in the evening may make you feel sleepy. And eating very little while at work may also contribute to fatigue. Instead, eat a "breakfast" in the evening before work and plan on eating at least two to three times at work. Bring along trail mix and fruit juice for a midshift snack and also pack a lunch of a sandwich or bean burrito and fruit. Eating every 3 to 4 hours will help you stay energized during work.

To prevent a postexercise energy dip, eat carbohydrate-rich foods within an hour of finishing your workout. If you are exercising at the start of your day, eat a solid breakfast such as hot cereal, toast with peanut butter, and fresh fruit before you head off to work. Then be sure to eat every 2 to 3 hours—crackers and cheese stick at midmorning, tuna sandwich and a salad for lunch, an afternoon snack of dried fruit and soy milk, and then dinner. If you cut back on the size of your three main meals—breakfast, lunch, and dinner—these snacks won't result in weight gain.

Tips for the Night Shift *(continued)*

Avoid caffeine. Loading up on caffeinated beverages such as soda may keep your eyelids open at 3 A.M., but come bedtime at 8 A.M., you may still be wide awake. Because caffeine has a half-life of 5 to 7 hours, hold off drinking anything caffeinated past midnight to give your body time to clear this stimulant by "bedtime."

Modify the protein and carbohydrate content of your meals. Studies show that high-protein foods such as fish, lean meats, and eggs may enhance alertness by altering brain neurochemical levels. So a meal higher in protein such as a tuna sandwich and milk may help you feel more awake as you head off for work. High-carbohydrate foods, on the other hand, alter levels of the brain chemical called *serotonin,* which contributes to feelings of sleepiness. An hour or so before going to bed, munch on breakfast cereal and fruit to help you wind down.

Keep exercise a part of your daily routine. When you wake up in the "morning" or before you head off to work, fit in a workout. Routine exercise has been shown to help reset your body clock, allowing people to sleep better and longer.

Drink more fluids. During a workout of 45 minutes, you can easily lose up to a quart (liter) of sweat. Most people take a few sips of water and rush back to work, not realizing their bodies need more fluid. That dull afternoon headache (which you thought was from your boss) is actually a sign of dehydration.

Check your urine color occasionally by urinating into a clear cup. Pale yellow (lemonade looking) urine means you're hydrated. An amber (apple juice appearance) means you're dehydrated. Drink enough fluid daily, anywhere from 4 to 8 cups to more than 14 cups, depending on your body size and sweat losses, to keep urine pale yellow. Also, hydrate yourself before your workout by drinking at least 1 to 2 cups of fluid. Then as you exercise, drink ½ cup every 15 to 20 minutes.

Check your alcohol consumption. While a glass of wine before retiring may help you feel relaxed and help you fall asleep, studies show that alcohol disrupts deep sleep patterns. Thus you may not be getting restful sleep and, consequently, may wake up in the hole.

More important, alcohol interferes with your body's ability to recover from a workout. When you head to the local bar for a few celebratory beers after that game of softball or long day on the links, your liver, which processes alcohol, gets distracted from refreshing spent glycogen stores. With alcohol present, this job is left undone and can lead to fatigue and poor performance.

Enjoy wine or other alcoholic beverages in moderation (one drink or fewer for women and two or fewer for men) at meals and at least 3 hours before bedtime. Avoid alcohol just after exercise, opting to first restock your fuel stores with a sports drink and a small snack.

GASTROINTESTINAL PROBLEMS

What to eat to avoid pit stops, heartburn, side stitches, and other exercise barriers.

A few years ago, during my long early morning runs, I could count on making at least one pit stop. I'd feel small rumblings in my lower abdomen and try to ignore them. But they'd get stronger, turning into a cramping sensation. At that moment I knew I'd have to either find a restroom or duck into the woods.

I was so embarrassed that I stopped running with my friends. Thankfully, after a bit of experimenting, I realized that skipping my traditional morning latte kept my intestinal track from overreacting to the hour-plus jostling. While I do miss my caffeine, I find that I feel

Quick Tip

If you love high-fiber foods, but experience horrific gas as a result, try using an intestinal enzyme, such as Beano. This over-the-counter product, available at most grocery stores, helps curtail gas production from offensive foods like beans and cabbage. Beano contains an enzyme that breaks down certain carbohydrates in these foods that our intestines barely touch but that bacteria go wild over. A few drops of Beano on your first spoonful of lentil soup or forkful of broccoli heads off gas production in the colon.

fully awake after a 10-minute warm-up, and, better yet, I don't have to plan my running route around bathroom access.

Diarrhea is just one of many different types of gastrointestinal (GI) woes that can turn a fitness pursuit into anything but enjoyable. Others include nausea, gas, and heartburn.

Unfortunately, fitness enthusiasts are slightly more prone to GI problems. Your GI tract needs fluids and blood supply to operate normally. Exercise diverts blood from your stomach and intestines to your working muscles, compromising your GI tract. Also, during hot weather, you may sweat more fluids than you replace.

Furthermore, your GI tract doesn't always appreciate the jostling motion of exercise. Deeper breathing can compress the stomach, for example, pushing acid into the esophagus, causing heartburn or nausea. And jostling can cause your intestine to spasm, bringing on a case of the runs. It can also cause your diaphragm to spasm, bringing on an intense side stitch or ache.

Now for the good news: In most cases, you can easily solve GI problems with the tips included in this section. However, if you chronically have digestive problems during exercise—and none of the tips in this section help—see your doctor. You may have a more serious underlying problem such as irritable bowel syndrome, an ulcer, or Crohn's disease.

Here's how to get your digestive tract back on track:

Be patient with fiber. When I examine the eating habits of those who complain to me about frequent pit stops or about all-too-frequent gas attacks, I usually find that they are following extremely healthful high-fiber diets full of fruits, vegetables, whole grains, and beans. Generally, such a diet is great for your health, but your digestive tract doesn't always appreciate it.

For example, fiber adds bulk to your stool, making pit stops much more likely during your workout. And the carbohydrate in many types of high-fiber foods—such as beans, broccoli, and onions—provides wonderful food for the bacteria that live in your colon. As these bacteria break down food, they produce hydrogen, carbon dioxide, and methane gas.

Because fiber is good for your health, you don't want to eliminate it from your diet. Instead, be patient. Many people who have fiber-related gas have recently increased the amount of fiber in their diet. It takes a while for the natural bacteria in your gut to adjust to your new diet. But don't worry, they will. Over time, the different types of bacteria will flourish in your gut, helping to more efficiently break down your food and create less gas as a result.

Try this experiment. As you wait for the bacteria in your colon to adjust to a high-fiber diet, experiment with different types of beans, vegetables, and fruits. Some may be less gas-forming than others. By switching around, you'll not only lessen gas production but also improve the variety of nutrients in your diet.

If you suffer from during-exercise pit stops, try this timing experiment. Try to eat your lowest-fiber meal just before your workout. And if you have an extra long or intense session coming up, eat lower-fiber meals the day before as well. Then, after your workout, load up on those healthful fruits and vegetables.

Eat friendly bacteria. As I mentioned, a number of types of bacteria live in your gut. While this may seem like a stomach-turning concept, keep in mind that these bacteria help to break down your food so that you can absorb needed nutrients. Like it or not, gut bacteria are good for you. You can't live without these good guys.

Unfortunately, these good guys are extremely sensitive, particularly to antibiotics. Many types of antibiotics can kill beneficial bacteria in your digestive tract, allowing other types of intestinal bugs to flourish, triggering a bout of diarrhea.

Fortunately, many types of foods such as yogurt and some types of milk contain natural and healthful bacteria that will survive the trip through your stomach and into your intestine. Eating these foods every day can help keep the bacteria in your gut at optimal levels.

Try liquid meals. Liquid meals such as Ensure, Slim Fast, and Carnation Instant Breakfast digest quickly, so they may not tax your intestines as much as solid foods eaten a few hours before your workout. No matter what you eat, give yourself 2 to 4 hours to digest any preworkout meal.

Decrease your caffeine consumption. This little drug may irritate your intestines and speed up bowel transit. Beware of some sports gels that contain caffeine. Also, just before exercise, avoid using aspirin and other medications that may irritate your intestines.

Avoid sugar substitutes. Called *sugar alcohols,* sorbitol and manitol are used to sweeten sugarless gum, candies, and other sugar-free products. Your body slowly digests these sugar alcohols. So when you consume large amounts of them, such as eating a pint or more of sugar-free ice cream, your colon bacteria ferment sorbitol and manitol, causing gas and abdominal distension and discomfort.

Stay well hydrated. Dehydration can starve your bowel of needed fluids. Your bowel responds by letting fluids pool in your intestine, which later comes out as diarrhea. So make an extra effort to drink up before and during your workout, especially in hot weather. You should drink ½ cup of fluid every 10 to 20 minutes, or a generous gulp at every water fountain you pass.

Avoid the common offenders. Coffee, alcohol, fatty and spicy foods, chocolate, and citrus fruits have all been associated with GI trouble. Avoid these foods in the couple hours leading up to your workout. And if you are a heavy coffee drinker, try quitting altogether.

Eat smaller meals. Large meals can take up a lot of room in your stomach, forcing stomach acid up where it doesn't belong. They also make your stomach heavier, more likely to bring on a side stitch. Finally, if you tend to eat a high-fiber diet, or are particularly partial to beans, broccoli, and cabbage, which are notorious gas-forming foods, you are better off eating small meals rather than gorging on larger amounts. By presenting small amounts of these gas-forming foods, less gas is produced and it's spread out more evenly during the day.

Switch to a nibbling lifestyle, if possible, and try to eat small meals surrounding your workouts. During longer workouts, take small bites on an energy bar or small nibbles of gel rather than downing the whole bar or gel at once.

Stay upright. Many people come home from a long workout, slurp down a huge meal, and then flop onto the couch. This supine position on the couch encourages all that stomach acid needed to digest that large meal to come up into your esophagus. Try to walk around or remain in an upright sitting position for a couple of hours after eating. If you do get heartburn, try downing a glass of milk or water. It should wash the acid back down into your stomach.

Get the salt you need. If you drink too much water before and during an ultraendurance event, you can dilute the sodium in your blood, which can make you feel nauseous. Sports drinks are your best bet since they contain some sodium. However, the salt added to foods you eat easily supplies the sodium you need (and then some), so there's no need to heavily salt your food.

Try ginger. If you feel nauseous after an endurance event, try ingesting some ginger. Real ginger ale (look for ginger listed as one of the ingredients) or a ginger tea made with ground ginger root may help ease nausea. Some people find that defizzed cola also helps.

Limit your lactose intake. Many people suffer from the inability to digest milk sugar, or lactose. Then your colon bacteria happily ferment the lactose, forming gas and giving you a bloated feeling. Milk, some yogurts, ice cream, and other dairy products may trigger gas trouble in lactose-intolerant people.

Delay eating after a tough workout. Because your working muscles are in greater need of oxygen and nutrients, heavy exercise reduces blood flow to the intestinal tract. As you recover from a session of exercise, your blood flow needs some time to readjust. That's why some individuals find eating soon after a workout creates greater gas formation or nausea as the intestinal tract may not yet be ready for work. Waiting 30 to 60 minutes to eat may help lessen gas production following that meal.

GOLF

The right foods to help you focus, calm your shaky hands, and endure an entire day of lugging your clubs.

Many people minimize the importance of performance nutrition when it comes to golf—and their game suffers as a result.

For example, my friend Diane often hit the links with a group of ladies literally at the crack of dawn. Because these excursions were so early in the morning, she regularly skipped breakfast.

Diane complained to me that her hands often shook during the game, and she generally grew tired before the 18th hole. I encouraged

Quick Tip

Practice makes perfect. That clichéd saying couldn't be more true about golf. While performance nutrition will certainly help your game, it's no substitute for time on the course. If you are doing everything right in the nutrition department, but your game continues to suffer, invest in some lessons. It could be that a simple adjustment in your form or your swing could make all the difference out on the course.

her to store shelf-stable food—such as boxed cranberry juice drinks—in her car, to snack and sip on her way to her golf outing.

At first, she scoffed at my advice. "Golf is a social outing, not a fitness routine," she told me. "What difference will food make?"

I told her to just trust me, and sure enough, her game improved.

Despite what many people think, golf *is* a form of exercise, especially if you carry your clubs. A full game of golf will keep you on the links for hours. During those hours you are burning calories, sweating fluids, and concentrating more than you do during a typical day at work. If you walk the course rather than ride in a cart, you'll cover 4 to 5 miles, depending on the course. You'll burn 400 to 500 calories by the end of the game. Lugging your own clubs adds about 100 to 150 calories to that burn. And swinging the club gives your back, hips, buttocks, and thighs a good workout.

Add all of that together, and you're in desperate need for proper performance nutrition. A day on the links requires you to be vigilant about fitness nutrition. Here are some tips:

Stay hydrated. Depending on the weather, you can lose a liter or more of sweat in an hour of golfing. If you're lugging your own clubs, your sweat losses can be even greater.

If you don't replenish lost sweat, your performance suffers. Feelings of light-headedness, fatigue, and even nausea are telltale signs of dehydration. Don't wait until you feel thirsty. Thirst typically lags behind true dehydration, signaling you to drink up long after you've gotten stuck in the sand trap.

To stay hydrated, drink about ½ cup of plain water or sports drink every 15 to 20 minutes. If you're worried about nature calling while out on the course, stick with sports drinks. The small amount of salt in the drink will encourage your body to retain fluids, decreasing urination.

Nibble as you go. Though it's not as rigorous as some other sports such as running, you do burn some calories playing golf. Depending on your body size, walking speed, club-carrying efforts, and course length, expect to use up anywhere from 150 to 400 calories or more per hour.

On a typical day, you usually eat every few hours, even when you're sitting at your desk at work. Now you're walking for miles and standing for hours. As your muscles and brain pull sugar out of your bloodstream, your liver falls behind on replacing it. Once your blood sugar falls, you lose your ability to concentrate and can even become shaky and light-headed.

To prevent a blood sugar drop, munch on fresh or dried fruit or a light sandwich, or drink a 16-ounce sports drink every 2 to 4 hours to stay energized. Many people lose their appetite when playing a long game of golf on a hot day. If you don't feel like eating during your game, then at least eat a small meal beforehand, even if that means shifting mealtimes, eating lunch at 10 or 11 A.M., for example.

Nix the caffeine. Caffeine (from coffee, tea, or soda) can cause feelings of anxiousness. That, along with even the slightest trembling or shaking, can take the control out of your swing.

If you're not a veteran coffee drinker, you're better off leaving the java alone. Of course, if you're a big coffee drinker, you don't want to

Your Preseason Program

To get your shoulders in shape for a long day of swinging your clubs, try this simple exercise three times a week during the off-season.

Hold a pair of dumbbells at your sides (2 to 15 pounds each, depending on your strength). Simultaneously lift both arms out to the sides, raising them until your hands are level with your shoulders. Lower and repeat 10 times. Take a 1-minute break, then do the same exercise, except only raise your arms 45 degrees, lower, and repeat 10 times. Take a 1-minute break and repeat again, this time raising your arms 90 degrees, lowering them to 45 degrees, and raising them back to 90 degrees, continuing to pulse up and down 10 times.

go off coffee cold turkey on the same day of a big game. In fact, avoiding caffeine only on the day of play may cause a performance disaster.

Caffeine from coffee, tea, colas, and other beverages acts as a stimulant, making you feel more awake (I'm thankful for that). The catch: Your body becomes addicted. A caffeine jolt in the morning, for example, is a typical ritual for many people. But if you go without your regular dose, withdrawal symptoms like headache and lethargy kick in within a few hours. The last thing you want while you're out there baking in the sun is a headache and low energy.

If drinking coffee or another caffeinated beverage is part of your daily routine, either abstain from caffeine every day or stick with it every day. Just don't combine the two methods. And don't *increase* your intake on the day of a game. If you plan to quit, don't go cold turkey. Instead, cut your regular dose with decaf over several weeks, starting with a 20 percent reduction the first week. Then switch to tea, which has less caffeine. Then switch to an herbal tea, which has no caffeine at all.

Forgo the beer. Indeed, there couldn't be a worse thing to drink if you want to keep your focus. Alcohol slows your reaction time and impairs your judgment, both skills that you need plenty of during a day on the links. You're better off celebrating your victory with a drink afterward instead of imbibing on the course.

If you must drink, at least alternate your beer with a bottle of sports drink to avoid dehydration.

HEADACHE

Whether caused by exercise or by some other trigger, here's how to stop the throb.

Headaches can make exercise anything but enjoyable. Many people complain of headaches particularly after exercise on a hot day, when the heat in their head coupled with the dehydration from sweating brings on a painful throbbing sensation.

Others feel a headache coming on well before exercise, and, for some of them, the stress relief provided by exercise helps obliterate the throb. For others, however, exercise only makes a headache worse, taking what was once just a dull ache and turning it into a throbbing monster.

Headaches can be caused—and cured—by a variety of triggers, and finding out what causes yours may take some detective work. Start your fact-finding mission by keeping a headache diary for a week or two, writing down your sleeping, eating, drinking, computer, and exercise habits along with the onset, duration, and severity of your headaches. That information will help you to spot patterns. For example, when you look over your diary, you may notice that your headaches always occur on a day when you've eaten a particular food.

Here are some more tips to help stop the ache:

Check your alcohol consumption. Alcohol can also trigger headaches in numerous ways. For example, the nitrates in red wine and the congeners in hard liquor such as gin and tequila can bring on a headache in people sensitive to those additives. Look for low- or no-nitrate wines and congener-free liquor. (It will say so on the bottle.) Also, alcohol is a diuretic, meaning it causes your body to excrete fluids. If you don't follow up with other liquids such as water or a sports drink, you can become dehydrated, which can also lead to a headache.

Look at your caffeine habits. When you drink a lot of caffeinated beverages, such as coffee, tea, and cola, your brain becomes addicted to them. Then, when you're too busy to down your daily cup of coffee, a withdrawal headache sets in.

Some people are also sensitive to substances in coffee and tea (also in red wine) called *tannins.* To avoid a headache caused by tannins, you may be able to switch brands and solve your headache issue, as some brands contain more tannins than others. Also, there are different types of tannins, and you may only be sensitive to some of them. Of course, this takes some experimentation. Look back through your headache diary. Were there days you didn't get headaches when you drank a different type of coffee or tea?

Another option is to slowly wean yourself off tea and coffee. However, don't just go cold turkey, because the caffeine withdrawal in itself will trigger a headache. So try to slowly cut back on the number of cups that you drink a day. You can also replace caffeinated coffee with decaf (replace about 20 percent of your regular coffee with decaf each week until you've slowly weaned yourself from caffeinated coffee).

Examine your meal patterns. Because your brain runs on the sugar glucose, simply skipping a meal can easily bring on a dull headache. These usually strike in the afternoon, after the effects of skipping breakfast or lunch take their toll.

Test your wheat sensitivity. A small number of people may be sensitive to the type of protein found in wheat, called *gluten.* For these people, gluten brings on a host of symptoms from intestinal trouble to headaches. One small study recently found that eliminating gluten

Quick Tip

If you get more than two headaches a week, ask your doctor about a new class of migraine medications called *triptans.* Sold under the brands Imitrex (sumatriptan), Maxalt (rizatriptan benzoate), Zomig (zolmitriptan), and Amerge (naratriptan), among others, these prescription drugs stop the mechanism in your brain that triggers a headache. Those who take them find that the drugs can stop a headache within ½ hour. They work especially well for people who have become addicted to over-the-counter painkillers and suffer withdrawal headaches as a result.

from the diet can reduce the incidence of headaches. To find out if you are gluten sensitive, take a look at your headache diary. Do your headaches surface on the same day that you eat wheat products such as pasta, bread, and anything else made from wheat flour? If so, try eliminating gluten from your diet. This isn't as much of a hardship as it may first seem. You'll find wonderful substitutes for wheat foods at your local health food store and often at the grocery store. Look for pastas, crackers, cereals, and breads labeled "gluten free." Often these products are made from other power grains such as quinoa, spelt, oats, and barley.

Stay hydrated. Because your brain is 75 percent water, a dull headache can result from dehydration. Following your exercise session, drink at least 2 cups of fluid. But don't stop there. Drink plenty of fluid at work—water, sports drink, herbal tea, or fruit juice. Your body still loses fluid as the day wears on, especially if you are working in a dry heated or air-conditioned office. You're drinking enough water when you empty your full bladder four to five times daily.

Consider a riboflavin supplement. Some research suggests that supplementing with high doses of this water-soluble B vitamin may reduce the incidence of migraine headaches (the type characterized by throbbing pain on one side of the head). Because this research is so preliminary, we're really not sure why riboflavin supplements may work.

Riboflavin is safe in high doses, as your body simply excretes the excess in your urine (turning it bright yellow). To see results, research shows you need 400 daily milligrams for at least three months.

Cut way back on fat. Some research shows that cutting fat intake to fewer than 20 grams a day may ease migraine headaches in some people. A lowfat diet may ease headache symptoms indirectly by helping to better balance your consumption of different types of fat. Most of us eat too much saturated fat (found in animal products), trans fat (found in hydrogenated or processed foods), and omega-6 fats (found in cooking oils) but too little omega-3 fats (found predominantly in fish). Because our distant ancestors ate much more omega-3 fats and much less of the other types of fat, researchers suspect that this modern-day fat imbalance may lead to a host of ailments, including headaches.

Rather than cutting your fat consumption down to a stark 20 grams, I recommend first boosting your consumption of omega-3 fats by eating more fish and flaxseed (and products made from them). Then, if you continue to get headaches, cut back on trans fats by avoiding fried foods and processed foods that list "hydrogenated" or "partially hydrogenated" oil on the label. Finally, if you haven't already, switch to fat-free milk, nonfat dairy products, and lean cuts of meat.

Check your magnesium intake. Some research has found a connection between headache incidence and marginal magnesium status in some people. Though few people are low in this mineral, you might want to look at your headache diary to see how many high-magnesium foods you generally eat in a day. High-magnesium foods include green vegetables, beans, nuts, cocoa and chocolate, whole grains, and molasses.

HEART DISEASE

Everyone—men and women—should take steps to prevent our number one killer.

When it comes to health issues, many people file heart disease under the "problems for men" category and osteoporosis under the "problems for women" category.

This thinking couldn't be more off target. Heart attacks rank as the leading cause of death for both men and women, and the number of deaths are growing, particularly among women. The heart attack rate for women grew by 36 percent during the 1980s and 1990s but only by 8 percent for men, according to a study done by the Mayo Clinic in Rochester, Minnesota.

In fact, more than eight times as many women die from heart attack as from breast cancer.

Surprised? You're not alone.

Heart Disease 101

Heart disease starts as early as childhood. Your arteries become clogged with cholesterol-and-fat buildup called *plaque* through a series of steps. Interrupting those steps or at least delaying them will give you an edge on heart health.

One of the first steps is high blood cholesterol.

Surprisingly, cholesterol, a waxlike substance, is not all bad. In fact, every cell in your body needs cholesterol for proper functioning. However, you can have too much of a good thing.

Because cholesterol, along with fat, doesn't dissolve in your circulation for easy transport, these substances have to take a ride inside microscopic transport vehicles called *lipoproteins* for delivery to cells.

LDL and HDL along with others such as VLDL are lipoproteins that carry cholesterol and fat throughout your circulatory system. I

Your Heart-Healthy Menu

Try the following menu to load up on natural heart disease fighters.

Breakfast

1 cup 9-grain cereal topped with 1 teaspoon chopped walnuts, 1 tablespoon honey, and 2 tablespoons dried cherries

1 cup blueberries with ¾ cup 1% milk

Lunch

1 cup bean salad made with 1 tablespoon olive oil and vinegar dressing

1 3-inch square cornbread spread with 2 tablespoons apple butter

1 cup fruit salad (strawberries, cantaloupe, grapes)

1 cup vanilla soy milk

Snack

⅓ cup soy nuts with dried papaya and pineapple

6 ounces mango juice

Dinner

4 ounces grilled tuna over 1 cup curried rice

2 cups spring mix salad tossed with ½ red pepper, 1 ounce goat cheese, 2 tablespoons raspberry vinaigrette

1 cup apple cobbler made with oats, brown sugar, and walnut topping

Nutritional analysis—calories: 2,000; protein: 75 grams; carbohydrate: 300 grams; calories from fat: 24%.

like to think of these lipoproteins as buses that transport their cholesterol and fat passengers to body cells or bus stops. The job of the LDL "bus" is to deliver cholesterol to body cells for use, and the HDL

Quick Tip

You may have heard that garlic contains heart-healthy substances. Thioallyls, substances also found in onions, have been shown to lower blood cholesterol levels. When garlic is eaten raw, cooked, or in powdered form, these various thioallyls appear to lower LDL levels and keep the blood thin, so risky blood clots are less likely to form.

Studies show that about a clove a day has cholesterol-lowering benefit. Try using garlic in your meals: a stir-fry with colorful vegetables (peppers, bok choy, snap peas) and garlic; crushed garlic tossed with pasta; or powdered garlic added to soups and stews. If garlic doesn't agree with your intestinal tract (some people report excess gas and cramping with abundant levels of garlic in the diet), you can take the equivalent in garlic pills found at health food stores.

bus picks up wandering cholesterol, bringing it back to the bus "depot" (the liver) for possible disposal from the body.

It turns out the LDL buses may not always make it to their destination and instead drive out of control and crash into your artery walls and litter their cholesterol passengers onto the walls. Over years of buildup, cholesterol hardens and blocks the flow of blood, causing heart disease. This is why you may often hear LDL called the "bad cholesterol."

Research clearly shows that people with high LDL levels (above 100 milligrams per deciliter) have a greater risk of developing heart disease. Vice versa, high HDL levels (above 40) help to lower heart disease risk. And a high total cholesterol level (200 and above) also increases your risk.

Beyond cholesterol, a host of other factors also contribute to heart disease, with high blood pressure leading the list. Every time your heart beats, it creates pressure to push blood through your arteries. Narrow arteries create more pressure as the same amount of blood rushes through a smaller space. This extra pressure can damage the lining of your arteries all over your body, leading to heart disease, stroke, dementia, and even blindness.

Blood pressure is measured with an arm-cuff device and is recorded as two numbers: systolic, which is the pressure exerted as the heart beats; and diastolic, which is the pressure exerted as the heart relaxes between beats. A reading of 140/90 (systolic/diastolic) is considered high.

What You Can Do

A heart-healthy diet and regular physical activity play a tremendous role in lowering and maintaining safe levels of cholesterol, as well as other heart disease risk factors.

Don't look at this as a prison sentence. There's no need to banish your favorite foods from your daily fare. Rather than approaching your situation with a what-not-to-eat attitude, focus on what lifestyle *additions* can knock down your cholesterol levels and boost heart health. Here are some tips:

Get in motion. Regular aerobic exercise, such as walking, jogging, or bike riding, helps lower levels of the artery-clogging cholesterol carrier (LDL) while boosting amounts of the good cholesterol transporter (HDL). Regular exercise, such as jogging, cycling, and weight lifting, also helps improve circulation, lowering blood pressure, a risk factor for heart disease. Adding regular activity to your daily routine, about four to five days a week for 20 to 30 minutes, has been shown to cut heart disease risk.

Get strong. Adding strength training, such as weight lifting or calisthenics that work both upper and lower body, also helps lower cholesterol levels while boosting the HDL good guys. Lifting two times

Are You at Risk?

To find out if you are at risk for heart disease, take this quiz by answering "yes" or "no" to the 10 statements and then tallying your score.

1. During the past year, my blood pressure was not checked.
2. I am older than age 45.
3. I am male, or I am female older than age 55.
4. My total blood cholesterol count is more than 200.
5. I smoke or used to smoke more than a pack or day, or I live with someone who smokes.
6. I am sedentary, getting less than 30 minutes of moderate activity, such as walking, a day.
7. My doctor has told me that I am overweight or obese.
8. I have excess weight around my middle.
9. My father or mother has been diagnosed with heart disease or high blood pressure, or has suffered from a heart attack or stroke.
10. I eat foods with added fats (chips, baked goods) and use dressings, margarine, oils, or fat-containing spreads on foods. I eat beef and other meats, eggs, and full-fat dairy products frequently.

Add up your number of "yes" answers and check the following to see what your score means.

0—Your risk is low.

1 to 3—Answering "yes" to any one of the questions means you are at a greater risk for developing heart disease and should do what you can to lower your risk.

4 or more—Make an appointment with your doctor for a review of your health—especially if you answered "yes" to questions 4 and 5, as cholesterol and smoking are major players in heart attacks.

per week for ½ hour (one set of eight to 12 different exercises) should do the trick.

Eat more monounsaturated fat. Reach for monounsaturated fats when cooking. Olive, canola, and peanut oil make great choices for stir-fries, salad dressing, and baking. Studies show that substituting monounsaturated fats for saturated fats (butter, lard, margarine, and vegetable shortening) lowers LDL cholesterol levels and cuts risk for heart disease.

Add soy to the mix. Tofu, soy milk, veggie burgers, and other foods made with soy protein protect your heart in several ways. First, daily servings of soy (aim for 25 grams of soy protein daily) help lower cholesterol levels. Also, substances in soy, called *isoflavones,* help protect your arteries from damage that leads to heart disease. They also make platelets less likely to stick together and form a clot that can lead to a deadly heart attack. Use soy milk on your breakfast cereal, add soy powder to smoothies, and use tofu as you would meat, eggs, or sour cream.

Reach for fiber. Adding more water-soluble fiber—found in beans (kidney, lentils, garbanzo, and others), fruits, and oat products such as oatmeal and oat bran—knocks down cholesterol levels. This special fiber traps cholesterol and its by-products in the intestinal tract, keeping cholesterol from entering your body. A bowl of oatmeal in the morning along with bean chili for lunch will get your cholesterol level moving in the right direction.

Pick fruit. Aim for four pieces of fruit daily (one medium-sized piece of fruit or ½ cup of juice). Vitamin C in fruit such as oranges has been shown to protect against the damage to artery walls instigated by LDL that leads to heart disease. The phytochemicals in fruits also act as antioxidants fending off damage that gum up your arteries.

Go fish. Add a serving of fish (3 to 4 ounces) at least once or twice a week to cut your risk of heart disease by as much as 35 percent. The fat in fish called omega-3s helps lower cholesterol levels and keeps platelets from sticking together and forming unwanted blood clots.

Fish oil capsules, which contain omega-3 fats, have been popular for some time. Makers of these supplements simply extract the fat from fish, particularly fatty fish such as salmon, mackerel, and sardines. However, the abundance of research shows that *eating* fish, rather than taking fish oil supplements, is protective against heart disease. Since the evidence in favor of fish-oil supplements for heart health is much weaker, scientists believe that other nutrients in the fish may have beneficial effects along with the omega-3 fats.

Snack on nuts. Almonds, walnuts, peanuts, and other nuts contain monounsaturated fats and vitamin E, which work to lower cholesterol levels and block damage to artery walls. Rather than snacking on chips, cookies, and other processed snack foods that contain hydrogenated fats (trans fats), which raise cholesterol levels, grab a handful of nuts.

Look for lean cuts of meat. Choosing lean meats along with lowfat or fat-free dairy products helps cut your intake of artery-clogging saturated fats. And you needn't eliminate eggs either, as studies show that eating eggs won't raise cholesterol levels as part of a low-saturated-fat diet that includes fruits, vegetables, and plenty of fiber.

Indulge in chocolate. Chocolate contains powerful phytochemicals called *polyphenols,* which work wonders for your heart. Polyphenols act as antioxidants, which keep LDL cholesterol from running amok on your artery walls. Keep serving sizes under control, as chocolate does come with calories. Try cocoa powder mixed with warm nonfat milk for a heart-healthy cup of hot chocolate.

Boost your veggies. Eating eight to 10 daily servings of vegetables and fruits helps lower cholesterol levels and helps prevent damage to artery walls from LDL buses driving out of control. Fruits and vegetables are also loaded with the mineral potassium, which helps to regulate blood pressure and counteract the effects of a high-sodium diet.

HIKING

Why you should always pack more than you need.

I learned one of my most important hiking lessons while at Yosemite National Park with my good friend and fellow nutrition expert, Kris Clark, and my kids, Natalie and Grant. We were packing for a 4- to 6-hour hike up one of the more challenging cliffs in the park, and I was stuffing enough energy bars and trail mix into my fanny pack to allow myself and my kids to eat about 100 calories every half hour.

I zipped up my pack and then glanced at Kris. She was stuffing enough food into her pack to feed an army—or so I thought. "Gosh, Kris, don't you think you're going a little overboard? You've got more than me, and I'm packing enough for three," I teased.

Fortunately, she didn't listen. Though my formula of 100 calories per half hour generally makes sense, I had forgotten to factor in lunch—and the fact that we'd be hiking through it. About halfway through the hike I was hungry, and so were the kids. I glanced at Kris, who had more than enough food. Thankfully, she was willing to share. Of course, then it was my turn to be teased.

Thus, my lesson: When planning any hiking excursion, take more food and water than you expect to consume! Every hiking trip—whether along the steep climbs of beautiful Yosemite, the large boulders of the Appalachian trail, or the wooded paths in your own backyard—requires careful preparation and planning. Taking a little extra time to pack the right essentials makes the difference between enjoying your hike and wishing you had stayed home.

Here's what to keep in mind:

Wear the right gear. If you've ever ventured into a performance-wear store, you know how expensive waterproof jackets and boots can be. They are worth every cent. There's nothing that can make a hike more miserable, more quickly, than cold, wet feet.

A pair of waterproof boots will allow you to cross shallow streams. They'll also help you trounce through snowcaps along the top of a mountain without your feet getting wet. Your waterproof jacket will also do wonders at keeping you dry. Plus, these jackets can be scrunched up into a tiny ball that fits into any pack, perfect for a high-altitude hike where you start out at 80 degrees and end up with 30 degrees and snow at the top.

Pack enough to feed every hiker on the mountain. Okay, maybe not that much, but you do want to bring along a bit more than you expect to eat. Depending on the terrain, trail incline, weight of your pack, and hiking speed, you can easily burn 400 or more calories per hour. Your muscles will burn stored carbohydrate energy, called *glycogen,* as well as stored fat. During several hours of hiking, your stores of glycogen can easily run out, leaving you feeling too drained to take another step, let alone get back to camp.

So take along enough food to provide about 150 to 200 calories every one-half to one hour. And, if you're going for a long hike, don't make the same mistake I did in Yosemite. Remember to pack the equivalent of breakfast, lunch, and dinner.

Pack as much water as you can carry. Fluids rank top on the list of necessities for an all-day hike. As you tromp on the trail, your body generates heat that must be dissipated so that your organs and muscles don't overheat and, literally, go into failure. Also, during warm weather, your body sweats more in an effort to stay cool. Finally, you lose more fluids at high altitudes than at ground level.

Under these conditions, you can easily lose about a liter of sweat per hour. Plan to pack enough water to supply ½ cup (250 milliliters) every 15 minutes. If you have a dog with you, remember that your furry companion also will need water. Many pet stores sell doggie backpacks that allow your pooch to tote its own food and water, rather than weighing you down even more.

Bring a water filter for hikes lasting 8 or more hours. The germs giardia and cryptosporidium and others that lurk in running stream water can bring on a terrible case of diarrhea and cramping. It's tough to carry enough water—because of the weight—to last more than 8 hours, so invest in a water filter or purifier. These gadgets are getting smaller and lighter, and most cost $50 or less. Also, do some research before heading out, to make sure a stream runs along the trail.

Focus on lightweight nonsquishables. Your backpack only has so much space, and you can physically carry only so much weight. So you want lightweight foods that don't take up a lot of space and that also don't get easily smashed by other objects in your pack.

Besides weight and durability, also consider the trash factor. If you're hiking responsibly, you should pack out trash—not leave it on the side of the trail. So bring along a plastic bag to stow trash for disposal later.

Ideally, you want food that is high in carbohydrate—to keep your muscles fueled. But you also need some fat and protein to keep you satisfied. Since fat packs more than twice as many calories per gram as carbohydrate, taking along some nutritious fat-rich foods helps cut down on weight in your backpack. Here are some good, lightweight options that won't take up a lot of room in your pack:

- Dried fruit, including raisins, apples, papaya, and others
- Beef or turkey jerky
- Nuts
- Trail mix, made from your favorite goodies, such as nuts, dried fruits, breakfast cereal, soy nuts, and, my favorite, chocolate chips and M&M's (Store trail mix in a sealable plastic bag. There's nothing worse than losing a twist tie and getting nuts all through your pack.)
- Dried fish (Give it a try—you may like it!)
- Energy bars and gels
- Peanut butter and cracker "sandwiches"

Your Preseason Program

There's nothing more uncomfortable than heading out for your first hike of the season only to feel a sharp pain between your shoulder blades under the weight of your pack, an uncomfortable tightness in your calves from wearing boots for the first time in months, and a burn in your butt and thighs each time you struggle to mount a boulder.

Good thing you can easily get in shape for hiking with two simple activities.

1. Take the stairs every chance you get. Climbing stairs simulates the motion of stepping up rocks. In the month before your first hike, agree to never take an elevator or escalator.

2. Wear your backpack often. When walking the dog, put on your hiking boots and stuff something heavy in your pack. Also, take your pack with you and wear it every chance you get. For example, take it to the grocery store and stuff it with your groceries, use it as your briefcase, or stuff it with your workout gear to haul to the gym.

Don't forget the salt. During long hikes, you can develop a rare but dangerous condition called hyponatremia. This condition, in which the blood sodium becomes diluted, is caused by sweating too much sodium or drinking too much water (or, more likely, both). This electrolyte imbalance causes a number of symptoms from fatigue to dizziness to nausea to death. The symptoms are similar to dehydration with one major difference. When you are dehydrated and you drink water, you tend to feel better quickly. When you have hyponatremia and you drink water, you feel worse.

Though hyponatremia can be caused by drinking copious amounts of water, don't opt for dehydration. Instead, consume some form of salt during your hike. The salt can come in the form of a sports drink or from the nuts or small pretzels in your trail mix.

Cooking 101

Trail mix is a hiking staple. Experiment by tossing together your favorite foods. My only caution: Don't load it up with food that's so irresistible (such as chocolate) that you are tempted to demolish the entire bag of mix during the first 20 minutes of your hike. Here's what I like to pack:

½ cup almonds
1 cup dried cranberries
½ cup raisins
½ cup dried papaya
¼ cup cashews
¼ cup roasted soy nuts (not a true nut but a stellar source of protein)
¼ cup shredded coconut (optional)

Combine all ingredients and store in a plastic container with a tightly fitting lid. Keeps about six weeks in the refrigerator. Makes 10 ⅓-cup servings.

Nutritional analysis (per serving)—calories: 167; protein: 4 grams; carbohydrate: 25 grams; calories from fat: 34%.

Pack light. For most, 50 pounds is the limit they can carry on their back and still feel comfortable. If you're on vacation, you may be carrying a little more than usual, such as a camera or some binoculars. Such items take up space in your pack. They also weigh quite a bit. So you'll have to make careful choices about what else goes in your bag.

Consider investing in a water backpack device, which works well for hiking and holds a substantial amount of water. These backpacks have an inner "bladder" with a convenient mouth tube that enables hands-free drinking. Also, many have other compartments to stash fuel like energy bars and trail mix.

Don't forget these essentials. Beyond food, you also should pack a few lightweight, small pieces of gear to ensure safety. I always bring a knife for emergency foraging, a whistle to blow to attract attention in case of emergency, a trail map, a compass, lip balm, sunblock (you're more likely to burn at higher altitudes), and a first aid kit that includes antiseptic and bandages.

Tie up your food. If you plan to camp in the wilderness, bring nylon rope to hang your food from tree branches. While it seems logical to stash food in your tent, think about what types of animals lurk in those parts. You don't want a bear sniffing around your tent in the middle of the night.

INJURY PRONE

The foods you need to bounce back quickly.

Not long ago, I found myself wheelchair bound, a result of numerous knee surgeries to repair a hole in my cartilage. I'd love to say that I injured my knee doing something impressive, such as skiing the Swiss Alps or even winning the three-legged race at a spring picnic.

But I did it in my kitchen. I slid on a slick spot and landed on my knee—hard. I didn't know it at the time, but that quick hard fall punched a hole in my cartilage. No wonder my knee continued to ache. The hole allowed bone to rub against bone.

I went to several doctors before fully realizing the extent of the damage. Every time my sore knee interfered with a bike ride, run, or swim, I felt frustrated. I felt even more frustrated as the soreness intensified, making me limp during my daily walk with the dog.

As I'm sure you can understand, I wanted to gain back a pain-free leg as quickly as possible. If you're reading this chapter, I'm sure you feel the same way.

To get better, I researched every way to heal my knee. In the process, I made some startling discoveries about what nutritional remedies not

How to Keep Off Creeping Weight

If you have been told by your doctor not to exercise, one of your first thoughts was probably "How am I going to keep from gaining weight?"

Relax. Even though you are not exercising—or exercising as much—your metabolism is still burning calories, between 5 and 15 percent more than usual, to patch your tattered body. Also, for most injuries, total downtime usually lasts two weeks.

If you restrict calories too much during this two-week window, you may end up lengthening your recovery time because your body won't have enough energy and protein to both repair your injury and complete other bodily functions. How can you prevent weight gain and still ensure a sound recovery? Don't cut more than 250 to 500 daily calories, and if you notice that you're losing weight, immediately start eating more.

only help heal an injury but also can prevent one from starting in the first place. Whether you're suffering from a pulled calf muscle, torn rotator cuff, sprained ankle, or broken leg, use the following tips to help mount a strong defense against muscle tears and strains:

Eat more. Chronic dieting puts your body in prime injury-waiting-to-happen mode. Your body needs calories. When it doesn't get enough, it raids your protein stores, which doesn't leave enough protein for basic muscle repair. End result: muscle tears.

If you're trying to lose weight—and you're not injured—cut no more than 500 daily calories from your diet. If you are injured and want to avoid weight gain during your downtime, see sidebar, "How to Keep Off Creeping Weight."

Make protein a mainstay. You need 80 to 100 grams of protein a day to maintain your muscles and other soft tissues. A small 3-ounce serving of chicken provides about 25 grams, a glass of milk 10 grams, a soy burger 14 grams, and a hard-boiled egg, 6 grams. Try to include a high-protein food with every meal.

Focus on zinc and iron. Fitness enthusiasts are notoriously low in these two important trace nutrients found predominantly in red meat. Though research hasn't linked zinc and iron deficiency with increased injury rates, I've noticed the connection when working with injured athletes, and so have many of my sports nutrition colleagues.

You need 15 milligrams of zinc and 18 milligrams of iron a day. Most people don't consume nearly that much, which is why I recommend eating a zinc-and-iron-fortified breakfast cereal or taking a multivitamin that contains both minerals.

Bone up on calcium. If you have a stress fracture or a broken bone, consuming enough of this important mineral will help, along with a healthy diet that includes adequate protein, vitamin C, and other essential nutrients.

However, don't go overboard. At high doses, about 1,000 milligrams in one sitting, calcium reduces the absorption of the mineral iron. Your daily supplement should supply no more than 500 milligrams. If you eat dairy products (about two to three servings daily) or regularly drink calcium-fortified orange juice or other calcium-fortified products, you are probably meeting your calcium needs and don't need a supplement.

Remember to rest, too. You must give a stress fracture a six-week time-out from physical stress so it can heal. All the calcium in the world isn't going to cut that rest time any shorter.

Load up on orange vegetables. They're loaded with beta-carotene, which is converted to vitamin A in the body. Your body uses vitamin A to make new epithelial tissue, the cellular covering along most of the internal and external surfaces of your body such as your lungs, skin, and blood vessels. New research shows that your body isn't as efficient at converting the carotenes from fruits and vegetables into vitamin A as we once thought, which means you need to eat even

Cooking 101

Some fitness enthusiasts are chronically malnourished—and injury prone—not because they are skimping on calories but because their busy lifestyles prevent them from cooking nutritious meals. The good news is that cooking healing foods doesn't have to take that much time. One of the quickest and easiest ways to boost the nutrition of your diet is to make a big pot of soup once a week and ladle yourself a bowl a day until it's gone.

Try this zinc-and-protein-packed stew. It's loaded with what you need to heal.

2 cloves of garlic, crushed
1 medium onion, chopped
1 tablespoon olive oil
2 medium carrots, sliced
2 medium russet potatoes, cut into bite-sized pieces
1 15-ounce can vegetable broth, low-sodium
1 bay leaf
Fresh ground pepper (to taste)
6 to 8 ounces of fresh catfish fillet, cut into bite-sized pieces
1 small can of clams with juice
1 small can of oysters
2 ounces canned anchovies (optional)
2 medium tomatoes, chopped

more of them. You need two servings of leafy greens and yellow and orange vegetables every day during your recovery. Also, drinking vitamin A–fortified milk is a good idea.

Don't skimp on fruit. Your body needs plenty of vitamin C to make collagen, an adhesive-like protein found in your bones, connective

Cooking 101 *(continued)*

In a large soup pot, sauté garlic and onion in olive oil. Add carrot slices and potatoes. Brown for 5 minutes. Pour broth over vegetables. Add bay leaf and ground pepper and then add enough water to cover potatoes. Bring to a boil and then simmer until potatoes are soft but not mushy. Turn up the heat to medium-high and add catfish. Simmer 3 to 5 minutes. Add clams, oysters, anchovies, and chopped tomatoes. Cook another 3 to 5 minutes. (Do not overcook as this tends to toughen clams and oysters.) Serves 6.

Nutritional analysis—calories: 223; protein: 23 grams; carbohydrate: 23 grams; calories from fat: 17%. (Supplies 86% of the Daily Value of vitamin A, 62% of iron, 50% of zinc, 45% of vitamin C, and 9% of calcium.)

tissues, and blood vessels. When you're injured, collagen is the stuff that glues the injured area back together. Women need 75 milligrams and men 90 milligrams of vitamin C a day. If you eat five to seven servings a day of berries, cantaloupe, oranges, and other fruit along with vegetables like tomato, broccoli, and pepper, you'll easily exceed that requirement.

Add supplements to the mix. Once you've injured a joint in your body, you're at a higher risk for developing osteoarthritis down the road. Fortunately, the supplements glucosamine and chondroitin sulfate have been shown to help lower inflammation, prevent osteoarthritis, and promote cartilage growth. It's not certain whether glucosamine, an amino acid, or chondroitin, one of the substances that make up cartilage, can work alone or need to be taken together. So, for now, take 1,200 to 1,500 milligrams of each daily—best divided into three doses. Why so often? These supplements have a short half-life in the body. Frequent supplementation ensures that they are prevalent at all times when you need them. (Note: If you are on anticoagulents, do not take chondroitin but consult your physician.)

MENOPAUSE

How to stay healthy and fit when your hormones take a dip.

Many women refer to menopause as the "change"; however, I've always felt the colloquial term for menopause should be plural, "the changes."

As estrogen and other hormone levels drop during menopause, your body goes through a series of changes, not just one. You're probably already well aware of the changes you can see and feel, such as hot flashes, fatigue, insomnia, erratic menstruation, and mood swings. Fortunately, some of those menopausal symptoms will subside once your hormone levels stabilize.

However, many other changes, if not treated with proper nutrition, will continue to escalate. For example, when hormone levels drop, your bones dramatically begin to weaken as the amount of minerals they lose each day outnumbers the amount of minerals that they absorb. (For more on bone health, see "Osteoporosis.")

This bone loss is most dramatic during the first few years of menopause; however, it continues at a slower rate as years progress. Between menopause and age 80, most women lose a third of their bone mass.

Besides weaker bones, menopause also leaves you vulnerable to heart disease. Before menopause, high estrogen levels help to keep cholesterol levels under control. However, as estrogen drops off during menopause, women often see a drop in HDL (the good cholesterol carrier that transports cholesterol out of your body) and a rise in LDL (the bad artery-clogging cholesterol carrier).

Quick Tip

Many health food stores and online pharmacies and even some chiropractors are hawking a supplement that they call "natural progesterone." Manufacturers claim that the product, made from wild yams, contains natural progestogens.

However, there's a difference between natural progestogens and the hormone progesterone that tends to take a dip at menopause. Wild-yam supplement makers extract a hormone called DHEA from yams. In order to make it into a supplement, they bring DHEA through numerous chemical transformations, creating a form that's highly unlikely the body will be able to use. Because no research shows that these supplements work, I suggest you instead talk to your doctor about hormone replacement therapy (HRT) that contains synthetic progesterone to see if you may be a good candidate (but even this prescription has health risks).

After menopause you gain weight more easily as muscle mass deteriorates and your basal metabolic rate slows, lowering the number of calories you burn during a typical day.

Your body fat distribution also starts to shift, with more of it gravitating toward your middle rather than your butt and thighs. This fat around the middle is more dangerous to your health than fat elsewhere in the body, as abdominal fat has been associated with diabetes, heart disease, and cancer.

And while all of that sounds pretty grim, it doesn't have to be. The following simple changes to your eating and exercise habits can help keep you healthy and fit for years to come:

Eat soy daily. This little bean is truly a miracle food when it comes to menopause. Research from Bowman Gray Medical School has found that consuming 20 grams of soy protein a day can decrease hot flashes.

Other research has found that 25 grams of soy protein a day can lower blood cholesterol levels and may also help strengthen bones.

The magic ingredient in soy may be its phytoestrogens, natural compounds that weakly act like the female sex hormone estrogen. Eating more of this plant estrogen may help counterbalance the dramatic drop in hormone levels that occurs with menopause. Experiment with different soy products by substituting soy sausage, burgers, and links for their pork or beef counterparts. Also, use silken tofu instead of cream for soup and mix soy nuts into your favorite trail mix.

Boost your vegetables and beans. In addition to soy, many other whole foods contain estrogen-like compounds that can help ease the estrogen fluctuations during menopause that cause hot flashes and other symptoms. Fruit, vegetables, beans, and flaxseed top the list. Try to maximize your consumption of these foods by including a fruit or vegetable (or two) with every single meal, adding beans to soups and salads, and adding flax meal into baking recipes.

Avoid spicy foods. Certain foods may be more likely to trigger a hot flash possibly because they set off a temperature regulation mechanism in your body. For example, in your premenopause years, you probably felt warm after eating spicy foods. Now those same warming foods trigger the reflex that leads to a hot flash. Because hot flashes usually ebb once estrogen levels stop fluctuating, you don't have to give up spicy foods forever. However, you might want to cut back for a few months or only eat them at home when you can comfortably remove some clothing to cool yourself down.

Cut back on caffeine. Because caffeine raises your blood pressure and heart rate, it can also trigger a hot flash. However, going cold turkey with caffeine will result in sluggishness and a withdrawal headache. So slowly cut back by switching to half regular, half decaf coffee beans. As you get used to this mixture, keep adding a little more decaf and a little less regular beans, until you come to a point where the caffeine no longer produces a hot flash.

Talk to your doctor about herbs. Many women explore the world of herbs at menopause, in search of a magic potion that can cure their ills. Unfortunately, little research has been done on many of these herbs, so it's tough to know whether they really help.

It's okay to try herbs such as St. John's wort, black cohosh, chasteberry, Don Quoi, ginseng, and others, but talk to your doctor first. We're only starting to learn how these herbs interact with medications. For example, we now know that Don Quoi has blood-thinning effects. If you take that herb while taking a daily aspirin or prescription cholesterol-lowering medications, you run the risk of excessive bleeding with a simple cut or of hemorrhages in the eye and elsewhere. Many prescription medications that your doctor may prescribe after menopause make you more sensitive to sunlight, and this photosensitivity can be heightened even more by particular herbs, leaving you prone to burns, premature aging of the skin, and skin cancer.

Lift some weight. One of my friends recently went through an early menopause in her 40s. She had been trim and fit her entire life, but after menopause, she began looking more like an old woman. She also complained of little energy, her muscles were noticeably smaller, and fat was starting to fill out her middle.

I started her on a weight training program with an exercise ball, and soon her outlook dramatically reversed. The weight training helped her to build back most of the muscle she had lost, which increased her metabolism. Soon the extra weight around her middle disappeared. The muscle also helped boost her energy, so everyday tasks such as carrying groceries were not as tiresome. A few months after starting my ball workout, she told me she had tried snowboarding, an activity she never would have attempted had she not gained the energy through weight lifting.

Besides building muscle and boosting energy and metabolism, weight training also helps to strengthen bones. If you haven't weight trained before, now is the time to start. There are numerous ways to build muscle, from exercise machines at the gym to dumbbells to calisthenics, but I love fitness balls because you can exercise on one in any room of your home—or even in your backyard. For a complete ball workout, check out my book *Bounce Your Body Beautiful.*

Mix it up. You may notice a drop in exercise performance and motivation with menopause. Injuries are also more likely with age and tend to heal more slowly.

All of those reasons make cross training a must. Switching back and forth between different types of exercise helps keep you mentally entertained, reduces your risk of overuse injuries by spreading out the work over several muscles, and gives you an extra performance edge. Switching between different activities may also help you increase your calorie burn by keeping your muscles constantly surprised.

Finally, when you try new activities such as yoga or Pilates classes, you meet other women, some of whom might be going through menopause as well. Such classes often provide a great support group.

MOTIVATION

Nutrition strategies and fitness tips that keep your fitness program on track.

As a lifetime fitness enthusiast, I truly do love to exercise. However, even I have days when sleeping for 5 or 10 more minutes sounds much more enjoyable than getting up for an early morning run or swim. On such days, I tell myself that I'll feel better physically and mentally once I start running. Usually that's enough to encourage me to crawl out of bed—as well as the fact that I've never been wrong. Exercise *always* makes me feel good.

The first step to overcoming such mental fitness obstacles is admitting and recognizing that you have them. Sure, some days both your mind and body will look forward to your workout. Other days, however, one or the other—or both—simply haven't bought into your training plan.

Here are ways to keep those low physical and mental motivation days to a minimum:

Check your eating habits. I notice that when many people start an exercise program, they are very vigilant about what they eat. But the romance often wears off, and soon old habits return. With them return unwanted pounds, which can make your hard exercise efforts feel fruitless. I don't know about you, but a few pounds of extra weight is enough to make me wonder whether my 1-mile swim in the pool is doing any good.

Take a look at what you are eating. Perhaps you've reverted to snacking in the evening, which can easily add a few hundred calories that you had worked so hard earlier in the day to burn off. Jot down everything you eat in a given day and examine your food choices. Are you piling on unnecessary calories? Are you making the smartest food choices?

Eat more often. Many people feel too tired or too unmotivated to work out either because of too few or too many calories.

When you skip meals or don't eat often enough, your muscles and brain don't have enough fuel. When your brain runs low, it doesn't want to move, which doesn't help your motivation.

Then again, when you eat too much, such as a huge lunch, you may rather take a nap in the afternoon than exercise. That's because your body diverts some of your blood volume to your stomach—and away from your brain and muscles—to aid with digestion.

To avoid either problem, try to eat five small meals a day: a moderate breakfast, lunch, and dinner coupled with two small snacks, at midmorning and midafternoon. The smaller, more frequent meals will give you a constant supply of energy, fueling your motivation all day long.

Drink a glass of water. When you are dehydrated, your brain suffers, making you not feel like exercising. Start your day with a glass or two of water, and follow up with a glass at every meal. Carry water bottles with you everywhere to encourage yourself to drink.

Quick Tip

To see more motivating results from a weight lifting program, add some pounds. Increase your current lifting weight by 10 percent and stick with this for a few weeks, and then up the weight another 10 percent. This, along with changing the type of lifting exercises, will create noticeable results in muscle toning and strength.

Push the clock. Most people lose weight easily at the beginning of a fitness program. But that weight loss eventually begins to level off if you stick with the same exercise habits. Once those results drop off, motivation often follows.

To keep your results and motivation going, push yourself a little more every time you start to hit a plateau. Consider adding another 10 to 15 minutes to your workout time or adding another exercise day to your schedule. This combined extra exercise time will help you melt away some unwanted weight.

Push the speed. Increasing the intensity of your workout will not only burn more calories per workout but also boost your fitness level and make your workouts more interesting. For example, if you walk for your form of aerobic exercise, try adding faster bursts of walking or jogging or even skipping once every 5 or 10 minutes. Alternate 10 minutes of regular walking with 5 minutes of faster walking or jogging.

Try new moves. Variety does much more than keep exercise interesting. It also helps you lose weight. When you do the same exercise over and over, your muscles get used to the exercise and are able to perform it more efficiently. However, if you periodically change your program, you keep your body and mind constantly challenged. You might alternate between running, cycling, and a teacher-led dance routine, for example. For one or two days a week, give a new activity a try. Instead of walking, go for a bike ride, hop in a pool and swim laps, or, if you belong to a health club, give an aerobics or a kickboxing class a whirl. Or you might switch from lifting free weights to using fitness and heavy balls.

Put on your exercise clothes. If you feel anything but enthused about a particular workout, simply put on your exercise clothes. You can even watch TV while wearing them, but chances are, once you have them on, you'll find some way to exercise in them.

Tell yourself you'll only do 10 minutes. Instead of dreading your normal half hour or longer workout, just tell yourself you'll only do 10 minutes. Head out the door for that short walk, run, or bike ride. Chances are, once you've warmed up, you'll exercise for longer than you anticipated. Even if you don't, however, know that even 10 minutes is better than nothing.

Exercise in the morning. Studies show that more afternoon and evening exercisers blow off their workouts than morning exercisers. It's easy for the general stress and fatigue of a workday to encourage your brain to think you don't have the energy for your workout. Also, throughout the day, numerous people compete for your time, and one of them may easily win out over your exercise plans. Perhaps this is why morning is the most popular time for regular exercisers.

Do it with a friend. Making your exercise session into a social session gives you more reasons to look forward to your workout. Additionally, promising your friend that you'll both meet at the pool for a swim makes you accountable to each other so you'll both be more apt to exercise.

Exercise as you work and play. Don't forget that many enjoyable activities such as gardening, swing dancing, playing tag with your kids, and chasing your dog around the yard all count as exercise.

MUSCLE BUILDING AND WEIGHT LIFTING

The secret to stronger muscles may lie in the number of meals you eat each day.

I once heard a man lament during his gym workout: "I just can't seem to build any muscle. I keep watching what I eat and I lift weights consistently, but my muscles never seem to grow."

He was making a common mistake. He was dieting and trying to build muscle at the same time.

Muscle needs calories to grow, about 5,000 for every pound of muscle. When you vigilantly watch what you eat in an effort to keep off fat, you also hinder your muscles from growing larger. Fortunately, if you are hitting the gym regularly, adding 500 to 1,000 calories to your daily diet will go straight to your muscles, not to your fat cells.

Here are some tips to help you do just that:

Snack often. Many of those who have trouble putting on muscle tend to be nonnibblers. Food just doesn't turn them on. So they find they must consciously force themselves to eat in order to consume enough calories to fuel the muscle-building process.

If you're not "into" food, then you'll have a tough time adding the daily 500 to 1,000 calories you need to build more muscle. Instead of stuffing yourself sick during each meal, switch to a snacking lifestyle, eating as often as every 2 to 3 hours, totaling seven to eight minimeals a day.

Focus on high-calorie foods. Those of you who've struggled your entire life to put on weight need to eat all of the foods that we lifelong dieters are trying to avoid. Nuts and peanut butter make great high-energy snacks. So does dried fruit such as raisins, dried apricots, and dried papaya. Smoothies can also make for a high-energy snack, especially if you add a scoop of soy or protein powder.

Lift slowly. Research has shown that the more slowly you lift a weight, the more effective your muscle building. In other words, if it normally takes you 2 to 5 seconds to do one repetition of a bench press, try making the repetition last 10 to 12 seconds.

Besides more fully and quickly fatiguing your muscles, this type of slow lifting forces you to focus on proper form, helping to prevent injury. However, this type of lifting workout is too hard for most beginners, so only switch to it once you've established a solid weight lifting base.

To switch to the super slow method, you'll probably have to lower the amount of weight you lift or the total number of repetitions of a particular exercise at first. Listen to your body. Your goal is muscle fatigue. When you can't lift the weight one more time, you've worked your muscle to the limit.

Don't push it. Many lifters try to push their fitness by suddenly adding a lot of weight, a lot more exercises, or a lot more repetitions or sets (or all three) than usual during one workout, in an attempt to thoroughly "rip up" their muscles. They base their workouts on the theory that muscles grow stronger when they have to repair small tears inflicted during a workout. However, recent research shows that this theory is seriously flawed. It's true that your muscles grow in response to a challenge. However, when you overchallenge your muscles and literally rip them up, you actually take longer to recover from a workout and experience fewer results. It's okay to feel mildly sore the day after a workout, but if you still feel sore 48 hours later, you've overdone it.

Mix it up. During the first few months of a weight lifting program, most people get results quickly and easily. Your muscles get hard and start to grow. Seems like each time you hit the gym, you're able to lift heavier weights, and the fat melts away.

However, at some point, most people hit a wall. Your progress drops off and your muscle size seems not to budge. That's because once your body adapts to a particular motion, it doesn't have to work as hard to accomplish the task. So mix up your weight lifting moves.

For example, instead of always bench-pressing to work your chest, try chest flies, push-ups, or incline bench presses. Instead of always doing bicep curls, try preacher curls or concentration curls. Instead of always doing dips for your triceps, try kick backs and skull crushers. Also, alternate between two sets of 15 reps, three sets of 8 reps, and a drop set of 8 hard and then an immediate set of a light 15.

Rest. When it comes to weight lifting, more isn't necessarily better. Your muscles do most of their growing when you are resting, not while you are in the gym. Various studies have found that working the same muscle without a 48-hour break between sessions is actually counterproductive. So never lift more often than every other day for the same muscle groups. And consider taking a few days off. Surprisingly, fewer sessions may net you bigger results.

Focus on quality protein. Studies show that weight lifting boosts protein needs an estimated 50 percent or more above the U.S. RDA.

Your protein requirement is based on your body weight. The RDA for protein is 0.36 gram per pound of body weight—about 65 grams for a person who weighs 180 pounds. But the extra 50 percent bumps the requirement up to about 100 grams daily for a 180-pound athlete. Your body uses the extra protein for building and repairing muscle tissue and also burns small amounts for fuel.

Chances are you already get this much protein from food alone. Most people easily meet their increased protein needs simply by eating foods such as fish, lean meats, soy, eggs, beans, and dairy products. For example, a 3-ounce serving of fish or lean meat (the size of a deck of cards) has 21 grams of protein. The only athletes who fall short of their protein requirement are usually strict vegetarians. (And even they can get enough protein from their meals with some careful planning.)

Don't forget carbohydrate. Too many body builders put all of the emphasis on protein, but carbohydrate is just as important. You need carbohydrate to fuel your lifting sessions. Worse, if you burn all of

Cooking 101

As I mentioned, one of the keys to building muscle during your workout is arriving at your workout with food in your belly. Those who work out on an empty stomach usually do so first thing in the morning. You'll be happy to know that you can easily consume the minimum 6 grams of protein and 35 grams of carbohydrate with the following quick and easy meal suggestions:

- Eat a small Balance Bar or some other type of energy bar that contains both protein and carbohydrate.
- Swallow a smoothie made with strawberries, banana, nonfat yogurt, and a carton of egg substitute.
- Drink two glasses of lowfat or nonfat milk.
- Eat a carton of fruit-flavored yogurt.

your stored carbohydrate during a lifting session, your body starts eating up protein, which makes your muscles smaller, not bigger.

More surprisingly, loading up with carbohydrate before hitting the gym may also help you recover faster and build bigger muscles during the hours following your workout, research shows. That's because carbohydrate ingestion stimulates the hormone insulin, which can shuttle those amino acids to your muscles. Combining carbohydrate with protein as a snack before your lifting sessions is probably the most effective way to build bigger muscles.

Shoot for 15 to 20 servings of carbohydrate a day. This may sound staggering, but the average bowl of Shredded Wheat cereal with a banana counts as five servings. Two sandwiches (with four slices of bread) make four more. A pasta salad and baked potato for dinner offer nine more servings. Snacking on bagels and muffins easily brings you to 20.

Consider creatine carefully. Weight lifting depends on creatine phosphate for fuel, and you can burn almost all of it during a session. When taken over several weeks, creatine supplements do help build muscle size. In one study, from Truman State University, weight-trained men taking creatine for six weeks experienced significant gains in lean tissue, approximately 4 pounds, compared to men taking a placebo.

However, once you stop taking creatine, the performance benefits disappear. Also, researchers don't know what happens to your own body's ability to make creatine if you stay on the supplements for months. In other words, will supplementing with creatine hamper your own daily production? Considering that creatine supplements come with a hefty price tag, the temporary boost hardly seems worth it. For more on this supplement, see chapter 4.

MUSCLE CRAMPS

How to stop the pain before it starts.

If you've ever experienced a muscle cramp, then you know all too well how painful and sometimes dangerous these muscle spasms can be. A foot cramp during swimming, for example, can make you abandon your stroke and instead grab on to a lane line to drag yourself to the pool wall. A calf cramp during running or touch football can drop you to your knees. A foot or calf cramp in the middle of the night can wake you from sleep and cause you to moan in pain.

Studies show that some 30 to 50 percent of athletes who participate in endurance activities occasionally suffer from exercise-induced muscle cramps.

These painful muscle spasms usually strike during a long session of exercise or soon after you finish. Unfortunately, they often cut workouts short and can deter some people from exercise altogether.

Quick Tip

If you wake during the night with a foot or leg cramp, a simple stretch can help soothe it away. Just reach for your toes and pull them toward your knee, stretching your arch, Achilles tendon, and calf. The stretch will help to stop the contraction in your muscle, stopping the cramp.

The cause of exercise-induced cramping has been long debated. For many years researchers placed the blame for cramping on dehydration and loss of electrolytes such as sodium and potassium due to heavy sweating on hot days. This fluid-electrolyte theory is still popular, but new evidence challenges this belief, especially since many people suffer from cramps during exercise in cooler temperatures and without major losses of sweat or electrolytes.

New research, based on a technique that measures electrical activity of muscles both during and after exercise, shows that muscles cramp only when they are fatigued. Fatigue brings on a series of internal changes that cause your muscles to enter a state of enhanced excitability. Once in this state of heightened activity, a muscle will suddenly shorten—or cramp—when faced with repetitive movements that cause it to contract.

Once cramped, the muscle stays tightened, then usually relaxes after 5 to 15 seconds. In other words, even if you do nothing, the cramp will go away within 15 seconds. However, without preventative measures, your muscle remains in a state of high excitability, allowing the cramp to easily return minutes later.

Another type of muscle cramp can occur at night as you sleep. These annoying and equally as painful leg cramps occur most often in the 50-plus crowd. Also, people with high blood pressure and those taking certain medications such as diuretics are more likely to suffer from them. The true cause of these troublesome cramps has eluded physicians for some time, and effective treatment is even harder to pin down.

Warding off muscle cramps during exercise and during sleep involves keeping muscle fatigue at bay. Here are some training and eating strategies that will help:

Get in shape slowly. Good overall conditioning for exercises such as long-distance running will ensure that you're not overtaxing your muscles. Work up to longer efforts by upping your duration slowly, increasing your duration or intensity by no more than 10 percent each week. That will ease your muscles into longer efforts and help you avoid undue fatigue and possible cramping.

Cut workouts short. If you are still plagued with cramps during longer exercise efforts, even though you are not dramatically increasing your distance or intensity, it's time to cut back. Shorten your workout intensity or duration until you're cramp-free. Then increase the distance or time slowly.

Stretch it out. During a cramp, passive stretching of the cramped muscle, such as pulling your toes toward your knee when you have a calf cramp, will bring almost immediate relief because the stretch interrupts the excitability cycle and helps the muscle get some rest. Stretching cramp-prone muscles on a regular basis will help lengthen them, lowering their excitability level. Prepare your muscles, especially those involved in previous cramping episodes, with passive stretching before exercise, and introduce more stretching throughout your daily fitness routine. If you often cramp in the middle of the night, stretch before going to bed.

Stay fueled. Drink fluids and consume carbohydrate (such as a sports drink) during longer workouts (generally, those lasting 60 minutes or more). Eating a banana, a handful of dried fruit, an energy bar, or an energy gel and drinking plenty of water during a workout will help delay muscle fatigue. However, despite popular belief, bananas don't offer anything special that specifically prevents or cures muscle cramps brought on by exercise, since loss of potassium is an unlikely cause for cramping.

Eat salt during endurance efforts. If you sweat excessive amounts of salt, you may need more sodium than a typical sports drink provides. You'll know if you are a "salty sweater" simply by examining your workout clothing. If they are caked with a white, dusty substance after exercise, you're losing a lot of salt in your sweat.

Consume extra electrolytes by munching on salted crackers or pretzels. For the less than 1 percent of the population that suffers sodium-related total body cramping, Gatorade has recently created a product called Gatorlytes, an electrolyte pack of sodium, potassium, and other minerals to add to your sports drink bottle. It's available only through athletic trainers and organized sports teams.

Consider quinine carefully. The standard treatment for night cramps is a prescription drug called *quinine,* but it's typically less than 50 percent effective. Also, dosing with quinine is not without risks, which include side effects such as dizziness, irregular heartbeat, and dangerous drops in blood pressure. Additionally, quinine use has been associated with an increased chance of stumbling or falling due to dizziness or vertigo.

Take a B-complex supplement. Though quinine may hold little promise for you, a simple B-complex supplement may ease problems dramatically. Researchers from the divisions of Cardiovascular Medicine and Clinical Pharmacology at the Taipei Medical College in Taiwan studied the effectiveness of a B-complex vitamin supplement against a placebo in elderly patients suffering from recurring nocturnal cramping. The men and women either took a B-complex pill (containing vitamins B_{12}, B_6, and riboflavin, or vitamin B_2) three times daily or a look-alike placebo for three months. They also kept a diary to record the frequency and severity of nighttime cramping.

At the end of the three months, those taking the B vitamins suffered significantly fewer and less severe cramps compared to those on the placebo. About one-fourth of the subjects had complete remission of nocturnal cramping, while another 50 percent had significant reduction in number of cramps. The placebo group, on the other hand, showed no improvement during the entire three months.

While at a loss for an explanation for these dramatic results, the researchers point out that those taking the B vitamins suffered no side effects. The daily dose amounted to 7.5 milligrams of B_{12}, 90 milligrams of B_6, and 15 milligrams of riboflavin. These amounts greatly exceed the recommended needs, and while these vitamins are water-soluble and excess is easily excreted in the urine, you should talk to your physician before supplementing with these B vitamins in these amounts.

MUSCLE SORENESS

Foods that feel like massage to your muscles.

You probably have heard the phrase "no pain, no gain" before. It was very popular during the 1980s, when fitness fanatics felt that the only way to gain more fitness was by pushing beyond your comfort zone and inflicting a great deal of discomfort.

Fortunately, we now know that the no pain, no gain theory is seriously flawed. In fact, this theory has probably been responsible for more exercise burnout, injuries, and motivation problems than any other training concept.

True, to some extent, you will feel some soreness when trying to push your fitness to the next level. That's because lifting a heavier weight at the gym or walking another loop around the block forces your muscles to work harder than usual.

Sometimes this extra effort inflicts small micro tears in your muscles. In theory, these small tears are not bad. Since your muscles want to help you perform that same task again—without discomfort—these small tears encourage your muscle fibers to grow. As the muscle fibers readjust, you may feel slight postexercise soreness or a burn.

However, if you push yourself too far beyond your limits, those tears become larger. To repair these tears, your immune system responds with inflammation. The swelling puts pressure on nearby nerves. And you say "ouch." These larger tears are tougher to quickly repair, causing you to feel sore for numerous days and preventing you from exercising at your full capacity.

Pushing yourself too far beyond your limits also encourages the formation of free radicals. These rogue molecules are missing an electron, making them extremely unstable. In your body, free radicals can cause a lot of damage, and they are thought to be the culprit for numerous health problems, including heart disease and cancer. When too many of these free radicals form during exercise, they can overwhelm your body's natural defenses and damage your muscles and other soft tissues, causing inflammation and pain.

Fortunately, eating the right foods can not only counteract free radicals, it can also help patch up muscle tears, helping you get back on your feet faster.

However, there's one important caveat. Proper nutrition can only help if you are combining it with proper training. Listen closely to your body during exercise. If you feel any pain, particularly around a joint such as your knee, stop. Follow the golden 10 percent rule of never increasing your distance or intensity more than 10 percent each week. Finally, train with a hard-easy approach. That means taking every other training day easy or even completely off. Your muscles take about 48 hours to recover from a tough exercise session. If you keep pounding them into the ground, they never fully recover and you can end up overtrained. (See "Overtraining" for more information.)

Assuming you are training properly, use the following tips to prevent muscle soreness:

Cooking 101

After a grueling exercise session, try making a smoothie packed with different types of fruit. The fruit will supply needed antioxidants to your muscles, and the smoothie itself tastes wonderful just after exercise. Try blending the following:

½ cup ice
1 cup frozen blueberries
½ cup soy milk
½ cup orange juice
½ cup vanilla yogurt
2 teaspoons honey

Nutritional analysis—calories: 330; protein: 10 grams; carbohydrate: 66 grams; calories from fat: 14%.

Eat more whole foods. Fruits, vegetables, and whole grains contain important nutrients called *antioxidants*. Antioxidants lend electrons to those destructive free radicals that I mentioned earlier, keeping the rogue molecules away from your precious cells. In the past, people have tried to fend off free radicals by taking high doses of particular supplements. But new research suggests a more diverse approach.

Fruits, vegetables, and whole grains contain hundreds of different antioxidants. For example, the carotenes that give vegetables their yellow, orange, and red hues make up just one type of antioxidant. But there are more than 400 different carotenes, each of which extinguishes different types of free radicals. So instead of focusing solely on just one antioxidant vitamin, eat as many different fruits, vegetables, and whole grains as you can. Make sure to eat eight to 10 servings of fruits and vegetables a day—the more colorful and varied, the better—and at least six or more servings of whole grains such as barley, millet, quinoa, and wheat. Besides produce and grains, many other foods also supply antioxidants, including black and green tea, red wine, dark beer, and dark chocolate.

Take a vitamin E supplement. This powerful antioxidant may help protect you from the oxidative damage caused by endurance exercise. I'd love to say you can get all the E you need from foods, but that's very difficult to do. After all, 400 IU is almost 1,000 percent of the RDA. During periods of heavy training, consider taking a vitamin E supplement that contains no more than 400 IU. Take your supplement with a meal, since your body needs a small amount of fat for optimal absorption.

Eat fish twice a week. A type of oil found in fish—called omega-3 fatty acids—acts as a natural anti-inflammatory, and some research shows that an omega-3 fatty acid supplement of 1 to 1.5 grams a day may reduce muscle pain. Rather than taking supplements, which can be expensive, I suggest eating a fatty fish such as salmon twice a week. This same amount of fish is also good for your heart health.

Try these supplements. The same supplements that may help reduce pain from osteoarthritis may also help reduce pain from muscle damage, though more research is needed to prove the connection. Glucosamine and chondroitin sulfate might work by producing substances in ligaments, tendons, and joint fluids called *glycoproteins,* which may speed healing. Studies show that taking about 1,500 milligrams daily of each of these supplements helps lessen pain and improve joint function.

Aspirin and other nonsteroidal anti-inflammatory drugs also alleviate pain, but side effects such as stomach upset and bleeding make these drugs less desirable over the long term. Glucosamine and chondroitin sulfate take time to work their magic, so take them regularly for at least two months to see results. If you want to give these supplements a try, follow the package instructions, and consult your doctor if you are already taking prescription medications.

ON-THE-GO EATING

Fitting in good nutrition when you don't have time to cook.

I know all about the on-the-go lifestyle. I frequently travel to meetings and engagements out of town. Once I flew halfway around the world to Japan for a two-day meeting and then flew right back and headed straight to work, without a breather.

Even my days in town are packed full of activities. But I don't let my busy schedule get in the way of wholesome fitness nutrition. Over the years I've perfected numerous ways to stick to my exercise schedule and healthy eating routine no matter how hectic my day, what part of the world I might find myself in, or how often I find myself eating out at restaurants.

No matter how busy you are—or how much you travel—the following self-tested tips will help you to fit in nutritious meals, eat the required amount of fruits and vegetables, and keep off unwanted pounds:

Always eat breakfast. Your brain is counting on you for needed fuel and nutrients to launch your workday, so never skip breakfast, no matter how pressed for time.

An ideal start-your-day-right meal supplies a good source of protein, carbohydrate, vitamins, minerals, and fiber. However, you don't need to spend a lot of time in the kitchen to satisfy all of those requirements. For example, ready-to-eat breakfast cereal such as raisin bran topped with milk (cow's milk or soy) and fresh berries offers an ideal quick-and-easy breakfast. It takes less than a minute to pour the cereal and milk into a bowl and drop a handful of blueberries or raspberries on top.

Other fast-and-nutritious morning meals include:

- Toasted whole grain bread spread with peanut butter and topped with sliced banana.
- Blender drink of yogurt mixed with orange juice, banana, and a squirt of honey (makes for great sipping on a morning commute).

- Leftover vegetarian pizza with a glass of milk.
- Goat cheese spread over a whole wheat tortilla topped with tomato slices.

Don't overlook dried fruit. Dried fruit offers one of the easiest and fastest ways to sneak in produce. Most techniques used to dry fruits only remove moisture and small amounts of vitamin C. The rest of the minerals, such as potassium, iron, and calcium (dried figs are a great source), phytochemicals, and vitamins stay put. Aim for a variety of dried fruits daily. Since they require no refrigeration, you can pack dried fruits in your briefcase or stash them in the car.

Make the most of frozen dinners. Surprise! Frozen dinners offer good nutrition, providing you choose your dinners carefully and round out your meal by adding a vegetable, such as a salad (quickly made from a bagged mix) or chopped raw veggies (prechopped at the store). Also, nix any dessert that comes with the dinner, and instead finish off your meal with fresh berries topped with a touch of light whipped cream or yogurt. Frozen fruit, such as blueberries, peaches, and strawberries, sweetened with a drizzle of honey, also makes an easy vitamin-packed dessert.

Now for your frozen dinner. To pick out the most nutritious types, look for those with:

- 300 to 500 calories per dinner.
- No more than 10 to 15 grams of total fat and 2 to 5 grams of saturated fat per frozen entrée or meal.
- 5 or more grams of fiber.

Watch your portions. Unless you're eating at an expensive nouveau cuisine restaurant that serves up tiny, artfully presented portions, you'll find that most restaurants pack your plate with much more than you would otherwise normally eat.

Ask for smaller portions, opting for a half-portion meal or even just two appetizers rather than a main course. While paying the same

Quick Tip

Every on-the-go person at one time or another succumbs to pressure and ends up in a food emergency. This often happens on an unusually busy day toward the end of the week, on the day that you sleep in and don't have time to make your lunch. Because it's late in the week, you've already exhausted your supply of fruit and nuts that you keep in your briefcase. By midafternoon you're so hungry you could eat your foot, so you head to the only sustenance nearby: a vending machine.

This doesn't have to be the end of your nutritional efforts. Scan what's available. First, look to see if you can buy fruit juice from the soda machine. Then, look in the vending machine for items that supply at least some nutrition, such as an apple, peanut butter and crackers, a bag of nuts or trail mix, yogurt, or whole grain crackers.

price for a smaller meal is hardly a value, it's worth not wearing the extra calories around your waist.

Get someone to wait on you. Avoid buffet- and cafeteria-style restaurants if you can, opting instead for sit-down restaurant meals where you order from a menu. According to nutrition-anthropologists, when we see lots of food, we're programmed to eat more, taking a taste of every selection. During our prehistoric days, this feasting helped humans survive periods of famine. But in a cafeteria- or buffet-style restaurant, this feasting only leads to one thing: weight gain.

Make the most of the salad bar. You want to eat at least five servings of fruit and vegetables daily, which makes a restaurant or grocery store salad bar one of your best nutritional allies. Select a variety of dark green lettuces, fresh cut-up vegetables, beans, and sprouts and top it all off with an oil-and-vinegar dressing or just plain vinegar.

Plan ahead. When traveling, get an idea of where you are staying and what is available at the hotel or nearby. Ask about the hotel's fitness room or local health clubs and rates. Does the hotel have an in-house restaurant? If so, ask for a menu to be e-mailed or faxed so that you know what types of fare you can expect.

Some extended-stay hotels offer kitchenettes with a refrigerator, microwave, and stove. If you have this option, it's worth it. When you get to your destination, make a quick stop at a grocery store and stock up on a few breakfast items: whole grain cereals, fresh fruit, and lowfat milk or soy milk. This way you can bypass that morning restaurant meal of pastries and fatty omelets, which usually add up to unwanted calories and fat. You can also keep one or two frozen entrées on hand along with bagged salad mix or precut vegetables for a healthful dinner.

Take your sneakers everywhere. You're more likely to keep fitness a part of your busy schedule—whether on the road or even at home—if you have easy access to your fitness equipment. A pair of sneakers allows you to take a stress-releasing walk in a nearby park whenever you can sneak out for a break.

When I travel, I bring along my own equipment to do weight training exercises. This doesn't mean you have to lug a set of dumbbells in your luggage. I take along rubber tubing and bands, often used in physical therapy for rehabilitation of injuries. The bands and tubes come in different thicknesses or strengths, providing varied levels of resistance. When you pull on the tubing with your hands (or your legs), the tube provides resistance to help you tone your muscles. In this way, you can do a variety of exercises that strengthen your arms (triceps, biceps), back, shoulders, and legs.

Look before you order. When eating out, peruse the menu for grilled fish, fresh vegetable side dishes or salads, and healthful vegetarian entrées. In fact, before you take a seat in the restaurant, ask to see the menu. This allows you to opt for another local eatery with better choices if needed.

Make time for fitness. Your day can easily be overrun with meetings. So plan your time for fitness, such as the morning or just before an evening business dinner, and stick with your plans.

If you schedule some sort of exercise into your day—walking with relatives, strolling at the mall, a visit to a health club, jogging in the park—then you're more likely to do it. Also, plan on being physical earlier in the day, since commitments tend to stack up as the day moves on and there may be no time left for your workout.

Stay moving on your travel day. When in transit, it can be difficult to fit in formal exercise, such as a jog or an aerobics class. However, you can still stay in motion. Walk around airport terminals while you wait for your flight. If driving, stop and take walking "stretch" breaks. This should help keep you from feeling sluggish, besides burning extra calories.

ORGANIC LIFESTYLE

Choosing to go organic is often an environmental decision. Can it also improve your health?

Many people opt for organic produce, milk, eggs, and meat as a revolt against factory farming, which has caused the demise of small family farms across the country. Others opt for organic because they worry that widespread use of herbicides and pesticides on crops may leach into the soil, contaminating groundwater. These same environmentally concerned folks also worry that crowding hundreds of animals into a small space contaminates the local soil, air, and water with by-products from methane gas and excrement.

Finally, there are those who reach for organic foods for health reasons. Such folks worry that pesticide residue on produce makes its way onto their plates, raising their risk of cancer. They also worry that the routine antibiotics and hormones given to poultry and cattle create tainted meat and milk.

With so many fears, it's no wonder the organic industry is booming. But is going organic better for your fitness than eating conventionally grown foods? In my quest for the dirt on organic foods, I've unearthed information on why buying organic, at least some of the time, may be best for you. First, though, let's take a look at what "organic" actually means.

Organic 101

Until recently, there was no way to know for sure if the free-range chicken you bought at the grocery store truly grew up with area to roam freely or if an organic vegetable truly had no pesticide residue. As many as 49 different states and various private organizations were certifying foods as organic, but each had its own definition and standards, some of which were much less strict than others.

The federal government, however, has put an end to this confusion by enforcing new federal guidelines that allow you to feel confident that what you're buying is truly organic.

The U.S. Department of Agriculture recently established a new set of rules for certifying organic foods. For a food to carry the USDA organic seal, it must:

- Consist of at least 95 percent organically produced ingredients. (This leaves room for ingredients such as baking soda in bakery goods that don't fit the organic definition.)
- Not be genetically engineered or modified.
- Not be grown on soil fertilized with sewage sludge.
- Not be irradiated (a process using radiation that kills bacteria and other harmful organism in meats, spices, and other foods).
- Be raised with 100 percent organically grown feed (for beef, pork, dairy, and eggs).

- Be given outdoor pastures (for livestock and poultry).
- Not be given hormones or antibiotics.

Under the new rules, foods with 50 to 95 percent organic ingredients won't bear the USDA seal but may state "contains organic ingredients" on the label.

Organic Food and Health

Few studies have compared organically grown produce to standard fare grown with the use of pesticides. Even fewer have looked at the differences between animals raised in feedlots versus those raised while grazing in open pastures. Since food handling, seasonal variations, and other factors can have an impact on the nutrient content of foods, scientists have long said the difference between organic and conventionally grown foods is too close to call.

But a handful of studies have found a slightly greater vitamin and mineral content in some organically grown foods. Some of the organic farming techniques, such as crop rotation and use of animal manure, do add back nutrients, such as minerals, to the soil. What has not been adequately assessed is whether organically grown foods have higher levels of phytochemicals, such as the polyphenols found in grapes, which have health-promoting benefits.

Some research has found that cows who graze on grass produce milk with more conjugated linoleic acid (CLA) than those who eat grain, hay, or silage. CLA is a fatty acid that may hold promise as a cancer fighter as well as provide other health benefits.

Many of those who raise organic beef and other meats claim that animals that roam and graze on grass build more muscle and less fat than those kept confined in a feedlot and injected with growth hormones. However, research has yet to prove that claim.

Organic produce, grains, and meats do contain a lower level of pesticide residues compared to conventionally grown; however, they

Quick Tip

Opting for organic meat and poultry may help to reduce a growing problem o(tibiotic resistance. Antibiotics were a wonderful invention many years ago, he(us to survive a host of once fatal illnesses. However, antibiotics never kill every single bacterium. The few that survive adapt and become resistant to antibiotic treatment.

Overprescribing of antibiotics by doctors coupled with the rise of antibiotic home-cleaning supplies as well as overuse of antibiotics in farming (they are routinely given to cattle, hogs, and chickens kept in crowded conditions to prevent bacterial infections from spreading rapidly) has created numerous strains of antibiotic-resistant germs, such as the germ that causes strep throat.

If you choose organic foods, you're taking one positive step in fighting this war against antibiotic-resistant bacteria. However, don't stop there. Make sure that the cleaning agents you use at home are not the antibacterial type. Also, whenever given antibiotics by your doctor, finish your prescription to completely kill all of the bacteria in your body.

are not totally pesticide-free due to residual chemicals in the soil, water, or air.

Though all foods—whether organic or conventional—must not exceed federal limits set for pesticide residues, a few conventionally grown types of produce may be riskier than others. In particular, a handful of fruits and vegetables, including spinach, apples, peaches, and strawberries, particularly if eaten by children, tend to have levels of pesticide residue deemed risky by some consumer groups. So for these and other produce that may be eaten unpeeled or in greater amounts during parts of the year (in-season produce, for example), opting for organic may be your safest bet.

Ma Most of Organic

se these helpful tips when buying and preparing organic or conven- onally grown produce to help you save money and minimize pesticide esidue exposure along with contamination risk for bacteria such as harmful *E. coli* (which lurks in both organic and conventional produce):

Wash everything. Wash all produce—organic or conventional—in cool running water. Scrub it lightly with a vegetable brush to help remove dirt and bacteria. However, don't soak your fruits or veggies in a detergent or dilute bleach solution, as these substances may be absorbed through the surface.

You can also try a produce rinse available at most supermarkets, such as Healthy Harvest. Sold in a spray bottle, it is designed to remove wax, dirt, and pesticide residue. Most produce rinses are water mixed with a small amount of a biodegradable surfactant, designed to act like a detergent to remove surface residue.

Get rid of the first layer. Most pesticide residue only exists on the top layer or skin of a fruit or vegetable. Remove outer leaves from leafy vegetables like lettuce, bok choy, and cabbage, and remove the peel of suspect fruits and vegetables. While peeling strips some fiber and nutrients, it does remove most of the pesticide residue.

Store it right. Keep your produce stored properly in a plastic bag, free of water, in the produce bin of your refrigerator. You may want to purchase a produce "life extender" such as Extra Life or Fridge Friend, both of which neutralize the ethylene gas production given off by some produce that speeds the rotting process.

Head to the farmer's market. On average, organic produce runs 20 to 50 percent more in cost than conventional. However, local organic farmers usually will sell their produce directly to you at lower prices than grocery stores. You can find these local farmers at a local farmer's market. Also, ask around to find out if a local organic farm offers a food co-op. For these co-ops, you usually buy a share of the crop preseason. Then each week, the farmer provides you with a large bag of whatever produce has ripened that week.

Go online. Many small farms now have their own e-commerce Web sites that allow you to place an order with a credit card. They often ship next-day air and run seasonal specials. In some areas in the country, online shopping may be your only way to track down organic meat.

My favorite mail order organic grocer: Diamond Organics (www.diamondorganics.com). I often order their field greens (Mesclun) salad complete with edible flowers and have it shipped to friends for a welcome fresh surprise.

OSTEOARTHRITIS

Aching joints shouldn't bring an end to your fitness habits.

Many people erroneously blame their exercise habits for the pain in their knees or other joints. For example, they will make comments like, "I used to run until it destroyed my knees" and "If I had never taken aerobics classes, I wouldn't have arthritis."

However, repeated studies have found that exercise—even more vigorous types of exercise such as running—is actually good for your joints. The repetitive movement of exercise strengthens and stretches the bones around your joints, allowing you to move more fluidly without pain.

In fact, exercise is often used to treat arthritis.

To understand why, you first must understand how your joints work. The joints in your body serve as junctions where two bones meet. Ligaments hold the two bones together as well as allow them to move. Within many of those junctions, particularly your knees, hips, elbows, and shoulders, there's a small space—called the *joint capsule*—between the two bones. Within that space, you'll find three types of "cushions" that help to keep the ends of the two bones from rubbing together. Cartilage functions like a shock absorber, whereas synovial fluid and bursa sacs act like the air bags in your car.

When you have the most common form of arthritis, called *osteoarthritis,* the shock-absorbing cartilage begins to wear away, allowing the bones to come in contact with one another. Though an injury, such as the type inflicted during a sudden twisting movement during a game of basketball, can lead to osteoarthritis if left untreated, the most common culprit is age-related degeneration. If you live long enough, osteoarthritis is a given. It affects about 85 percent of those older than 70.

Another less common type of arthritis, called *rheumatoid arthritis,* is caused by an overly active immune system. In this form of arthritis, your immune cells erroneously attack your joints, as if they were germs, causing pain and inflammation. If you have rheumatoid arthritis, seek a physician's advice on the best medications to reduce the swelling and suppress your immune system.

If you have osteoarthritis, follow these tips:

Do the right exercise for you. Some people with arthritis can perform most types of exercise without discomfort. However, if your joints hurt when you exercise, switching to low-impact types of exercise such as cycling, rowing, swimming, and water aerobics may ease the pain. Water exercise provides an ideal environment because the buoyancy of the water holds up your body, taking all of your weight off your joints and allowing you to exercise pain-free. Make sure to thoroughly warm up for at least 10 minutes before each session, and only exercise to the point of discomfort, not beyond it. Finally, make sure to stretch every day to keep your joints supple.

Don't believe everything you hear. Plenty of people tell me that they are taking the supplement MSM (methylsulfonylmethane) to ease joint pain. Supplement makers claim, among other things, that MSM blocks the pain message in your nerve fibers, preventing the sensation from getting to your brain. They also claim that it acts as a natural anti-inflammatory.

However, as of yet, there are no clinical studies done on people showing that this supplement reduces the pain associated with osteoarthritis. Also, the safety of this supplement just isn't known. If you see a benefit after taking this supplement, that's great, but to be honest, I'm not convinced it works. If you plan to give it a try, talk with your doctor about the pros and cons of this supplement as well as how it may or may not interact with other medications you're taking.

Consider SAMe. First used to treat depression, SAMe (S-adenosyl-L-methionine) also shows promise as a joint pain soother. One study found that as little as 200 to 400 milligrams taken three times a day (half the dose recommended to treat depression) reduces symptoms of osteoarthritis. The supplement may work by lending molecules to parts of the body that need them. SAMe may provide a particularly good option for people who need prescription NSAIDs (nonsteroidal anti-inflammatory drugs) to control their pain. NSAIDs tend to have a blood-thinning effect, which may rule them out if you are already taking other medications that thin the blood (such as certain heart medications). Since SAMe doesn't have the same blood-thinning effect, it serves as a good alternative.

If you are already taking SAMe for depression, don't increase the dosage. However, if you are not already taking SAMe, check the bottle to find out how many milligrams are in each pill. Because most SAMe supplements are formulated to treat depression, you'll probably only need to take half the bottle's recommended amount. SAMe is not very stable, so look for bottles that are opaque (to reduce light exposure) and don't leave the top off your bottle once you get it home.

Look to vitamin E. Certain research shows that this antioxidant vitamin reduces some of the inflammation associated with arthritis when

Quick Tip

If you have a family history of rheumatoid arthritis, consider switching your wake-up beverage from coffee to tea. The Iowa Women's Health Study recently found that women who drank four or more cups of decaf coffee a day were two times more likely to develop rheumatoid arthritis than those who drank less than that amount. Also, women who drank more than three cups of tea a day were 60 percent *less* likely to develop the condition.

taken in amounts of 400 to 1,000 IU. Though vitamin E is a fat-soluble vitamin and this is many times its Daily Value, it has been shown to be safe up to 1,000 IU. Higher doses may have a blood-thinning effect, so avoid this supplement if you are taking a daily aspirin.

Focus on fruit. A small amount of research shows that vitamin C, abundant in brightly colored fruits and some vegetables, may ease the pain of arthritis, particularly when combined with vitamin E supplements. However, you can easily meet your vitamin C requirement by consuming the recommended five to nine servings of fruits and vegetables each day.

Opt for Gluco. Two supplements, called *chondroitin sulfate,* a component of cartilage, and *glucosamine,* a building material for special cells that make cartilage, may alleviate joint pain caused by wear and tear. Studies show that taking about 1,500 milligrams daily of each of these supplements helps lessen pain and improve joint function. Aspirin and other nonsteroidal anti-inflammatory drugs also alleviate pain, but side effects such as stomach upset and bleeding make these drugs less desirable over the long term. Since chondroitin and glucosamine actually work by building new cartilage, pain relief takes time. Expect to wait as long as two months before you feel a difference.

OSTEOPOROSIS

Both women and men should take steps to keep bones strong.

Many people think osteoporosis is an old ladies' disease. It's not.

Yes, older women are more prone to osteoporosis, but this disease also affects one in eight men. Also, you build all the bone mass that you will ever have before age 35, so preventative measures offer the most results when undertaken at a young age. In other words, osteoporosis is something that everyone should think about—not just the elderly.

To understand how to prevent osteoporosis, however, you first must understand how your bones grow.

Your bones are active tissues that constantly break down and rebuild themselves. About one-seventh of your skeleton is replaced each year. However, the amount that your bones break down doesn't always equal the amount that they build back up, which, over time, results in bone loss.

During the first three decades of life, your bones usually undergo more rebuilding than breaking down, helping your bones to grow stronger. As they rebuild, they pack themselves solid with minerals, giving you a high bone mineral density.

After age 35, this process begins to shift, with more breaking down taking place than building back up. Each time your bones build back up, they don't pack themselves as solidly with minerals. The fewer minerals in your bones, the weaker your bones become, allowing fractures to occur more easily.

If you don't build up enough bone before age 35 or you lose bone too quickly after age 35, you end up with osteoporosis.

Is Soda Bad for Your Bones?

Did you ever have a grade school science teacher who submerged a tooth or bone in a beaker of soft drink, let it soak, and then removed a rubbery, mineral-depleted mass? I often hear about such science experiments from my students, who wonder if their six or more sodas a day caffeine habit will turn their bones to rubber.

I often tell them that, yes, drinking this much soda might weaken their bones, but not for the reason their science teachers led them to believe.

Soda, particularly cola, has added phosphoric acid, which is a source of dietary phosphorous, an essential mineral for bone health. This acid also contributes to the low pH, or acidity, of sodas. If you soak a tooth (or piece of bone) in acid solution, the integrity of the tooth enamel and mineral structure will be damaged. But when you drink soda, it washes by your teeth quickly. Once in your body, the acid is quickly neutralized by your own digestive juices, which act as a buffer. In other words, your teeth and bones never come in contact with soda the same way as that notorious science experiment. Soda, by itself, doesn't weaken your teeth or bones.

However, drinking lots of soda can weaken your bones if you substitute your soda for milk. According to some research, a high phosphorous intake coupled with low calcium intake may contribute to losses of calcium in the urine (a sign the bone is losing this vital mineral).

You can certainly enjoy soda in moderation, such as one daily 12-ounce serving, provided you are getting the calcium you need from other sources. But if soda has become your major thirst-quenching beverage, it's time to reintroduce milk to your daily dietary repertoire.

Prevention Starts Early

As you may have already guessed, the mineral calcium plays an important role in helping bones to remain strong, but you shouldn't wait until you're 60-plus to take supplements.

Studies on children show that calcium supplementation can increase bone mineral density. Other studies show that older women who regularly consumed milk during adolescence have greater bone mineral density and, in turn, have lower fracture rates than women who consumed no or very little milk.

To build and keep strong bones, adults younger than age 50 need 1,000 milligrams of calcium and men and women 51-plus need 1,200 milligrams. Of course, with some calcium savvy, you can get all you need of this bone-strengthening mineral from foods. However, taking a supplement gives you extra insurance.

Start by powering up on calcium with foods such as dairy products and calcium-fortified foods or beverages like orange juice or soy milk. Count 300 milligrams of calcium for every serving, such as 1 cup of milk (whole, lowfat, or nonfat), 1 cup flavored yogurt, 2 ounces of cheese (preferably reduced fat to save on calories), and 1 cup of calcium-fortified orange juice or soy milk. Plain yogurt (nonfat or regular) offers more calcium, at 450 milligrams per cup.

Other sources of calcium tip in at lower levels: tofu (made with calcium sulfate), 250 milligrams per ½ cup; canned salmon with bones, 200 milligrams per 3 ounces; frozen yogurt, 100 milligrams per ½ cup; turnip greens, 100 milligrams per ½ cup cooked; dried figs, 80 milligrams per 3 whole; and broccoli, 50 milligrams per ½ cup cooked.

Here's an example of a day's menu that supplies just over 1,000 milligrams of calcium:

- **Breakfast.** 1 cup plain yogurt topped with fruit, whole grain toast
- **Lunch.** Lentil soup topped with 2 ounces of reduced-fat cheddar cheese
- **Snack.** Three dried figs and iced herb tea
- **Dinner.** Stir-fry made with ½ cup broccoli and ½ cup firm tofu over rice

I also recommend taking a supplement, particularly on those days when you skimp on the calcium powerhouse foods. Supplements vary in the form of calcium and the amount per tablet. Calcium carbonate is the most common supplement available; it is also found in calcium antacid tablets. It's less expensive than other calcium supplements, such as calcium lactate, and well absorbed. If you're younger than age 50, take one 500-milligram supplement with a meal, particularly a meal that's low in calcium (often lunch or dinner). If you are 50-plus and are starting to develop signs of osteoporosis, take two 500-milligram supplements, one with lunch and the other with dinner.

Beyond Calcium

A host of other vitamins, minerals, and phytochemicals work to help keep bones strong. Here are some tips for eating a bone-strengthening diet:

Don't forget D. Vitamin D is crucial for calcium use in the body. Your only major dietary source for this vitamin is vitamin D-fortified milk. While we can make this vitamin when our skin is exposed to sunlight, during the dreary winter months we often don't meet our sunlight exposure quota of 20 minutes (fair skin) to 2 hours (dark skin). A supplement (no more than 100 percent of the RDA) may be in order for some people, especially the elderly who don't get outside much.

Get C and K, too. Vitamins C and K both play a role in healthy bone formation. Eating daily servings of citrus fruits, berries, tomatoes, peppers, and other vitamin C–rich produce along with green leafy vegetables such as spinach, collard greens, broccoli, and asparagus for vitamin K will ensure ample intake of these bone-building nutrients.

Keep tabs on protein. Very high protein diets coupled with low calcium intake may increase calcium losses from the body. This is why high-protein, low-carbohydrate weight loss diets may jeopardize your bone health (not to mention your heart health). It's best to keep

Osteoporosis—Are You at Risk?

Research has linked the following factors to an increased risk of osteoporosis. Some factors are out of your control ("Fixed Risk Factors"), but others are not ("Lifestyle Risk Factors").

Fixed Risk Factors

- Female sex
- Caucasian, Asian, or Hispanic ancestry
- Family history of osteoporosis
- Age over 40
- Menopause
- Diabetes
- Forced bed rest or immobilization
- Slender build

Lifestyle Risk Factors

- Inactivity or sedentary lifestyle
- Excessive exercise to point of amenorrhea
- Low calcium intake
- Low vitamin D intake (low sunlight exposure)
- Dieting to cause excessive slimness
- Smoking
- Alcohol abuse
- Excess sodium intake
- Excess fiber intake
- Excess caffeine intake

protein intake moderate, about 50 to 100 grams daily depending on your body size and exercise levels.

Ease up on alcohol. Studies show that excessive alcohol intake may compromise bone health and increase risk of bone fractures. Keep alcohol consumption moderate, with one drink or fewer per day for women and two or fewer for men.

Keep exercising. Physical activity strengthens bones just as it tones and strengthens muscles. And just as your muscles shrink when you don't use them, so do your bones. During spaceflight, for example, astronauts can lose 4 grams of bone calcium in four weeks' time due to the lack of gravity and weight bearing on their bones.

Conversely, physical activity, particularly weight-bearing sports, stimulates an increase in bone mass. For example, walking about 1 mile daily has been shown to improve bone mineral density in postmenopausal women, and strength training or weight lifting has been shown to increase bone mineral density in older men and women.

Quit smoking. Women smokers, especially those who are postmenopausal, have greater fracture rates than nonsmoking postmenopausal women. Some research suggests that smoking may bring on menopause at an earlier age by altering hormone levels, which leads to a greater cumulative loss of mineral from the bone. Also, smokers generally have a lower body weight and activity level than nonsmokers, both of which contribute to reduced bone mass.

Load up on fruits and vegetables. Though fruits and vegetables are poor calcium sources, studies show that people who regularly eat them have greater bone mineral density. The high potassium content and nonacidic nature of these foods are believed to promote an environment that inhibits loss of calcium from the bone. Aim for five to nine servings of fruits and vegetables a day.

Add in some soy. Soy foods, such as tofu, soy milk, and tempeh, also protect against bone mineral loss, but in a different way. Substances called *isoflavones* (a type of phytochemical) act weakly like estrogen. In this capacity, soy isoflavones are thought to promote greater bone mineral density. Aim for 30 grams of soy protein a day from soy burgers, soy sausage, soy ground round, tofu, soy nuts, soy milk, and other soy foods.

OVERTRAINING

When performance suffers, examine your training and eating habits.

As a nutrition expert at a university, I see my share of overtrained athletes. For example, a track athlete recently sought my advice just one year after his best track season ever. He had trained hard all fall for cross-country and anticipated yet another successful spring track season.

Yet his expectations never materialized. Rather, his running slowed, injuries cropped up, and he generally felt tired all the time. He complained that, despite consistent and intense training efforts, he just couldn't run up to his potential.

His story was a familiar one to me, as I'd seen it many times before. In fact, 60 to 65 percent of elite endurance runners go stale at some point, as do 5 to 15 percent of all athletes.

For these athletes who so recently were performing at their peak and then who suddenly tumble to their worst performances ever, I generally offer the same advice: Take some time off. They often question my judgment at first. After all, if you want to improve your performance, you should train harder, not train less, right? Not always.

Your muscles and body adapt to the demands of exercise during your rest periods, not during your training sessions. During your recovery time, your body repairs and strengthens sore muscles, restocks your glycogen fuel tanks, and generally takes a mental and physical break.

Are You Addicted to Exercise?

A certain percentage of those who overtrain may be addicted to exercise. Similar to an eating disorder, exercise addiction involves compulsively exercising to lose weight and burn calories. An exercise addict justifies extreme day-after-day workouts with the philosophy that hard work creates strong athletes. You may be an addict if:

- You force yourself to exercise even when you don't feel well.
- You tend to go as fast and hard as you can during every single session.
- You feel stress or anxiety if you miss a workout.
- Your need to exercise interferes with your family or social life or distracts from work at the office.

See "Disordered Eating" for help with exercise addiction.

When you go hard day after day, never recovering with a day off or a light workout, your body doesn't get a chance to recover. Your muscles remain tattered. Your fuel tanks don't fully restock. Your immune system even falls behind, with the numbers of important germ- and disease-fighting cells taking a dip.

Over time, serious problems may develop. Your heart will beat less efficiently, increasing your heart rate and oxygen consumption during exercise. Your body stops burning as much fat for energy, slowing your metabolism. Blood lactate levels rise, making you feel the burn earlier during an exercise session. Levels of the stress hormone cortisol also rise.

End result: Exercise feels harder than it should. You fatigue faster than usual. Your motivation wanes. You catch frequent colds. You experience trouble falling and staying asleep. You're moody, irritable, and depressed, and you basically feel run down.

Generally, the harder you push yourself, the weaker you'll get. That is, unless you take some time off.

Here's how to bounce back:

Take a break. As I mentioned, the best cure for overtraining is less training. The amount of time off you need depends on how long and how much you've overdone it. If you've only felt tired for a couple days in response to a weekend-long run or bike ride, one or two days of rest will do it. If you've noticed symptoms for a few weeks, you may need five days off. If you've been struggling with fatigue for an entire season, you may need more than a month off.

You may not need to completely abstain from exercise, however. But you will need to take a complete break from your current form of exercise. Switch to a different exercise pursuit, particularly one that focuses on different muscles in the body. For example, if you run, try swimming. If you cycle, try rowing.

Also, choose a fun sport that involves other people, as those most prone to overtraining are athletes who train alone. When you train in your new sport, hold back a little. Try not to go all out. Focus on fun rather than performance and you'll do just fine.

Eat more fat. Researchers at the University of Buffalo suspect that essential fatty acids found in fish may help bolster immunity, especially the dip in immunity common with overtraining. Omega-3 fatty acids also tend to reduce inflammation, whereas other types of fats may promote it.

Many athletes cut fats from their diets in order to stay slim, which may keep them from consuming enough of these important fats. Eat fatty fish such as salmon twice a week. Follow up with nuts, nut butters, and flaxseed products on a regular basis.

Check your protein consumption. Though research has yet to prove a connection, many of the overtrained athletes I've counseled tend to eat very little protein. When you skimp on this important nutrient, your muscles never fully recover from exercise. Protein also helps keep immunity strong. Try to include a protein source with each meal, such as milk or soy sausage at breakfast, sliced turkey at lunch, and fish at dinner.

Load up on fruits and vegetables. I think I've probably suggested eating more fruits and vegetables in every chapter of this book. That's because these foods truly do act like medicine in your body. Fruits and vegetables contain high amounts of antioxidant nutrients, important in repairing muscle damage and bolstering immunity. Aim for at least five servings a day.

Take a multivitamin. A multivitamin provides some insurance that you'll get the nutrients you need. Look for one that contains roughly 100 percent of the RDA for the 13 vitamins and 15 minerals listed in chapters 5 and 6.

Monitor your heart rate. When you return to your regular form of exercise, gauge your heart rate to help you avoid a second bout of overtraining. The day after any hard bout of exercise, take your pulse for 1 minute in the morning just after you wake up, before getting out of bed. Then get out of bed and take your pulse again, this time while standing.

If the difference between the two numbers is greater than 15 to 20 beats, then you are not fully recovered from yesterday's workout. Take the day off or modify your workout so it's very light, giving your body time to recuperate.

A training log can also help you monitor your training habits. Write down the intensity and duration of each workout, as well as how you felt during the workout. If you find yourself writing "felt tired" during a string of days in a row, you're overdoing it and need to scale back your training.

Spice it up. Your brain is an important training partner. Bore your brain and your body will soon follow. Keep your workouts interesting by alternating shorter, more intense workouts with longer, low-intensity ones. Add in cross training, too, particularly types that involve other people.

Destress. Emotional stress takes as much a toll on your mental and physical health as overdoing it out on the field. In fact, many athletes go stale when training hard during a time when other factors of life are also stressful, such as when changing jobs or struggling to pass a class. Examine your home and work life for modifiable stressors. When training hard, try to cut back on other types of life stress as much as possible.

Eat more. Those who overtrain tend to burn more calories than they consume, which sets off an imbalance that eventually leads to poor glycogen stores. Pay attention to what you are eating, making sure to eat immunity-boosting fruits, vegetables, and whole grains in the optimum amounts for your age. (See my customized daily food and activity pyramids in chapter 10.) Snacking rather than eating fewer larger meals may help dramatically by keeping calories consistent throughout the day.

Check your recovery and training eating habits. Are you eating 100 calories for every ½ hour of endurance exercise? Are you prefueling your muscles 2 to 3 hours before your workouts with a light meal? Are you recovering with a meal that includes protein and carbohydrate within ½ hour of your workouts? Workout fatigue is often a direct result of failing to follow solid fitness nutrition. If you answered "no" to any of those questions, reread chapter 9 and change your eating habits accordingly.

PMS

It's not all in your head.

Just about all women experience some symptoms—such as breast tenderness, anxiety, insomnia, water retention, GI distress, headaches, muscle aches, and fatigue—just before their periods. For an unfortunate half of all women, these symptoms are severe enough to affect our work performance and our relationships, severe enough to make us cancel our exercise plans.

And though your male friends or family members may joke about your symptoms, know that premenstrual syndrome (PMS) is real. In fact, for those women with very severe symptoms (about 3 to 5 percent of the population), the medical establishment has recognized it as a disorder, giving it the name premenstrual dysphoric disorder (PMDD).

For your doctor to diagnose you with PMDD, you must experience five or more of the following symptoms before the onset of your period:

- Feelings of sadness
- Feelings of tension or anxiety
- Mood swings
- Bouts of teariness
- Irritability and anger
- Disinterest in daily life
- Trouble concentrating
- Fatigue
- Food cravings
- Poor sleep
- Feeling out of control
- Bloating, breast tenderness, headaches, and other physical symptoms

If you experience five or more of these symptoms, talk to your doctor about the prescription medication Serafem (fluoxetine hydrochlorine), which contains the same active ingredient as Prozac.

The drug may help bolster levels of beneficial brain chemicals to ease PMS symptoms.

PMS and PMDD are probably a result of both psychological and hormonal factors. During the phase just before your period starts, the hormones estrogen and progesterone are at their highest and then drop dramatically. Both of these hormones regulate the brain chemicals serotonin and gamma-aminobutyric acid (GABA), both responsible for soothing anxiety and bringing on a state of calmness.

When hormone levels drop, so do levels of these important brain chemicals, making you feel anxious. Research shows that women who experience excessive PMS have lower levels of these hormones during the PMS phase than women who don't.

Many other hormonal fluctuations may also contribute to PMS, including the stress hormone cortisol (fluctuating levels of which may cause either depression or anxiety), prolactin (the hormone responsible for your tender breasts), and numerous peptides (responsible for water retention and weight gain).

Here are some tips to help ease the bloating, aches, mood swings, and other symptoms associated with PMS and PMDD:

Eat wholesome foods. Not a bad strategy any time of the month, but particularly the week or two before your period, reach for whole foods (fruits, vegetables, whole grains, meats) instead of refined foods (snack crackers, potato chips, white bread). Whole foods are high in magnesium and vitamin B_6, a vitamin that's notoriously low in many women's diets.

In one study, a 200-milligram magnesium supplement helped to ease mild PMS symptoms such as anxiety. Vitamin B_6 aids the transformation of an amino acid into that important brain chemical serotonin. So ensuring you consume enough of this important vitamin may also help ease feelings of anxiety, among other symptoms. In a recent study, women who took a 50-milligram daily B_6 supplement were able to lower anxiety levels. High amounts of this vitamin can cause neurological damage, which is why I don't recommend a separate B_6

Why We Crave Chocolate

It's nearly universal. Just about all women crave chocolate right before and during their periods. Though none of us knows precisely why, we suspect the sugar in chocolate helps to make women feel calm. Besides, the sugar and fat combination provides a melt-in-your-mouth decadent taste that can bring on cravings at any time of the month.

supplement. Rather, make sure your multivitamin contains 100 percent of the RDA for this vitamin and magnesium, and follow up with a wholesome array of foods.

Go fish. In one study, Danish women who consumed lower levels of omega-3 fatty acids—the type of fat found in fish and flaxseed—had more menstrual pain than women who consumed higher amounts. Try to eat a fatty fish, such as salmon, twice a week, substituting it for foods high in saturated fat, such as meat loaf.

Take an "escape." A drink called PMS Escape, sold over the counter, actually may have some merit. It contains complex carbohydrate and has been shown to decrease symptoms of anger, depression, tension, and confusion in women who drink it. The drink also may help reduce food cravings and mood swings.

The drink probably works because carbohydrate consumption increases levels of the hormone insulin, which, in turn, helps the amino acid tryptophan get past the blood brain barrier and into the brain, where it converts into serotonin, the calming brain chemical. However, eating or drinking any type of carbohydrate—before you feel like bingeing—will do the trick. Consider having a baked potato every day in the few days leading up to your period.

Get moving. Sedentary women tend to report more severe PMS symptoms than women who exercise. Exercise may help by keeping hormonal levels constant as well as by encouraging the brain to produce more of the feel-good chemicals serotonin and endorphins. Get regular exercise throughout the month, not just when you have PMS.

Try this herb. The herb chasteberry comes from the dried berries of the chaste tree (*Vitex agnus-castus*). A study of 170 women, published in *British Medical Journal,* recently found that the herb lowered symptoms such as breast tenderness, headaches, and anxiety. The berry may work because it contains substances that mimic sex hormones, helping to ease the hormonal fluctuations that accompany PMS. Those in the study took 20 milligrams of the standardized herb extract once a day. Most supplements come in 225- and 400-milligram capsules, so read labels carefully to find one with the right dosage. If you are on hormone replacement therapy or birth control pills, talk to your doctor before taking this herb, as it may lower the effectiveness of those medications.

RUNNING

Many runners know exactly what they should be eating and when they should be eating it—it's the *how* that trips most people up.

Because you support your body weight and move it against gravity, running burns more calories than many forms of exercise, making it an incredibly efficient workout.

For example, a 150-pound person burns approximately 340 calories during 30 minutes of jogging at a moderate 10-minutes-per-mile pace and about 460 calories during 30 minutes running a faster 7½-minutes-per-mile pace. Some studies have shown that running also blunts your appetite immediately following exercise. Researchers theorize that running increases body temperature, which makes you feel too hot to eat for an hour or so following exercise.

However, you have plenty of other reasons to run beyond weight loss benefits. Many runners report feelings of euphoria, called *runner's high,* during and just after their runs. Running and other forms of intense exercise encourage your brain to secrete feel-good chemicals called *endorphins,* which give you this "all-is-right-with-the-world" feeling. Running also helps to build bone mass, particularly in your lower body, where the constant jarring of your foot hitting the pavement encourages bones to absorb and hold on to minerals.

Finally, running ranks as one of the most convenient forms of exercise (along with walking). You need only a good pair of running shoes to get started.

However, because of the intensity of running, you must pay careful attention to performance nutrition and hydration. Here are some tips:

Get over the pasta thing. Pasta and bagels both serve as a perennial food source for many runners. Just about every race in the country holds a prerace pasta party, and bagels often line the food tables after the finish line. Runners focus on these foods because they are high in muscle-fueling carbohydrate. However, there's much more to the carbohydrate world than bagels and pasta, both of which qualify as refined foods.

Experiment with other grains, particularly unrefined types. Unlike refined grains, whole grains contain a wealth of nutrients that help to protect your muscles from damage as they fuel them for exercise. Try oatmeal at breakfast, a quinoa and vegetable salad at lunch, or vegetable and barley soup at dinner. And don't forget that fruit and vegetables all contain muscle-fueling carbohydrate, too.

Carbo-load before races and long runs. Since glycogen stores empty quickly during moderate to long training runs and races, you must eat more carbohydrate in the days leading up to your big run to adequately stock your muscles. For men, this means eating 12 or more

Your 5-K and 10-K Menu

A training run of 2 to 5 miles burns 200 to 500 calories. And running bumps up your protein needs by an additional 15 to 25 grams to rebuild muscle, make new blood cells, and more. Here's a daily menu that provides the nutrients you need.

Breakfast

1 cup oatmeal with ¾ cup 1% milk or fortified soy milk
1 whole grain English muffin spread with 2 tablespoons jam and 2 teaspoons soft margarine
1 banana

Snack

¼ cup trail mix (made with soy nuts, nuts, raisins)
1 cup green tea flavored with 2 teaspoons honey

Lunch

1 bean burrito (1 tortilla, 1 cup black beans, ½ cup rice, 1 ounce cheese, salsa)
1 sliced tomato
1 cup fresh fruit salad
2 oatmeal cookies

Snack

Glass of water
1 energy bar

Dinner

1 cup pasta topped with ¾ cup red sauce (made with 3 ounces ground turkey or soy substitute)
2 cups green salad with 2 tablespoons reduced-fat dressing
2 1-ounce pieces of chocolate

Nutritional analysis—calories: 2,580; protein: 97 grams; carbohydrate: 380 grams; calories from fat: 27%.

Your Half-Marathon Menu

As a half-marathoner, you'll need more calories, carbohydrate, protein, and a host of other nutrients than those who run 5- and 10-Ks. The extra carbohydrate will fuel your training, and the extra protein will repair small muscle fiber tears. Also, as you bump up your miles, you'll need more healthful fats—especially omega-3 fats—for a healthy immune system.

Breakfast

Egg pita (2 scrambled eggs and 2 tablespoons salsa inside a whole wheat pita)
1 cup fresh fruit salad
1 cup cranberry juice

Snack

1 carton lowfat yogurt with 1 tablespoon honey and 2 tablespoons chopped almonds

Lunch

1 salmon salad sandwich (2 slices whole oat bread, 2 ounces canned salmon with 2 teaspoons reduced-fat mayo, ½ cup chopped celery, 1 chopped dill pickle, ¼ cup chopped cilantro)
1 apple sliced and spread with 1 tablespoon chunky peanut butter
2 fig bars

servings of grains and nine or more servings of fruits and vegetables daily. Women should aim for at least nine or more servings of grains daily, making most of these whole grain choices, and also should eat about seven or more fruit and vegetable servings daily.

Don't forget protein. Many runners focus solely on carbohydrate when it comes to eating for performance. However, new research

Your Half-Marathon Menu *(continued)*

Snack

4 dried pear halves

2 cups sports drink

Dinner

3 ounces grilled chicken served over 1 cup brown rice

1 cup steamed cauliflower and broccoli with 1 tablespoon grated Parmesan cheese

½ cup boiled red potatoes tossed with ¼ cup chopped parsley and 1 teaspoon olive oil

½ cup lowfat frozen yogurt topped with 1 cup fresh strawberries and 2 tablespoons chocolate sauce

Nutritional analysis—calories: 2,680; protein: 111 grams; carbohydrate: 459 grams; calories from fat: 18%.

shows protein may be just as important. Research shows male endurance athletes appear to break down more protein as fuel during a strenuous session of exercise than women do. This translates to a slightly greater need for protein in male endurance athletes compared to women, but both genders require more than the RDA. When you don't eat enough protein, your available stores go to fuel, leaving little left for muscle repair and general body maintenance.

Eat quality protein sources at every meal, aiming for two to four 3-ounce servings of lean meats, soy, eggs, fish, or poultry along with bean and grains and two to three daily dairy servings. Also include protein sources, such as soy nuts or drinkable yogurt, as snacks.

Your Marathon Menu

Training for a marathon seriously ups your nutritional ante. Not only does your increased mileage boost your calorie needs, but you'll need to eat even more carbohydrate to recover from those training runs, especially ones exceeding 90 minutes. Additionally, you must pay special attention to eating wholesome foods that are rich in vitamins and minerals such as iron, zinc, and B vitamins.

Breakfast

2 cups fortified cereal with 1 cup 1% milk or fortified soy milk
1 whole grain bagel spread with 1 tablespoon almond butter
12 ounces orange juice

Snack

4 fig bars
12 ounces tomato juice

Lunch

1 roasted turkey sandwich (3 ounces roasted turkey meat, 2 hearty slices whole grain bread, ⅙ of an avocado sliced, 2 teaspoons reduced-fat mayo, 4 tomato slices, 2 teaspoons mustard, 1 ounce provolone cheese)
1 cup vegetable soup
1 cup red grapes
4 ginger snap cookies

Stay away from high-protein diets. Runners and other endurance athletes often ask me about the Atkins and other high-protein diets, wondering if these eating plans can help them to lose weight. Yes, you may lose some weight by eating a high-protein diet, but don't count on having much energy for training.

Your Marathon Menu *(continued)*

Snack

1 cup cold rice mixed with ¼ cup vanilla-flavored soy milk, a dash of cinnamon, 3 tablespoons raisins, and 2 tablespoons chopped pecans

Dinner

3 ounces lean beef stir-fried with 1½ cups total of baby spinach, corn, snow peas, and broccoli, all served over 1½ cups whole wheat soban noodles

3 potstickers

3 fortune cookies

Snack

3 cups air-popped popcorn

12 ounces cranberry-grapefruit juice

Nutritional analysis—calories: 3,340; protein: 141 grams; carbohydrate: 540 grams; calories from fat: 20%.

These diets often suggest you cut carbohydrate intake to less than 50 to 75 grams a day (most runners need at least eight times that much). This forces your body to use protein to manufacture sugar for brain fuel. As a result, you develop what's called *ketosis*, a partial breakdown of body fats that ultimately increases fluid loss. So during the first several days of a high-protein diet, you easily lose 5 or more pounds, almost all of it from water. This may be motivating, but only a small amount of the loss comes from body fat.

The worst part—for runners—is the lack of energy. The low-carbohydrate intake allows the glycogen stores in your muscles to approach empty. After a week or so on the diet, you must make a trade-off—you can either give up running or you can agree that this low-carbohydrate thing is for the birds (or, more accurately, cats, who survive best on a high-protein diet).

Drink more. If you run outside in the heat, you need to drink more than the typical eight glasses a day. Scorching temperatures increase your sweat losses during your runs, boosting fluid needs by 50 percent to more than 100 percent. Aim for at least 12 cups daily. Plain old tap water and bottled waters, such as still or sparkling mineral waters, provide your best source of fluids. If you're looking for flavor, try iced decaffeinated tea (black, green, or herbal) flavored with lemon, lime, or fresh peppermint leaves.

During runs, hydrate with ½ cup of fluids every 10 to 20 minutes, drinking water, sports drink, or fitness water.

Focus on vegetables. Vegetables are naturally low in calories and pack a nutritional punch with vitamins such as B_6 and folate (vital for healthy blood cells) and minerals such as magnesium, which plays a pivotal role during exercise. Most runners fall short on this mineral, so dish up an extra-large serving of leafy greens, such as baby spinach, romaine lettuce, or asparagus. Try a new vegetable every week and aim for at least four servings daily.

Eat according to your mileage. Your calorie needs as a runner vary depending on the mileage you put in on the roads. For example, someone who runs 10 to 25 miles a week needs about 2,200 to 2,600 calories, 330 to 375 grams of carbohydrate, 70 to 85 grams of protein, and 50 to 80 grams of fat a day, whereas someone putting in 30 to 50 miles a week needs 2,700 to 3,300-plus calories, 440 to 600 grams of carbohydrate, 90 to 110 grams of protein, and 60 to 95 grams of fat each day. See the sample daily menus for 5-K and 10-K, half-marathon, and marathon distance training.

Recover with a smoothie. Your body needs calories, carbohydrate, protein, and other nutrients following your workout. Eat within the hour and be sure to include both carbohydrate and protein.

Here are some good options:

- A fruit smoothie made with a tablespoon of protein powder
- Eggs (or egg substitute), whole grain toast, and juice or fresh fruit
- Leftovers from dinner—pasta, soup, chili, casserole, or (my favorite) vegetarian pizza with goat cheese

Don't skimp during your taper. Many runners taper both their training and their eating during the week before a big race. For the training, the taper allows your muscles to rest and restock fuel stores. However, there's no reason to taper your eating.

Many runners worry that a week of less-than-usual activity coupled with usual eating habits will result in weight gain. Usually it will; however, in this case, it's a good thing. With rest, your muscles get the signal to store up extra glycogen—part of the reason you taper in the first place. But since glycogen gets packed away in your muscles with water, you'll put on a few pounds as a result. Just remember, those pounds aren't from bulging fat cells—they're from heavier muscle and water.

SKIN HEALTH

Ways to keep that healthy glow well into your golden years.

Fit people look good. Regular exercise helps bring blood circulation to your skin, giving you a healthy glow.

However, exercise also poses a threat to your skin health. Because many types of exercise place you outdoors, they involve spending more time than usual in the sun, your skin's archenemy.

Sunlight penetrates the top layer of your skin, the epidermis, causing it to thin. The thinner your skin, the more easily the rays penetrate deeper, to the underlying dermis, causing even more damage, including wrinkles, age spots, and cancer.

Though many of us worry about wrinkles and age spots, the fear of skin cancer—both disfiguring and deadly—should top our list of concerns. One in two Caucasians who live to age 65 will develop one of the following three types of skin cancer:

- **Basal cell.** These small, fleshy bumps, usually on the head, neck, and hand, can eventually bleed, crust over, and disfigure your skin. However, this type of cancer rarely spreads to other parts of the body.
- **Squamous cell.** These red, scaly patches usually appear in the rims of the ears, face, lips, and mouth. Though not as dangerous as melanoma (see below), this type of cancer can spread, with fatal consequences.
- **Melanoma.** This deadliest form of skin cancer spreads quickly, so early detection is a must. Melanomas start as a mole or dark spot, usually as a direct consequence of a severe sunburn.

Some people have more natural protection from sunlight than others. Those lucky people have skin that contains more melanocytes, pigmented cells that produce melanin, or color, causing skin to tan rather than burn. This coloring provides some natural protection from UV rays, offering some protection against both cancer and wrinkles. The lighter your skin color, the less melanin you have, and the less your natural protection against the sun.

However, none of us is immune from the sun, and all of us should wear sunscreen when outdoors. For daily exposure, use a moisturizer, foundation, or sunscreen with an SPF (sun protection factor) of 15. For long-term exposure, such as for a game of golf or day of beach

Quick Tip

Numerous skin care lotions and other products advertise that they contain vitamins C and E, green tea extract, and other known antioxidants. However, antioxidants are unstable by nature. Because they want to lend their electrons, they tend to do so right away. The longer a product remains on the shelf, the less active the antioxidants it contains.

Rather than spend lots of money on these products that may or may not contain the antioxidants your skin needs, head to the skin care pharmacy in your kitchen. Try relaxing with orange slices on your face. Or use wet green tea bags. The antioxidants will seep into your skin as you relax. Plus, taking a time-out from your hectic schedule to relax with tea bags or fruit will help soothe stress, one of the worst skin-agers next to sunlight.

volleyball, use a sunscreen with an SPF of 30, making sure to reapply it every 3 hours.

In addition to your skin, don't forget to protect your eyes and hair, as sunlight can damage all parts of your body. Your eyes in particular suffer cumulative effects from sun damage, so wear sunglasses with a 100 percent UV protection and a broad-brimmed hat when outdoors.

Besides sunscreen, nutritional strategies can also help protect your skin, with some research estimating that dietary factors are responsible for 20 percent of skin protection. Here's what you can do:

Boost your consumption of yellow and orange produce. Beta-carotene, the precursor to vitamin A, sits on the surface of your skin cells, where it gladly lends electrons to help neutralize free radicals stirred up by sunlight. One study found that 25-milligram daily beta-carotene supplements helped to protect skin from sun damage. However, to gain this protection, you don't need supplements. Simply eat several daily servings of yellow and orange fruits and vegetables. Green leafy vegetables such as spinach are also rich in beta-carotene. (These green vegetables would actually look yellow-orange if the green color from the chlorophyll didn't overpower the orange beta-carotene.)

Reach for foods rich in vitamin E. Another important antioxidant, vitamin E also protects your skin cells from damage when consumed in amounts at 500 IU a day. To boost your vitamin E intake, focus on whole grains, wheat germ, vegetable oils, and nuts.

Eat more fish. Fatty fish such as salmon is rich in omega-3 fatty acids, an important healthful fat that protects you from heart disease, inflammatory diseases, depression, and cancer, among many other health problems. Studies also show that eating more fish and other foods rich in omega-3 fatty acids can also reduce inflammatory skin conditions such as psoriasis and generally help give your skin a healthy glow. Try to eat fish twice a week.

Bolster your citrus intake. Citrus fruit, peppers, spinach, and many other fruits and vegetables are all rich in vitamin C, yet another skin-protective antioxidant. Besides protecting your skin from damage, vitamin C also helps to fuel collagen production. Collagen is the substance in skin responsible for keeping your skin smooth, supple, and youthful. Eat several servings of fruits and vegetables a day.

Eat a wholesome diet. Different antioxidant nutrients exist outside and inside various skin cells. For example, carotenoids (such as beta-carotene and lycopene) stick to the surface of your cells, protecting the cell surface against radiation from the sun. The mineral selenium works with an antioxidant enzyme, which also protects the skin cell's surface.

Inside your cells, numerous antioxidant enzymes also fight off radiation damage, assuming your diet is rich in the minerals that make them work, such as manganese, copper, and zinc.

That's probably why the most convincing study on skin health found that a diet rich in all of those nutrients—copper, manganese, zinc, vitamin C, beta-carotene, and vitamin E—provides the best protection. In that study of older people living in Greece, those who ate diets rich in legumes, olive oil, and vegetables had less wrinkling and skin damage than those who ate low amounts of those foods but consumed a high amount of meat, dairy, and butter. Diets rich in prunes, apples, and tea also have skin-protective effects.

SNOW SPORTS

Foods to help you stay warm and maintain energy for multiday skiing, snowboarding, and snowshoeing vacations.

Unless you're lucky enough to live near a mountain or an open, snowy area, you probably plan skiing (downhill and cross-country), snowboarding, and snowshoeing around your vacations, jetting off to Colorado, Vermont, California, Washington, New Hampshire, and other snowcapped states for long weekends or even full weeks of outdoor fun.

This means you'll suddenly be performing back-to-back bouts of downhill or cross-country, sometimes spending all day on the slopes. You not only want to eat right to fuel your current day's activity, but you also want to recover quickly so you can perform your best tomorrow and the next day, and the day after that.

And even if you do live near the slopes—making snow sports a more frequent activity—the same rules apply to help you stay warm, energized, and focused. Here are some tips to increase your performance, mental edge, and comfort when out on the slopes:

Eat a huge breakfast. Particularly if you plan to spend many hours outdoors, fuel up with as many as 800 calories of low-glycemic, sustained-release foods such as scrambled eggs along with whole grain bread and a bowl of oatmeal with nuts sprinkled on top.

Your Preseason Program

Many people don't ski all year long, and then they go on vacation and ski five days straight and wonder why they feel so sore. "I've been biking and running. Isn't that enough to stay in shape for skiing?" they ask me. Sadly, it's not.

Few other sports work the specific leg and abdominal muscles used in skiing and snowboarding. However, that doesn't mean you have to take the pain during every vacation. Do the following fitness ball exercise to keep your skiing and snowboarding muscles in shape all year long. For this exercise, you'll need a large fitness ball, available at most sporting goods stores.

1. From a kneeling position on the floor, with the ball behind you, place your hands on the floor and then place one shin and then the other on top of the fitness ball. Bend your knees and pull the ball in toward your hands, until your knees are directly under your hips and your hands are under your shoulders.

2. Slowly swivel your hips back and forth from left to right to left. You won't have to move them far to feel your abdomen, sides, and thighs work to keep you balanced on the ball. Repeat 10 to 15 times to each side.

3. For a greater challenge, try the same motion, but with your legs extended and feet flat on the ball.

And don't worry about such a large meal making you feel sluggish. By the time you suit up, get to the lift or trail, and get started, you'll have digested enough of your breakfast to fuel your workout, not thwart it.

Take along snacks. You never know when your buddies will talk you into attempting one extra pass or when you may inadvertently take a wrong turn on a trail, causing you to spend more time outdoors than you expected.

My friend Bill often tells me stories of his foibles. On a recent cross-country skiing excursion in the Sierras, he decided at the last minute to stuff extra food into a pack that he snapped onto his dog's back. Sure enough, Bill got lost and—during the many hours that followed—was thankful that the black Lab had carried extra food.

Even if you don't think you'll need it, stash a few energy bars, some beef jerky, a bag of trail mix, and a peanut butter and jelly sandwich in the pockets of your ski jacket or backpack. You'll be happy you did if you run into trouble on the mountain.

Eat often. Every once in a while, you're presented with an out-of-the-ordinary, blessed-from-above snow sport experience. You know the one—where a blizzard dumped numerous inches of snow the day before and then quickly left the area, allowing you to ski or snowshoe to blue skies and 60-degree temperatures.

However, we all know such days are few and far between. The norm for snow sports: cold, wind, and sometimes, well, snow.

Eating helps keep our body temperature up, preventing a case of the chills. Snack at regular intervals, either in the lodge if you're skiing downhill or as you move along the trail during a cross-country skiing or snowshoeing excursion. Consume 30 to 60 grams of carbohydrate (the amount in one energy bar or a handful of raisins and dried cranberries) during every hour of outdoor exercise.

Try to consume these carbohydrate snacks at regular intervals, starting within your first ½ hour. If you wait 3 hours to snack, you'll already feel chilled and may already be low enough on blood sugar that your brain stops functioning at its best, allowing you to make a bad decision, causing a wreck on the slope or a wrong turn on the trails.

Eat a recovery meal. Respect your sport. Yes, skiing, snowshoeing, and snowboarding are all fun, social sports. But they are also all rigorous. You burn as many calories out there on the slopes or trails as you would during a long bike ride or run.

If you don't replace those calories within ½ hour of heading indoors, you risk slowing your recovery. Your body restocks muscle fuel most efficiently during that ½-hour window. If you miss that window, you'll wake the next day with only partially stocked muscles, muscles that will quickly run on empty during your skiing or snowboarding experiences.

To help increase your staying power throughout the week, celebrate when you come in from the slopes with a hearty meal or at the very least a snack that contains a mixture of protein and carbohydrate. Good options usually available at the ski lodge include bean soup with corn bread, chicken burrito and fruit salad, or a hot turkey sandwich.

Drink up. Very few snow sport enthusiasts think to bring fluids along with them, possibly because they think they don't lose fluids in cold weather. Sure, you may not sweat as much as you would when exercising on a hot day, but you are losing fluids, primarily through your breath. The thin, dry air at high altitudes causes your body to expel more fluid with every breath than you do at sea level.

If you are snowshoeing or cross-country skiing, bring along a backpack with a built-in water carrier. These carriers contain light bladders to hold your water, so they won't weigh you down as much as carrying individual water bottles. They also provide a convenient drinking spout that you can clip to your collar near your mouth for easy access.

For downhill skiing and snowboarding, you can stash water bottles at the bottom of the slope or head indoors periodically for a large glass of water. You can also carry water with you on a waist pack, which won't interfere with your skiing.

Wear sunscreen and sunglasses. Many of us only think to protect our skin from the sun during warm weather. However, you can also get burned in cold weather, particularly at high altitude, where the sun's radiation is stronger. Also, sunlight bounces off the white surface of snow, magnifying its effects and causing you to burn in odd places such as the underside of your nose.

Protect your skin and your eyes from the damaging effects of the sun by wearing sunscreen—and reapplying it every few hours—as well as sunglasses with 100 percent UV protection.

SOCCER

Sprint longer and faster with these tips.

A typical game of soccer requires a lot from the human body. To chase down or block the ball, you must sprint all-out—over and over and over again.

As you complete multiple sprints, you continually shift and contort your body. Soccer engages just about every muscle in your body to sprint, cut, head the ball, kick, and remain balanced.

You often do all of this running while baking out in the hot sun on a shadeless field. And, if you're at a soccer tournament, you do all of this once in the morning, take a rest, and do it all over again a couple more times in the afternoon, spanning numerous mealtimes.

This repeated sprinting over the course of a game and particularly over the course of an all-day tournament can easily drain the stored glycogen (carbohydrate fuel) in your muscles. Doing so on a hot day can also dehydrate you, making performance fueling and hydration extremely important not only for your performance but also for your health. Dehydration quickly can lead to heat illness, particularly in children whose bodies don't dissipate heat as efficiently as adults.

Here are performance nutrition and hydration tips to help you improve your game or the game of your soccer son or daughter:

Teach your kids wholesome eating. High-energy children need a high-energy diet full of vitamins, minerals, and other nutrients to fuel their exercising bodies. Such a diet often differs tremendously from what children normally consume without parental supervision. Your child's daily diet should include:

- Several servings of breads, cereals, pasta, corn, and other grain products for B vitamins crucial for energy metabolism as well as fiber, carbohydrate, and a variety of minerals including iron.

- Five servings of fruits and vegetables, which supply carbohydrate, fiber, and vitamins C and A, along with minerals such as potassium and magnesium.

- Three to four servings of dairy, which give your child the calcium, protein, and other nutrients needed for growth.

- Two to four ounces of meats, eggs, or nonmeat alternatives such as beans and peanut butter. These foods provide protein and important minerals such as iron and zinc that also help your child grow.

Warm up with the right foods and drinks. Eating and drinking liquids before practice or a game is crucial. Without fueling up with calories and fluids, you or your little soccer star risk fatigue and dehydration during practice or a match. Try to eat a carbohydrate-rich meal or snack 2 to 4 hours before practice or a game. Cereal topped with fruit and milk or a light sandwich and milk make great pregame meals. Avoid fatty foods such as bakery treats, fries, or other fast foods, which digest more slowly than high-carbohydrate foods, making you feel sluggish during the game or practice. Foods high in fat may also upset your stomach. Two hours before a game drink 8 to 16 ounces of water, less for children and more for larger adults. This will help offset sweat losses during a game or practice, especially on a hot day.

Eat lightly. To prevent an all-day soccer tournament from exhausting your glycogen stores, eat your regular meals—breakfast, lunch, and dinner—during the tournament between matches. Snack every 2 to 4 hours between games, focusing on high-carbohydrate, lowfat foods such as breads, bagels, fruits, and sports drinks. Also, down a sports

Your Preseason Program

The numerous short bursts of running during a game of soccer place a heavy demand on your quadriceps, the muscles along the front of your thighs. A month before soccer season, start conditioning these muscles by performing walking lunges three times a week.

Do your lunges outside on the sidewalk where you'll have plenty of room. Lunge as you walk forward. For example, step forward with your right foot and then sink down, bending both knees at 90-degree angles. Then press up through your right foot as you bring your left foot forward, again sinking down into the lunge. Continue walking forward until you've lunged 10 to 15 times on each leg. You can also try side lunges, to condition your inner thighs for the cutting movements during soccer. To do them, step forward at a diagonal, planting your front right foot at 3 o'clock and then your left foot at 9 o'clock.

Once you can easily do two sets of 10 to 15 lunges, try them while holding hand weights.

drink during halftime of each match to help replenish glycogen stores and bolster performance during the game.

Drink up. You can lose a serious amount of sweat during a game or practice. If you don't replace these losses, your body experiences trouble dissipating heat, which can result in serious heat illness such as heatstroke. Replace those fluids by drinking water or sports drinks frequently, at the pace of a quart for every 45 minutes of play.

Don't wait until you feel thirsty to start drinking, as thirst often lags well behind dehydration, particularly in children. You may need to prompt your child from the sidelines to keep taking swigs from his or her water bottle.

Allow children to pick their favorite sports drink flavor. Research shows that children will drink more if they like the taste of the drink.

Numerous sports drink companies cater to children with interesting colors, flavors, or names, so this isn't hard. Also give children fluids in convenient containers such as sports bottles or wide-mouthed bottles that children can drink from easily.

Pack smart. Don't rely on food vendors at the tournament. Usually used as a fund-raiser, the food sold at most soccer tournaments—corn dogs, chili fries, doughnuts, hot dogs, candy bars—is the exact opposite of what you or your child should be eating. It's okay to patronize the vendors as long as you can find smart, high-carbohydrate foods, such as fresh fruit, a light sandwich, or a granola bar. Stay away from any food that contains a lot of fat, as fat slows digestion and can make you feel sick out on the field.

Stay on the safe side by packing high-carbohydrate snacks in your gym bag to eat throughout the day, such as energy bars, trail mix, bagels, and sandwiches with light fillings (such as hummus and low-fat cheese). Eat your food in between games, but don't overdo it. You don't want to feel heavy and stuffed during your next match.

Continue to drink. After the game, continue to replace sweat losses by drinking copious amounts of water and sports drink. It's okay to celebrate after the game with a beer or two (adults only!), but wait until you've completely replaced your sweat losses with a nonalcoholic beverage. A good rule of thumb: You're not allowed to have your beer until you empty a full bladder of pale urine.

SPINNING

Fuel up for class and you'll spin faster and harder.

Many cyclists, myself included, use spin classes as a way to stay in shape for road or mountain bike riding, when it's either too hot or too cold to ride outdoors. Others simply use these classes to stay in good aerobic shape and never plan to take the act outdoors.

Whatever your reasons for coming to class, spinning provides an excellent workout. In a typical spin class, a group of riders mount specially made stationary bikes. An instructor takes the group through a group ride, shouting when to speed up and when to slow down your cadence as well as when to add resistance and when to lower it. Invented by someone named Johnny G, the special spin bike includes a large flywheel on the front. The wheel gains momentum as you spin, making the spin bike a much closer cousin to the outdoor bike than a typical stationary bike.

Spinning burns as many as 600 calories during a 1-hour class, depending on your intensity and body size. It also helps to tone your thigh muscles. And though spinning can dramatically help you maintain your fitness for road, track, or mountain bike riding, it truly counts as its own form of exercise and demands unique fitness nutrition principles as a result.

Here are some tips for increasing your performance:

Fuel up for class. As with many of those who take aerobics classes, many spinning enthusiasts make the mistake of not thinking of spin class as "athletic." As a result, they fail to fuel up with calories before or during the class.

This lack of calories translates into lack of energy as your muscles run short on carbohydrate to fuel your sprinting and climbing. You respond by setting the bike resistance at a lower intensity and spinning less quickly—after all, no one knows you're slacking but you. In return, your body burns fewer calories during your workout.

Fuel up for an evening spin class by eating a small snack about 2 to 3 hours before class. Half an energy bar or 1 cup of sports drink can make a dramatic difference in how energetic you feel come class time.

Pack a snack in your car. If you spin first thing in the morning at 6 or 7 A.M., I can understand why you might not want to get up a few hours early to fuel yourself with a light carbohydrate snack. However, that doesn't give you an excuse to spin on empty. Pack shelf-stable

Quick Tip

If spinning is your only form of exercise, you may develop overuse injuries in your thighs and back if you don't couple it with resistance training. During your resistance training workouts, focus particularly on your hamstrings, along the backs of your upper thighs, buttocks, and inner thighs. Good exercises include hamstring curls and lunges. Also, make sure to give your upper body a workout with weights or tubing since spinning focuses mostly on leg conditioning.

foods such as a breakfast bar or bottle of sports drink into your gym bag or glove compartment and then consume them on your way to the gym. Just 100 calories will make the difference between dragging through your workout and spinning with confidence.

Bring a water bottle. I often glance around during spin class and am amazed by all of the empty water carriers on the bikes. Because you're indoors at a gym with a constant 65 to 70 degree temperature and no wind, you can easily sweat more during a spin class than you would on an outdoor ride.

Plus, most people are already dehydrated by the time they get to class. For example, you don't drink all night long while sleeping, which is why your urine first thing in the morning is more intense in color than daytime urine from compacting the same amount of waste into a smaller amount of water. When you show up for that 6 A.M. class, your blood is already thick and viscous. You need fluids to get your blood to flow more easily, your brain to think clearly, and your muscles to release heat more readily. The same goes for postworkday spin classes. By the end of the workday, most people are dehydrated from breathing in dry air all day long.

In either case, you'll need a minimum of one 16-ounce water bottle worth of water during your class. Drink from it liberally, during every rest break or slower spinning sequence. Don't wait for the instructor to prompt you.

Consider filling your bottle with sports drink. Research shows that consuming some carbohydrate during intense sprinting efforts helps to boost performance. Fill your water bottle with sports drink, particularly if you forgot to eat a midafternoon snack or didn't have time to nibble while on the way to your morning session.

When I suggest sports drink to people who take part in spin classes, they sometimes complain that they want to burn calories, not consume them. Yet the 120 calories in 16 ounces of sports drink goes a long way, helping you to burn more calories during your class.

When you spin on empty, your tired body responds by slowing your cadence. Because your hunger fuels your fatigue, you may not notice that you're merely going through the motions. Yet spinning slowly on less resistance lowers your calorie burn no matter how you look at it.

Make class worth your while by consuming the calories your brain and muscles need. Your faster cadence and increased resistance will not only burn more calories, it will also better condition your heart, increase the strength in your legs, and better prepare you for road and mountain bike riding. You'll also feel better mentally as your brain gets needed energy for a positive attitude!

Get connected. Most spin bikes contain special pedals that allow you to either slip your sneakers under toe clips or clip special cycling shoes to the pedals. Once connected, you'll work your legs through the entire revolution, as you press down on the pedal as well as when you pull up. Investing in a pair of hard-bottomed cycling shoes and learning how to snap them into the pedals allows you to do this smoothly, helping you to increase your spinning cadence and maximize your workout.

Move around. The best spin instructors take you through a balanced workout that includes some sitting, some standing or "jumping" out of the saddle, some climbing, and some sprinting. If your instructor merely tells you to sit and spin for 45 minutes straight, search for a new class. Or do your own moves during the existing spin class by standing with resistance, sitting with resistance, standing and sprinting, and sitting and sprinting. The more varied your spin workout, the better prepared you'll be for road or mountain bike riding.

Customize your bike. All spin bikes include an adjustable seat and adjustable handlebars. Not setting either correctly will at the least lead to discomfort and bad form during your workout and at the worst lead to injury. Set your seat at a height that allows your leg to remain slightly bent at the bottom of your pedal stroke. Your foot should disappear from view at the top of your pedal stroke. Set the bars at a height that allows you to lean forward from a sitting position with a slight bend in your elbows.

STRESS

Comfort eating that's easy on your soul—and on your waist.

During times of stress—whether from work, family, or world events—I head for the kitchen, often to the freezer, where I keep my stash of premium Häagen-Dazs ice cream. During serious stress, I also head to the cupboard, where I keep my large supply of chocolate.

I'm willing to bet that you can relate.

Most of us use food to lift our spirits, and for good reason. Many comfort foods, such as chocolate and mashed potatoes, contain ingredients that act like antidepressant and antianxiety medication to our brains.

Here's how this food-mood connection works. In response to stressful situations, tiny glands near your kidneys produce the hormone cortisol. This hormone is thought to stimulate eating by signaling a center in the brain called the *hypothalamus,* which, among other things, monitors body cues that signal the need to eat.

Your brain and other organs in the body make numerous chemicals that can alter your mood. Studies done on both animals and people show that eating certain foods can alter levels of these chemicals thereby affecting mood. Additionally, some foods may contain unique substances that can have soothing effects.

Here are some of the most common types of food we turn to in times of stress, as well as what the research says about how they may alter brain chemicals:

- **Carbohydrate.** According to some research, eating foods rich in carbohydrate, such as mashed potatoes, boosts insulin levels, which, in turn, facilitates the entry of an amino acid called *tryptophan* into the brain. Once in the brain, tryptophan gets converted into a brain chemical called *serotonin.* Known to have a calming effect, increased levels of serotonin may ease feelings of stress or anxiety. However, researchers point out that some people may be carbohydrate responders and some not. Those with a tendency toward depression may feel most calmed by carbohydrates.

- **Sugar.** Though sugar is a type of carbohydrate, it probably soothes stress through a different mechanism. Studies done on animals suggest that levels of the hormone cortisol, released in response to stress, may be altered when you eat sugar. In one study, laboratory rats that were forced to swim in cold water and given sugar water to drink had lower levels of cortisol than rats offered plain water.

- **Chocolate.** A favorite comfort food of mine (and millions of other people), chocolate may improve your mood due to a diverse collection of biologically active compounds. Small amounts of caffeine and another similarly acting stimulant called *theobromine* in chocolate gives the brain a little wake-up call, which may mildly improve mood. Another compound in chocolate called *phenylethylamine* (PEA) acts on brain cells to lift depression. Chocolate's feel-good effect may be a combination of these compounds along with its delicious, melt-in-your-mouth taste.

- **Familiar foods.** Macaroni and cheese, apple pie, meat loaf, biscuits and gravy, and even green bean casserole with those little crunchy onions on top are just a few of the comfort foods that many people seek out during times of stress. Since flavors and aromas of food often elicit memories, it makes sense that taking a bite of apple pie or slurping on a bowl of mom's chicken soup brings back feelings of safety and calm.

Comfort-Eating Tactics

So, as you can see, food can act as powerful medicine to your brain. I'm all for feeling good, but too often, self-medicating with food gets out of hand. You've probably been there: What starts out as a few bites of ice cream or a snack of one or two cookies to calm your nerves or lift your mood turns into an unplanned eating frenzy. This overindulgence may then leave you feeling too sluggish for exercise that day and, worse yet, may set off more overeating episodes down the road.

Mindlessly eating a pint of Ben & Jerry's on rare occasions is no big deal; but frequently using food as a mood booster can lead to unwanted weight gain. Here are some strategies that can calm your soul without weighing you down with unwanted calories:

Call a friend. Oftentimes talking about your bad day or stressful situation can help you calm down before you turn to food, or before you turn to *too much* food.

Write it down. Jot down your thoughts—what you wanted to say to your boss but couldn't—or anything else that may help you settle your nerves. Therapists often suggest keeping a journal, particularly

Cooking 101

My mashed-potato mood fix brings me back to simpler times of my childhood. Whether I make my own or order them at a restaurant, I always feel better with a warm helping of spuds. For this quick-and-easy recipe, I've omitted much of the fat of mom's old version (one that was loaded with butter and sour cream) by using fat-free products.

1½ pounds small red potatoes (clean outside skin with vegetable brush)
1 carton of fat-free yogurt
½ cup fat-free sour cream
Ground pepper to taste
4 tablespoons grated Parmesan cheese

Put cleaned potatoes in a pot and fill with enough water so that two-thirds of the potatoes are submerged. On medium heat, boil potatoes until very tender. Drain off water. Add yogurt, sour cream, ground pepper, and grated cheese. Mash potatoes with a masher kitchen tool or use a handheld mixer until all ingredients are blended. Serves 6.

Nutritional analysis—calories: 157; protein 7 grams; carbohydrate: 20 grams; calories from fat: 31%.

during stressful times. This way you get your feelings out rather than stuffing them down with food.

Hit the road. Going for a walk or some other form of exercise is often the best medicine for stress. Studies show that a single bout of exercise can dramatically lift your mood. You also get time away to mull over situations, which may help you put your troubles or stress in perspective.

Find a distraction. Focusing on another task can keep you away from the cookie jar. Run an errand, repot that overgrown houseplant, or replace those worn laces on your walking shoes. Do anything that will take your mind off the stress and you away from a food stimulus that may lead to an eating-out-of-stress episode.

Go single. Rather than buying a carton of ice cream, opt for a single-serve cup or bar and savor it slowly. This way you control the calories.

Sip or dip that chocolate urge. When chocolate is the comfort food of choice, sip on hot chocolate made with fat-free milk (just ask at your favorite coffee shop). Dipping fresh fruit such as strawberries or pineapple chunks in sweetened cocoa powder is another satisfying and nutritious way to lift your mood.

Reach for the nutritious. I'm not suggesting a rice cake will calm your nerves, but try a slice of pumpkin pie or a fruit smoothie instead of cheesecake or a milkshake for some comfort along with a good dose of vitamins, minerals, and fiber.

Make over mom's. Take your favorite comfort food that mom used to make and give it a makeover. I made over mom's mashed potatoes (see sidebar, "Cooking 101," on page 369) recently and found a way to omit the full-fat sour cream but still end up with potatoes that were creamy and delicious—and low on fat. Cut back on added fat in recipes by using reduced-fat ingredients such as lowfat cheese in macaroni and cheese. Also add chopped vegetables to meat loaf for extra nutrition. Cut back on the added sugar in cookies and other recipes.

Satisfy salt cravings with alternatives. Some folks feel soothed with salty snacks like chips and snack crackers by the handful. Opt for salted air-popped popcorn for a big calorie savings, or try ready-to-eat breakfast cereal, mixed with soy nuts and pumpkin seeds, all drizzled with soy sauce and baked in the oven for a salty snack loaded with protein, vitamins, and minerals.

SWIMMING

Tips to help you burn more fat, gain more fitness, and boost your performance.

I love swimming, particularly in the summer. Here in California, scorching temperatures, even in the early evening, can make running and other types of outdoor exercise less than comfortable. During the hot summer months, I generally run less and swim more, looking forward each morning to diving into the cool pool water.

Swimming helps me to stay in top shape during the summer, providing a perfect alternative to running. Swimming laps continuously at a moderate pace burns about 270 calories in 30 minutes. Stepping up the pace burns approximately 340 calories for the half hour. Considering that many masters' swimmers spend an hour or more in the pool, you're looking at some impressive calorie burning.

And ditch that myth you may have heard about swimming not burning body fat or helping you to lose weight. It's simply not true. Swimming provides an excellent form of exercise for boosting your fitness and burning calories. Look at the body of any competitive swimmer for proof.

When it comes to building muscle strength, swimming provides an edge over many other fitness pursuits. After just a few weeks of regular swim workouts, you'll notice improved arm, shoulder, and back strength. Depending on the type of swim workouts you do, you can experience strength gains comparable to modest weight training.

However, to make this all happen, you must fuel yourself properly, avoid overeating when out of the water, and make the best of each workout. Here are some tips to make that happen:

Eat while you swim. If you swim intensely for more than 1 hour, you'll need fuel and fluids to get you through the workout. You need 30 to 60 grams of carbohydrate for every hour of exercise. However,

Your Preseason Program

To get in shape for an upcoming swim season or simply to get in even better shape for your current season, invest in some rubber tubing. Sold at most sporting goods stores, these elastic bands and tubes allow you to perform your swim stroke with added resistance, just as if you were using one of those expensive swimming machines.

Attach the tubing to a doorjamb or loop it around a table leg, or some other stable object. Place your hands in the handgrips, turn around so your back faces the tubing, and mimic your swim stroke, pulling the bands as you perform freestyle, breaststroke, butterfly, and backstroke. (Turn around and face the bands to do back stroke).

since you are in a pool, solid foods are out of the question, particularly as they tend to make many swimmers feel sick. Focus on liquid or semiliquid foods, such as sports drinks or energy gels. Keep your sports drink bottle by the edge of the pool and take generous swigs every 10 to 20 laps.

Don't wait until you feel thirsty to drink, however. Because you're in water, you may not feel thirsty despite your dehydrated status. Also, because the water washes off your sweat, you probably are losing more fluids than you realize. If you've never before consumed fluids and calories during a workout, try it. You'll find that you will last much longer and feel much more energized. If you have kids that swim, let them choose their favorite, brightly colored sports drink to encourage drinking.

Eat soon after swimming. During a typical workout, you can completely deplete the glycogen (stored carbohydrate) from various small muscles in your upper body. Because your body doesn't shift glycogen stores around—for example, by moving them from your legs to your arms—you must replace that spent fuel in order to swim tomorrow or the next day without fatigue.

Your body most efficiently restocks these fuel stores within the first half hour to hour after your workout. Unfortunately, because many swimmers shower, change, blow-dry their hair, and then drive home after a workout, they often don't eat until this important time window has elapsed. When you miss this important half-hour window, your upper body muscles often don't fully restock their fuel stores and you feel tired halfway through your next workout.

To help quickly restock these fuel stores, pack a snack into your gym bag that contains a mix of carbohydrate and protein, such as shelf-stable milk, a trail mix made with nuts and dried fruit, or a sports bar. The protein will help repair any muscle damage inflicted during your workout as well as help escort carbohydrate to your muscles more quickly.

When you get home, follow up with a full meal that contains a mix of carbohydrate and protein, such as a bean burrito or a tuna sandwich.

But don't overeat. When you exercise outdoors, particularly on a hot day, you generate a lot of body heat that tends to blunt your appetite. Following a swim, this appetite-suppressing effect is minimal, most likely because the water keeps your body cool. This doesn't mean that swimming makes you eat more or makes you prone to gaining weight. But you should monitor your hunger feelings after working out and pay attention to how much you eat, particularly if you are experiencing creeping weight gain.

Avoid the junk. Your eating plan for an all-day swimming tournament differs dramatically from your eating plan for practice. For a tournament, you'll burn significantly fewer calories than you do at practice as you'll only swim a few events rather than for 1 to 2 hours straight.

Many swimmers overeat at these tournaments, partially out of boredom. Eat normally for a tournament, your usual breakfast, lunch, dinner, and snacks. But don't gorge or add in lots of extras. Also, try to stay away from the food tables. Usually these fund-raising tables only sell junk food—brownies, corn dogs, and other foods that will make you feel like an anchor in the water. (These food tables are particularly tempting for children who swim.)

To keep boredom from leading to snacking, bring cards, a book, or some other activity to keep you entertained between events. Or, if you know the amount of time between events, leave the area altogether, heading to a cooler location out of the sun to relax. To help your children who swim to stay away from the tables, pack wholesome snacks in their swim bag rather than providing them with money to buy food from the snack tables.

Stay out of the sun. Hot, direct sunlight can fatigue you during an outdoor swim meet. Remember to bring sunblock and some sort of shade such as a hat or umbrella. Try to stay out of the sun as much as possible to keep energy levels high and to avoid dehydration.

Push yourself. To boost your fitness level, you must work out with your heart rate between 60 and 80 percent of your maximum heart rate. To determine your maximum heart rate for sports other than swimming, you would normally subtract your age from 220. For example, if you are 40 years old, your maximum heart rate would be 180 beats per minute.

However, since your maximal heart rate in the pool is about 15 beats lower than when your body is upright and out of the cooling effects of water, you'll use a different formula to determine your maximum heart rate in the pool, subtracting your age from 205 rather than 220.

Multiply your answer by 80 percent to get your target heart rate. Then, during your workouts, periodically take your pulse for 10 seconds, and multiply by 6 to get your number of heartbeats per minute. If you're well under your target heart rate, you'll need to push your pace a bit.

Because many swimmers tend to cruise at a pace below their target heart rate, this occasional pulse check will keep you on track in the pool. You can also push your pace by joining a swim group that puts on organized pool workouts.

TENNIS

Eating strategies that put more oomph into your swing—well into your fourth match.

I often go to tennis matches to cheer for my friend Diane. I'll find the shadiest spot near the court and then sit down, sip my sports drink, and watch the game unfold in front of me.

Each time I go to cheer her on, I'm always amazed by how many players use nothing but sporadic sips of water to get them through a game. When I ask why they don't use a sports drink or even eat small snacks, they tell me that they are just out there to have fun. For whatever reason, they don't think of sprinting from one end of the court to the other to whack a ball on a hot day as a form of exercise.

For example, one of Diane's tennis buddies complained that she always felt exhausted during her fourth game. She said it didn't matter how consistently she played. She just couldn't get through the last game without feeling fatigued. I asked her what she was drinking and eating. She told me she only drank water. When I suggested she try a sports drink, she thought I was nuts. She said she didn't play competitively, so why would she need a sports drink?

I told her I was the nutrition expert and she should just trust me on this. She gave sports drinks a try, and now she's playing through that fourth game full of energy!

You see, it doesn't matter how skillfully you lob the ball or how quickly you run around the court. You're still out in the heat for hours, baking on a hot, opaque court that tends to radiate heat.

Tennis players lose a lot of fluid through sweat. They also tend to play back-to-back matches and use the same muscle groups in one arm, one shoulder, and their legs over and over, which can easily deplete

Your Preseason Program

Tennis requires a lot of twisting as you lob the ball back and forth. To keep those rotating muscles in your abdomen, chest, and upper and lower back in shape, try this simple exercise: Hold a heavy ball at waist level with both hands, hugging the ball into your navel. Then quickly twist your torso back and forth 20 times. Then move the heavy ball, holding it just below chest level. Repeat the exercise.

To keep your shoulders in shape for whacking the ball, include lateral lifts in your strength training program, particularly during the off-season. Stand with your feet under your hips and hold dumbbells at your sides. Leading with your elbows and with your arms extended but not locked, raise the weights laterally to shoulder height, lower, and repeat 15 times.

If you tend to experience tennis elbow, also work in some triceps extensions. Stand with your feet under your hips and hold a pair of dumbbells at your sides. Lean forward from your waist about 45 degrees. Bend your arms so that your knuckles point toward the floor, but keep your upper arms by your side near your ribs. Then extend your arms as you raise the weights behind your torso. Once you fully extend your arms, lower and repeat 15 times.

stores of fuel in those specific areas, causing premature muscle fatigue. Finally, if you play multiple matches, you can run low on blood sugar, cutting off the important fuel source for your brain. Soon you experience trouble making quick decisions on the court.

Whether you're out there for fun or out there to win, use these tips to help you increase your staying power and concentration:

Drink more. The dark color of the tennis court coupled with lack of shade creates a hot environment for play. That means you'll lose lots of fluid through sweat, even if you're not the type of player who moves quickly from one end of the court to the other. Also, many people play tennis early in the morning, when they are already dehydrated from sleeping 8 hours without any sips of water. If you started the day with coffee, tea, or latte with a hit of caffeine, you magnified that fluid loss by boosting urine production. So beat the fluid drain by drinking 5 to 12 ounces of fluid during every 15 to 20 minutes of play.

Eat something. By now, most people know that endurance sports such as running and cycling require the consumption of calories to keep blood sugar levels steady and muscles well fueled. However, it wasn't until recently that we discovered that sports that require short bursts of intense activity coupled with fine motor skills (such as tennis and soccer) also benefit from the consumption of carbohydrate during a game or match.

In a study published in *Medicine & Science in Sports & Exercise,* those who consumed a carbohydrate sports drink (such as Gatorade) during a game that involved bursts of shuttle running (running quickly from one marker to another, about 5 to 20 yards apart) performed better than those who did not. These players improved their time during each shuttle run, which required fine motor skills similar to lobbing a tennis ball in a chosen direction, than those who didn't consume the sports drink. They also reported feeling less exhausted.

The carbohydrate in the drink works by keeping blood sugar levels steady, providing your brain with a constant supply of fuel, which allows you to make better decisions on the court. It also may help prevent localized carbohydrate depletion, particularly in your shoulder and arm muscles, helping you to play longer with more energy.

You might be able to make it through one game on only water. However, if you plan on playing numerous games, sip a sports drink instead of water. (Even if you plan on just one match, consider sipping a sports drink to see if your performance improves. It probably will.)

For numerous games, also eat something more substantial between bouts, such as a carbohydrate bar, a light carbohydrate sandwich (such as a jelly or honey sandwich), or dried fruit.

Respect the heat. If you play tennis only occasionally, hitting the courts periodically in the middle of the summer when a friend suggests a match, you can easily suffer from heat illness if you don't listen to your body and you neglect to drink the right amount of fluids.

Your body only slowly adjusts to heat. Just like you train your muscles to slowly become stronger and more aerobic, you also train your body's ability to release extra heat. When you suddenly hit the courts in the middle of the summer with no other form of outdoor activity, your body's heat-shedding capacity is out of shape. You can easily overheat, running the risk of serious heat illness.

Pay close attention to your body on hot days, particularly if the weather has recently changed, if you're out of shape, or if you've just switched from indoor to outdoor play. Start with just one shorter game. And if you feel light-headed, stop. Don't try to play through heat illness.

Pack for emergencies. Tennis is a very social sport. You may head to the courts with only a bottle of water to get you through one game. Yet you never know when you might run into a buddy who talks you into another match. Because the foods served at the tennis clubhouse are usually anything but ideal, always bring shelf-stable snacks in your gym bag for that just-in-case extra game. Good options include sports bars and gels. My tennis friend Diane is always stealing gels from me because she knows I have them just about everywhere in my house. They have kept her fueled during plenty of surprise matches.

VEGETARIAN EATING

How to get the protein and minerals you need without eating meat.

Vegetarians tend to eat more fiber and antioxidant nutrients and less fat than meat eaters, helping them to have lower body mass indexes, cancer rates, total cholesterol, and bad (LDL) cholesterol than meat eaters. They also tend to live longer than meat eaters.

However, not all vegetarian diets promote health and fitness. I've counseled many a vegetarian who simply gave up meat, dairy, eggs, and fish but neglected to build a healthful diet around those omissions. Rather than boosting consumption of fruits, vegetables, soy, nuts, seeds, and whole grains—all rich in the minerals, fiber, healthful fats, and nutrients we all need—such vegetarians instead survived on refined foods, such as pastas and breads made from white flour.

And even with a solid base, getting all the nutrients you need can still be challenging, particularly if you're a vegan vegetarian who eats no dairy, fish, or eggs. "Pesco-pollo" vegetarians, who eat fish and chicken, have little trouble meeting their protein, zinc, and iron needs, as those nutrients are abundant in fish and chicken. "Lacto-ovo" vegetarians, who eat dairy products and eggs, also experience little trouble. However, when you give up dairy and all forms of animal products, you must work harder to make up for the shortfall, particularly if you exercise.

Here are some tips to help you fuel your exercising body with the nutrients you need:

Combine your options. With the exception of soybeans, no one vegetable or grain provides all of the nine essential amino acids in the proper amounts your body needs. If you eat dairy products and eggs, getting enough protein won't be a problem. Those animal sources provide all of the essential amino acids you need in balanced amounts to make new proteins in your body. If you don't, then you must skillfully *combine* the right vegetables and legumes with the right grains.

You need 60 to100 grams of protein a day. The standard 3-ounce serving of lean beef provides 21 grams. To get that amount of protein through vegetarian options, you must eat both legumes *and* grains together. For example, a cup of curried chickpeas mixed with a cup of rice would amount to 21 grams of complete protein. So does a square of corn bread topped with a cup of cooked pinto beans.

Your Vegetarian Menu

This one-day menu supplies all of the protein, vitamin B_{12}, and minerals you need.

Breakfast

1 cup 9-grain cooked cereal topped with 1 ounce chopped almonds

¾ cup blueberries

1 cup soy milk

2 tablespoons honey

Snack

1 ounce trail mix (raisins, dried papaya, pumpkin seeds)

Lunch

1 bean burrito (¾ cup black beans, ½ cup rice, 1 ounce soy cheese)

¼ cup salsa

1 cup fruit salad

Snack

1 banana spread with 2 tablespoons peanut butter

½ cup cranberry juice

Dinner

Pasta with "meat" sauce (1 cup spinach pasta, ¾ cup red sauce, 1 veggie burger [soy] crumbled into sauce)

1 cup steamed broccoli

1½ cups dark greens tossed with 1 tablespoon olive oil vinaigrette

1 ounce dark chocolate

Nutritional analysis—calories: 2,300; protein: 85 grams; carbohydrate: 337 grams; calories from fat: 27%.

When possible, eat these complementary protein foods at the same meal. It's okay to eat an occasional meal of incomplete protein as long as you eat the complementary protein a few hours later or at your next meal. Eating 1 cup of cooked beans (legumes) along with approximately 1⅓ cups of cooked grain will provide the essential amino acids in the proper proportions.

Eat soy often. Soy foods provide your only nonanimal source of complete protein. Ounce for ounce, soy protein matches milk or meat when it comes to both protein quality and amino acid profile.

Several studies also show that soybeans help protect you against age-related diseases such as cancer and heart disease and even may curtail menopausal symptoms. Researchers believe the phytochemicals in soybeans (especially one called *genistein*) act as antioxidants. As such, they may slow the progression of aging. Try to eat 25 grams of soy protein a day, the amount in two veggie burgers.

Allow soy products such as vegetarian burgers, hot dogs, lunch meats, cheeses, sausage, ice cream, and others to make a regular appearance on your plate. Also, learn how to cook with tofu and tempeh, adding either to stir-fries or barbecuing them for a sandwich. Use miso to season any dish, and use silken tofu to add a creamy texture to soups. Add soy ground round to any Italian dish as well as to soups. Consider buying a soy or vegetarian cookbook to learn many more ways to work soy into your cooking.

Go fortified. Vitamin B_{12} keeps blood cells healthy and maintains the covering around nerve fibers. Deficiency contributes to heart disease and can eventually result in debilitating nerve damage. You only need a few millionths of a gram a day, but it's found exclusively in animal products.

If you drink milk and eat eggs, you're fine. Otherwise, to get enough B_{12} as a vegan vegetarian, you have to eat vitamin B_{12}–fortified foods such as soy milk or cereal, or you must take a supplement. Also, gravitate toward fermented vegetable products such as miso and tempeh, which contain some B_{12} from the fermenting bacteria.

Bone up on dark leafy greens. Collards, kale, turnip greens, and mustard greens all contain high amounts of calcium, an important bone-strengthening mineral most abundantly found in milk. You need calcium for bone strength, cancer prevention, and blood pressure regulation, among many other things. If you consume two to three servings of milk and other dairy products a day, you're getting all the calcium you need.

If you don't do milk, however, eat two daily servings of dark green leafy vegetables, such as collards, kale, turnip greens, and mustard greens. Also, eat generous amounts of legumes, tofu, the grains quinoa and buckwheat, nuts, and seeds. Use blackstrap molasses when you bake, to increase the calcium content of your bread, muffins, and other baked items. And drink calcium-fortified soy milk.

Combine iron-rich foods with vitamin C. You need iron to develop hemoglobin, which carries oxygen from your lungs to the rest of your body. While vegetables, whole grains, and legumes do all contain some iron, your body doesn't absorb it as well as it does from beef.

If you're a woman, you need to make a special effort to eat high-iron foods including whole grains, fortified cereal, legumes, dried fruit, and green leafy vegetables that are low in oxalic acid, which blocks iron from getting into your bloodstream. If you include a vitamin C–rich food at meals, you increase your iron absorption. You can get a good dose of iron in lentils, kale, collard greens, dried fruit, and fortified breakfast cereal. Eat two servings of iron-rich foods a day, combining them with vitamin C–rich foods such as orange juice and other fruits.

Always go whole. You'll get more nutrients, particularly the mineral zinc, from whole grain foods than from refined grain products. Zinc plays a huge role in your health and your energy level. Again, meat is the major source of this mineral. Plus the high amounts of fiber in your vegetarian diet will bind to some of the zinc in your digestive tract, preventing absorption.

To get enough zinc, eat several servings of wheat germ, whole grains, dried yeast, pumpkin, sunflower seeds, dark leafy greens, miso, and fortified breakfast cereals a day.

Also, stick with brown rice and whole wheat pasta and bread. Branch out to new grains such as quinoa, barley, oats, and amaranth. Quinoa, especially, is a power grain that contains a healthy dose of protein. All totaled, to get the nutrients you need, you should eat two daily servings of greens, eight servings of whole grains, and two servings of seeds or legumes.

WALKING

Foods that help you go the extra mile.

When you mention walking as a form of exercise, most people respond with a hearty, "I can do that." Generally, they're right.

Walking provides one of the most accessible forms of exercise. You need only a good pair of shoes and your own two feet to get started. Unlike other activities, you don't need a series of lessons. You don't need any complicated or expensive equipment.

Possibly because walking is *so* accessible and *so* natural, many walkers don't think of it as a serious form of exercise. Take my colleague Marilyn, for example. For most of her life, she hadn't done any form of exercise. But during her 50s, she began walking.

She started signing up for charity walking events, training for half-marathon and marathon distances to raise money for cancer research and other causes. She would do what she could during the week and then train with a group on the weekends, walking 2 hours or longer.

She came in one Monday after one of these weekend walks and told me that she didn't think she possessed the genetic endurance to walk a half-marathon or marathon distance. She was almost ready to give up. "I just can't manage it," she told me. "My body must not be meant to go that far."

As I do with just about everyone who comes to me with a fitness difficulty, I asked her what she ate and drank during her walks. She told me that she would eat breakfast, drive 30 minutes to Sacramento to meet her group, and then stop at various water stops for a sip of water. "Water's good," I told her. "What do you eat?"

"What do you mean what do I eat?" she asked. "I'm just walking."

It was a phrase that I'd heard numerous times before. I eventually convinced Marilyn to eat a small snack during her next walk. "Just try it as an experiment. If it doesn't work, then you don't have to do it again," I told her.

When she returned to work the following Monday, she was ecstatic. Her body could go the distance after all.

Whether, like Marilyn, you walk for hours or you simply walk around the block a few times a day, here are tips to walk with more energy and comfort:

Eat before you walk. You don't need to fuel up with a huge meal, but you do want some calories in your system, particularly if you plan to walk for an hour or more. For example, if you're walking first thing in the morning, try drinking a cup of juice before heading out the door.

Know your limits. Because your body burns a mixture of fat and carbohydrate during lower-intensity exercise such as walking, you can probably go for an hour or even 90 minutes without consuming calories, as your body will stay fueled by raiding your fat stores. (A nice plus!) However, go much longer than 90 minutes—particularly if you are power walking at a higher intensity—and you'll soon run low on blood sugar, especially if you didn't eat much beforehand.

Every walker's blood sugar limit is a little different. Some people burn more fat when they walk and consequently can walk for a longer period of time before hitting the wall. Others may need to consume

Your Preseason Program

If you're training for a long charity event but don't have a lot of free time to walk during the week, try to fit in as many "mini" walks as you can. Take the stairs—always. Going up simulates the act of walking uphill, and going down simulates walking downhill. Try to walk as much as you can at work, too. Go to a coworker's office rather than calling or sending e-mail. Walk your outgoing mail to the mail-room rather than a nearby mail bin. Take midmorning and midafternoon walk breaks instead of coffee breaks, using them to walk the halls or the parking lot.

some form of calories sooner. Just listen to your body. When you start to feel irritable, fatigued, and woozy, your blood sugar is low. A good rule of thumb for most walkers is to consume 100 calories an hour. Don't worry about these calories counteracting your weight loss. You'll burn three times that much during each hour of your walk. Make these calories high in carbohydrate for easy digestion, such as a sports drink, honey sticks, dried fruit, or a sports bar or gel pack.

Stay well hydrated. Aim to drink 5 to 12 ounces of fluid for every 20 to 30 minutes of walking. Carry a water bottle with you in each hand (just think of them as hand weights) or in a fanny pack water carrier. You can also walk on a route that includes water fountains or stash water bottles along your route the night before.

Work up your time slowly. Possibly because most people think of walking as "easy," many tend to take huge jumps in mileage all at once. For example, someone who has only walked for 20 minutes might try to suddenly walk for 2 hours. Or someone who has never walked for exercise before may show up at a charity event and try to walk for 4 hours without training.

Such jumps in distance almost always result in discomfort. Think about how tired you feel after shopping all day at a mall. Simply standing up for a long period of time when you're not used to it can be taxing on your body. Your feet get sore and your legs feel fatigued.

Combine that feeling with the act of walking, and you're creating a recipe for disaster. Because your muscles aren't trained, they may fall down on the job, causing injury and swelling. You may notice that your calves or heels hurt for days.

Instead, work up your mileage slowly, adding only 15 minutes at a time in distance. This will allow your muscles, your heart, and the rest of your body to slowly get in shape for longer distances.

Buy comfortable shoes. Buy shoes designed for walking rather than an old pair of tennis or running shoes. Quality walking shoes offer plenty of room in your forefoot, to prevent toenail mangling, along with a snug heel, to prevent blister-causing rubbing. No one brand works for everyone, so try on many types and walk around the store. As you test them out, pay attention to how they feel. Do they allow your foot to bend comfortably? Does your heel stay put or does it slide around? How do your toes feel? Do you feel any pinching or discomfort? Whatever you notice in the store will be magnified 100 times after an hour of walking, so trust your instincts.

Bring along blister relief. The best shoes in the world can't always prevent blisters caused by your shoe or sock rubbing against your skin. Sometimes your feet swell or your socks fit a little differently, allowing a blister to rear its ugly head. So always walk prepared. Johnson & Johnson and many other companies make numerous pads and other products that you can place on any hot spots before or during a walk, allowing you to walk pain-free. Stuff a few in your pocket before every walk—just in case.

Wear comfortable clothes. You want clothes that breathe and that fit loosely. Anything that rubs or fits your skin a little too tightly will definitely rub after an hour. Also, don't forget your sunglasses and sunblock.

Hold up your hands. Many people ask me if eating less salt will help keep their hands from swelling as they walk. Generally, salt has nothing to do with this problem. Your walking posture does. When you hold your hands at your sides for a long period of time, blood has a tougher time traveling up your arms against the forces of gravity. Some of it pools in your hands, causing them to swell. Holding your arms at a 90-degree angle and pumping them as you walk will help to prevent this. When you do notice them swelling, try holding your arms above your head for a few minutes, to encourage gravity to drain the blood back to your heart. Also, before your walk remove jewelry, such as rings or watches that may feel uncomfortable if your wrists or fingers swell.

WEIGHT GAIN

How to put on pounds without feeling stuffed.

One of my clients at U.C. Davis is a decathlete named Ryan. He's tall and lanky and burns so many calories during his workouts that he must eat more than 5,000 calories a day just to maintain his weight.

By the time Ryan came to me, he was frustrated. Whenever he tried to eat more, he felt sluggish and downright sick. He lamented that he couldn't put on weight no matter how much he ate.

I reassured him that I hear this concern often, both from underweight men and women. I explained that some people genetically experience a tougher time gaining and maintaining their ideal weight, just as others find themselves frustrated with trying to keep off extra pounds. All of us are born with one of three genetic body types:

- **Ectomorph.** A person with this body type has a thin body build with slender hips and little muscle size. If you're reading this section, you're probably an ectomorph.

Your Weight-Gain Menu

This day's worth of high-quality eating will give you an extra 500 to 1,000 calories (depending on your body size and exercise level).

Breakfast

2 eggs (or the equivalent as egg substitute) scrambled with 1 ounce diced lean ham and 1 ounce grated cheddar cheese

1 whole wheat bagel spread with 2 tablespoons peanut butter

1 cup fruit salad

1 cup orange-mango fruit juice

Snack

1 pita bread filled with 2 tablespoons hummus and cucumber slices

1 cup lowfat milk

Lunch

Turkey sandwich made with 3 ounces roasted turkey, 1 ounce provolone cheese, ⅛ avocado, and 2 hefty slices whole grain bread

1 banana

2 chocolate chip cookies

1 cup cranberry juice

- **Endomorph.** This body type is round and pear shaped, with a higher fat-to-muscle ratio than the other body types. Endomorphs will generally turn to "Weight Loss" for more information.
- **Mesomorph.** A person with this body type has broad shoulders, an hourglass shape, and a higher muscle-to-fat ratio than the other body types.

However, even if you're a genetic ectomorph, as Ryan is, you can still put on weight—without feeling stuffed.

Your Weight-Gain Menu *(continued)*

Snack

2 ounces trail mix (peanuts, raisins, dried coconut)

1 cup vanilla soy milk

Snack

2 ounces pretzel sticks dipped in 1 cup chocolate pudding

Dinner

4 ounces grilled fish over 1½ cups risotto

1 cup steamed broccoli with 1 tablespoon grated Parmesan cheese

1 whole grain roll with 2 teaspoons margarine

2 cups salad made with your choice of veggies and ½ ounce goat cheese, ½ ounce roasted almonds, and 1 tablespoon olive oil dressing

Snack

1 piece of berry pie topped with ice cream

Nutritional analysis—calories: 3,700; protein: 150 grams; carbohydrate: 458 grams; calories from fat: 33%.

I suggested to Ryan that he start eating numerous minimeals rather than two to three huge meals a day. All of us experience trouble shoveling in 1,000 or more calories at a time. That's why just about everyone feels sick and wants to take a nap after a huge Thanksgiving meal.

However, most of us can eat up to 700 calories without feeling stuffed. I suggested that Ryan eat seven or more small meals a day, every 2 to 3 hours. He soon began putting on muscle, and he never felt stuffed to the gills.

Most people don't need 5,000 calories a day to put on weight, however. To figure out how many meals you need to eat each day, use this rule of thumb: You generally need to eat 500 to 1,000 calories more a day to gain the weight you need. So, for most people, that's one to two extra meals beyond what they are already eating.

Include a hearty breakfast, lunch, and dinner plus at least two snacks (one just before bedtime). If you eat every few hours, you will be able to consume those extra calories without feeling stuffed.

Here are some additional tips for putting on weight:

Don't skip meals. When underweight clients tell me that they "eat all the time yet can't gain weight," I ask them to write down what and when they eat for several days. Many are surprised when we go over their food diaries together and I point out that they skipped breakfast or another meal on each of those days. Whether you're too busy to eat or you even "forget," a missed meal can mean 500 or more uneaten calories that could have gone to weight gain. Writing down what you eat holds you accountable, helping you to fit in every meal and snack.

Focus on nonfilling produce. Vegetables are good for your health, but most are so low in calories that they don't necessarily help you to put on weight. Vegetables are also high in fiber, which contributes to a feeling of fullness. To keep vegetables from filling you up, always eat them cooked rather than raw, which lowers the amount of volume they take up in your stomach.

Also, gravitate to fruit when picking produce. Most types of fruit contain more calories than most types of vegetables. Dried fruit offers your best option to help you gain weight because it packs the calories of a whole piece of fruit into a smaller size, allowing you to eat more calories from fruit without feeling as full. Fruit juice and fruit sauces (such as apple or cranberry sauce) also offer nonfilling fruit options.

Eat calorie-dense foods. Think of all the foods that dieters avoid—oils, nuts, peanut butter, and even desserts. They are yours for the eating. For optimum health, however, gravitate toward healthful versions of "fattening" foods by eating those made from monounsaturated fats, such as olive oil, nuts, and soy nuts, rather than those made from saturated or trans fats, such as processed and fried foods.

For example, try an oatmeal cookie spread with peanut butter for a high-calorie snack. The oats in the oatmeal and the monounsaturated fat in the peanut butter are both good for your heart. Another good option: guacamole. Avocados contain a ton of calories and fat, but the type of fat is the heart-healthy monounsaturated type. Use guacamole as a dip or even as a condiment on sandwiches.

Also, when choosing cereals, opt for higher-calorie granola-and-nut mixes rather than lower-calorie airy puffs. And don't shy away from the occasional beer along with some nuts and chips. Research shows that beer—particularly the darker, microbrewed variety—is also good for your heart (one to two beers per day for men, one per day for women).

Cut back on energy bars. Many of those who are trying to gain weight try to add calories by eating multiple energy bars each day. Though that's not a bad tactic, I've noticed that the monotony of eating the same food over and over throughout the day makes people less likely to actually eat. If you go the energy bar route, pick different types and different flavors to cut down on the monotony. Also, for variety, consider adding some other tasty, quick-and-easy high-calorie snacks such as trail mix made from dried fruit and nuts.

Always eat breakfast. Those who experience trouble gaining weight tend to be nonbreakfast types. They tell me that they just don't feel hungry until later in the day, and eating too early makes them feel sluggish. I often tell them to try a small liquid breakfast as a compromise, starting with a glass of juice and advancing to a calorie-packed smoothie. Depending on what you put in it, a smoothie can contain as many as 400 to 500 calories, yet taste so good and go down so smoothly that you don't feel stuffed at all. For a great, calorie-packed smoothie, try mixing 1 cup crushed ice with ¾ cup egg substitute, ¾ cup soy milk, 1 cup frozen berries, ⅓ banana, ½ cup fruit juice, and 1 tablespoon honey.

Eat more protein. Most people who want to gain weight don't want to gain just any old weight. They want to build muscle, and that requires protein. Studies show that weight lifting and other vigorous exercise routines, like running, cycling, and team sports, boost protein needs an estimated 50 percent or more above the U.S. RDA.

You need about 90 to 100 grams of protein daily, or about 0.7 gram per pound of body weight. For example, if you weigh 150 pounds, you should be eating 90 to 130 grams of protein a day. You can easily meet these protein needs by eating foods such as canned tuna, tofu, eggs, chicken, and lean meats. (See sidebar, "Your Weight-Gain Menu," pages 388 to 389, for more details.)

Hit the weight room. Beyond the extra food it takes to put on weight, you also need to add some exercise to avoid gaining weight where you *don't* want it: in your fat cells. You need to beef up your arms and legs by adding some muscle. This takes strength training exercises. If you've never strength trained before, go to a gym and enlist the help of an experienced personal trainer who can help get you started.

Develop a program that consists of eight to 10 different weight lifting exercises that target the major muscle groups in your body, such as the shoulders, chest, legs, back, arms, and belly. At a minimum, you should perform each exercise in a set of 10 to 15 repetitions. And you should lift weights two to three times per week.

WEIGHT LOSS

Eat big, eat often, and lose weight!

I know all about hunger. A few years ago, after my recovery from double knee surgery, I found myself with 10 extra pounds that I wanted to lose. I hated feeling ravenous and deprived, so I often gave in to my hunger, blowing my calorie-cutting efforts day after day.

To lose those stubborn 10 pounds, I knew I had to find a way to cut calories *without* feeling hungry. I decided to put science to work.

I dug up weight loss research done during the past several years. I saw that researchers had been busy, making major breakthroughs into why we feel hungry and what makes us feel satiated. After wading through the reams of research, I found that it all boiled down to a three-pronged eating approach: eat big (bulky food that has few calories), eat often, and eat some protein in between meals. And lo and behold, you eat fewer calories and lose weight!

It worked for me. Today I'm easily maintaining my weight and I don't feel hungry or deprived.

The "Big" Principle

For decades, researcher Barbara Rolls, Ph.D., from Penn State University, has extensively studied the mechanisms behind feeling hungry and feeling full. Her landmark research has revealed that the stomach (via feedback mechanisms to the brain) monitors the *volume* of food that comes in rather than the number of calories.

According to Rolls's stomach-volume research, you feel full after eating a big bowl of vegetable soup but not full after eating a small, yet calorie-rich, piece of cheesecake. Your stomach registers feeling full after eating 4 hefty cups of air-popped popcorn for 150 calories, but not after a mere handful or 1-ounce serving of cheese puffs at the same 150 calories.

Translated another way, eating foods with a low-caloric density (calories per gram of food) such as fruits, vegetables, and soups triggers feelings of fullness. But rich or calorie-dense foods don't trigger feelings of fullness as readily since they take up little space in the stomach. You can compute the calorie density of a food by dividing the number of calories per serving by the weight of the food in grams (found on the

The Big Switch		
Instead of	**Eat**	**Calories Saved**
½ cup granola	1 cup bran cereal	124
Cheese omelet (3 eggs)	Vegetable-egg omelet (2 eggs plus 1 egg white)	227
12 ounces soda	12 ounces fruit juice mixed with seltzer (1:1)	47
1 cup cream of broccoli soup	1½ cups vegetable and beef or chicken soup	106
Chili with meat	Vegetarian chili (beans and vegetables)	35
12 cheese crackers	½ whole wheat pita bread	89
1½ ounces cheddar cheese	½ cup lowfat cottage cheese	132
4 ounces ground beef, broiled or grilled	4 ounces fish, broiled or grilled	53
¾ cup ice cream	¾ cup lowfat yogurt	185

nutrition facts food label). The lower the number, the lower the energy density, and the more filling the food. Try the trade-offs for less filling calorie-dense foods (see table, "The Big Switch").

Here are four ways to add more big foods to your daily diet:

Pick big foods. Vegetables and fruit are your best bet. Most vegetables average only 20 calories per serving. (One serving equals ½ cup cooked or 1 cup raw.) Fruits supply just 60 calories per serving. (One serving equals ½ cup juice or one tennis ball–size piece of fruit.) Aim for seven to nine daily servings of fruits and vegetables.

Boost your fiber. The fiber adds bulk to food, helping you feel full longer. One recent study showed that adding 14 daily grams of fiber (the amount in a serving of Fiber One cereal) over a four-month period reduced calorie intake by 10 percent, resulting in a 4-pound weight loss. High-fiber foods include grains, vegetables, beans, and fruit. Add steamed vegetables to pasta dishes, beans to your casseroles, and fruit to shaved chocolate for a filling dessert.

Add water. Dr. Rolls's research also shows that eating foods with high water content, such as chicken soup, reduces subsequent calorie intake at the next meal compared to eating drier foods with the same number of calories, such as chicken casserole.

Slurp soup for a first course, particularly soups with lots of vegetables in a base of vegetable or lowfat chicken or beef stock. Smoothies made with fruit, nonfat yogurt, and lots of ice also make a filling, watery snack or quick meal. Not only does the water help you feel full, but the air blended into your fruit concoction also helps stave off hunger.

Cut the fat. Fat adds lots of extra calories to food, but very little weight or volume. Use nonfat dairy products, use cooking sprays instead of added oils, select lean meats, and avoid frying. Make sure to check the label of many reduced-fat or fat-free goodies like cookies and cakes, as added sugar may make up for the calorie savings.

Additional weight loss tips include:

Eat often. Studies show that eating more frequent meals and snacks rather than eating the same amount of food in one or two large meals a day leads to better regulation of circulating levels of hormones like insulin and other metabolites that affect your hunger level. This, in turn, may be why frequent meal eaters and snackers are able to better control their weight and have lower body fat levels.

In one study, those who nibbled a breakfast throughout the morning ate significantly less at lunch compared to when they ate the same breakfast as a single meal five hours before lunch. After eating the single meal for breakfast, subjects rated their feelings of hunger greater than when they spread their breakfast out over a few hours.

Aim to eat three meals daily with at least two snacks, one in the morning and the other in the afternoon.

Eat protein. Many studies have shown that eating a high-protein meal or snack lowers feelings of hunger and calorie intake. In one study, subjects were given a high-protein snack, such as a few ounces of

Your Weight-Loss Menu

Here's a day of eating for weight loss that won't leave you hungry.

Breakfast

1½ cups oatmeal topped with ¾ cup sliced strawberries

1 cup skim milk or light soy milk

Snack

1 apple

1 ounce of almonds

Lunch

1½ cups hearty vegetable and bean soup

1 cup fruit salad

2 cups tea with 2 teaspoons honey

Snack

8 ounces vegetable juice

1 ounce mozzarella cheese stick

Dinner

2 cups chicken pasta primavera (3 ounces chicken, 1 cup steamed vegetables, ¾ cup pasta)

2 cups green salad with sliced tomato and 1 tablespoon reduced-fat dressing

½ cup lowfat ice cream topped with 1 tablespoon chocolate sauce and ½ sliced banana

Nutritional analysis—calories: 1,600; protein: 85 grams; carbohydrate: 247 grams; calories from fat: 17%.

canned tuna served with vegetables, and then allowed to eat a dinner when they felt hungry. Following the protein snack, subjects felt less hungry than after a high-fat or high-carbohydrate snack and waited longer before eating dinner.

Protein suppresses hunger by slowing digestion and by altering levels of circulating metabolites that affect hunger signals to the brain. So rather than munching on just pretzels for snack, dip them in hummus. Or snack on soy nuts and fresh fruit or a handful of peanuts and fresh vegetables.

YOGA

Eat the right foods at the right times to boost concentration and calm.

My students who don't practice yoga sometimes snicker when I mention performance nutrition and yoga in the same sentence. "But you're *only* stretching," they might remark. "Why would you need to pay attention to what you eat before you stretch?"

I sometimes suggest that they perform an extra-credit experiment. "Take a yoga class ½ hour after eating a hamburger," I suggest. "After the class, come to my office and let me know whether you've changed your mind about yoga and performance nutrition."

However, since you're reading this, you no doubt already know how profoundly the wrong or right foods and eating plan can affect your practice. You also know that yoga involves much more than relaxed stretching. Many yoga poses—such as the Warrior series—are downright demanding. Others, such as sitting spinal twists, can compact and rotate your abdominal area, quite an uncomfortable sensation if you've just eaten a foot-long submarine sandwich. Still other poses, such as headstands and shoulder stands, require you to invert your body. Eat the wrong foods in the hours before practice, and they'll try to come back up when you defy gravity.

Beyond the actual yoga poses, pranayama deep-breathing exercises common in many yoga classes require you to fully expand and contract your abdomen, a process that goes much more smoothly if your stomach isn't weighed down with food. Finally, the process of digestion in general as well as some foods in particular can distract you from the inward, meditative focus that you seek.

With all of that in mind, here are some nutritional tips to help keep food from getting in the way of your yoga practice:

Eat 2 to 4 hours before practice. For just about every other fitness pursuit, I recommend eating a light snack within an hour before exercise to provide a fresh jolt of energy. Yoga, however, provides an exception. You don't want any food sitting in your stomach as you do poses, particularly inverted ones.

Many factors affect stomach emptying, including the size of a meal. You can probably practice within 2 hours of eating a light snack, such as half a bagel. However, after a heavy meal, you may need to wait as long as 4 hours.

If you practice yoga first thing in the morning, you may practice on an empty stomach. However, if you find that you experience lightheadedness, nausea, fatigue, or other signs of low blood sugar, try consuming easily digestible liquid nourishment before practice, such as half a glass of juice or sports drink. If you take a class in the evening, plan around it by eating (at 4 P.M.) a small snack such as a few pretzels, a piece of fruit, or a slice of bread spread with hummus. Then follow up with dinner after class.

Eat easily digestible foods before practice. Protein, fiber, and fat all slow digestion, making food sit in your stomach longer than if you ate pure carbohydrate. If you need a snack in the hours before practice, make it as pure in carbohydrate as possible, such as half a bagel or a piece of fruit. Carbohydrate foods move through your stomach quickly, ending digestion before class begins.

Avoid reflux-causing foods. Coffee, chocolate, mint, alcohol, and fatty foods all tend to relax the pyloric sphincter, the small muscular lid that keeps stomach contents from rising into your esophagus. Avoid these foods—and any other foods that you've learned from personal experience to cause heartburn—in the hours before practice. That will help ensure that your stomach acid and other contents stay put should you attempt a shoulder stand or headstand.

Avoid gas-promoting foods. Some yoga positions put pressure on your abdomen, pressing out any gassy contents. Also, as you relax your mind, you may also relax any muscular locks that you usually use to hold gas in. Combine any of those elements with the high-fiber, vegetarian diet that many yoga practitioners eat, and you've got a perfect recipe for flatulence.

Flatulence results from fermentation—or the chemical breakdown—of substances in food by bacteria that normally live in your lower intestine or colon. Carbohydrates found in beans, broccoli, onions, and other vegetables and fruits make wonderful food for colon bacteria, in the process producing hydrogen, carbon dioxide, and methane gas.

That said, a high-fiber, vegetable-rich diet is extremely good for your health, so don't feel you need to cut back on all of these foods all the time. It takes roughly 2 to 6 hours for food to make its way from your mouth to your stomach and through your GI tract. So, the meal you eat 3 to 4 hours before practice will most influence your gas production during class. Because everyone's intestinal bacteria are somewhat different, foods that create gas for you may not create gas for someone else, though known offenders include broccoli, beans, and onions. During those 3 to 4 hours before class, avoid foods that you've found from personal experience tend to cause problems.

Nix the smelly foods if you're taking a class. If you practice yoga alone at home, you may not have to worry about this. However, if you practice in a class setting with others, consider avoiding foods such as

The Fasting Myth

Thousands of years ago, deep thinkers and philosophers such as Socrates claimed that the process of eating distracted one from thinking and meditating, which may be why fasting has become so popular at various yoga centers today.

Many people look to fasting for gaining a sense of oneness, bolstering their concentration, cleansing their bodies, and jump-starting weight loss. However, science fails to support most of these claims.

In fact, fasting may do the opposite. Research shows that people who fast tend to have higher levels of fat-soluble contaminants such as pesticide residues in their bloodstreams than people who don't fast. That's because these contaminants leave your fat cells during your fast, but they don't leave your body. Rather, they simply circulate in your blood until you end your fast and then reposition themselves in different fat cells.

When you go without calories for 24 hours, your intestinal tract slows digestion, causing wastes to stay put. Your metabolic rate drops as your body tries to conserve calories. Within 36 to 48 hours, your body begins to burn muscle—including heart and liver muscle—as fuel. This slows your metabolism even more, a slowdown that lasts long after you reintroduce food.

Within 72 hours, your intestines, heart, and liver actually start to shrink. Your digestive enzymes drop in number.

garlic and onions that will cause your breath or body to stink during class. If you're worrying whether your classmates can smell you, you're not fully achieving the oneness and focus that you seek.

Eat mindfully. Some yoga centers promote silent meals designed mainly to help you carry your meditative practice into your eating. However, silence during meals may also enhance your yoga practice later in the day.

The Fasting Myth *(continued)*

Then, when you reintroduce food, your body can only slowly readjust. Digestion works slowly, as your intestines now lack the enzymes needed to break down food. Your intestines also have lost the muscular fitness they need to push food along. Since your body continues to burn protein as fuel rather than use it to build muscle, nitrogen levels rise in your blood.

At the end of a fast, your body has been anything but cleansed. In fact, fasting can be downright dangerous for pregnant and lactating women as well as those with already compromised health, such as someone with heart or kidney disease.

But can fasting be good for your mind? That depends on whom you ask. Many modern day yogis now say no, and I tend to agree. Because your blood sugar levels plummet, you'll feel shaky, dizzy, and nauseous—not positive sensations for meditation. I believe that people who receive beneficial mental results from fasting achieve them through gaining a sense of control over their bodies and by taking the time-out from life needed in order to focus on fasting.

If, despite everything I've said, you still decide to fast, pay careful attention to how you break your fast. Reintroduce foods slowly, eating only 100 to 200 calories during your first meal. Make those calories mostly carbohydrate, as your body will lack the ability to process protein and fat at that time. During the course of the next few days, refrain from eating large meals, to avoid taxing your intestines and your body's ability to process the nutrients.

Because some yoga poses compress the abdomen, they can trigger uncomfortable belching. Belches result primarily from gases released when swallowing air, referred to as *aerophagia,* and to a lesser extent from gases in beverages, such as carbonated drinks like soda. You swallow air by eating rapidly, chewing with your mouth open, or drinking beverages through straws.

Eating your meals mindfully in silence helps encourage you to slow down, chew your food thoroughly, and avoid swallowing air.

Stay consistent. During yoga, you want a clear, relaxed mind. And that's hard to get if your stomach is growling or if you simply don't feel quite right. Try to keep your dietary patterns consistent. A swing to one extreme may cause that funny feeling during class when you simply don't feel quite right. So if you hardly ever eat meat, don't all of a sudden have a steak. In the same vein, watch out for Chinese food and other high-salt meals, which may leave you not feeling your best.

Avoid stimulants. Avoid caffeine and alcohol just before class. While legal, both of these substances are strong drugs than can affect your concentration and calm.

INDEX

ABOUT THE AUTHOR

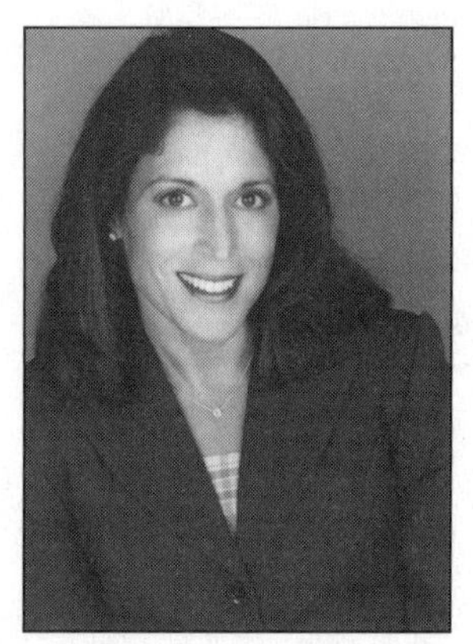

Liz Applegate, Ph.D., nationally renowned expert on nutrition and fitness, is a faculty member at the University of California, Davis. Her enthusiasm and informal teaching style make her undergraduate nutrition classes the nation's largest, with enrollment exceeding 2,000 annually. She is a recent recipient of the Excellence in Teaching Award from the University of California.

Dr. Applegate is also a columnist and nutrition editor for *Runner's World* magazine and on the editorial board of the *International Journal of Sport Nutrition and Exercise Metabolism*. She is the author of several books on fitness and nutrition and has written more than 300 articles for national magazines such as *Woman's Day, Better Homes and Gardens, Good Housekeeping,* and others.

A Fellow of the American College of Sports Medicine, Dr. Applegate is also a member of the Sports, Cardiovascular, and Wellness Nutritionists, a practice group of the American Dietetic Association, and on the board of directors of the American Council on Exercise (ACE). Frequently serving as a keynote speaker at industry, athletic, and scientific meetings, she has been a guest on more than 200 international, national, and local radio and television shows including *Good Morning America* and health segments on CNN and ESPN. Dr. Applegate serves as a nutrition consultant for the U.S. Olympic Team as well as NBA and NFL individuals and teams. She lives in Davis, California.